Study Guide for

Basic Pharmacology for Nurses

Fifteenth Edition

Valerie O'Toole Baker, APRN, BC
Assistant Professor
Villa Maria School of Nursing
Ganon University
Erie, Pennsylvania

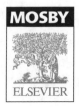

MOSBY

ELSEVIER

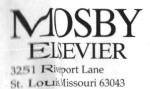

3251 Riverport Lane
St. Louis, Missouri 63043

STUDY GUIDE FOR BASIC PHARMACOLOGY FOR NURSES,
FIFTEENTH EDITION

ISBN: 978-0-323-05779-0

Notice

Knowledge and best practice in this field are constantly changing. As new research and experience broaden our knowledge, changes in practice, treatment and drug therapy may become necessary or appropriate. Readers are advised to check the most current information provided (i) on procedures featured or (ii) by the manufacturer of each product to be administered, to verify the recommended dose or formula, the method and duration of administration, and contraindications. It is the responsibility of the practitioner, relying on their own experience and knowledge of the patient, to make diagnoses, to determine dosages and the best treatment for each individual patient, and to take all appropriate safety precautions. To the fullest extent of the law, neither the Publisher nor the Author assumes any liability for any injury and/or damage to persons or property arising out of or related to any use of the material contained in this book.

The Publisher

International Standard Book Number 978-0-323-05779-0

Senior *Editor:* Lee Henderson
Senior *Developmental Editor:* Rae L. Robertson
Publishing Services Manager: Anne Altepeter
Senior *Project Manager:* Doug Turner
Publishing Services: Lisa Hernandez

Printed in the United States of America
Last digit is the print number: 9 8 7 6 5 4 3 2

To the Student

This study guide was created to assist you in achieving the objectives of each chapter in *Basic Pharmacology for Nurses, Fifteenth Edition*, and establishing a solid base of knowledge in nursing pharmacology. Completing the exercises in each chapter in this guide will help to reinforce the material studied in the textbook and learned in class. Such reinforcement also helps students to be successful on the NCLEX-PN.

STUDY HINTS FOR ALL STUDENTS

Ask Questions!

There are no stupid questions. If you do not know something or are not sure, you need to find out. Other people may be wondering the same thing but may be too shy to ask. The answer could mean life or death to your patient. That is certainly more important than feeling embarrassed about asking a question.

Chapter Objectives

At the beginning of each chapter in the textbook are objectives that you should have mastered when you finish studying that chapter. Write these objectives in your notebook, leaving a blank space after each. Fill in the answers as you find them while reading the chapter. Review to make sure your answers are correct and complete. Use these answers when you study for tests. This should also be done for separate course objectives that your instructor has listed in your class syllabus.

Key Terms

At the beginning of each chapter in the textbook are key terms that you will encounter as you read the chapter. The key terms are in color the first time they appear significantly in the chapter. Phonetic pronunciations are provided for terms that students might find difficult to pronounce. The goal is to help the student reader with limited proficiency in English to develop a greater command of the pronunciation of scientific and non-scientific English terminology. It is hoped that a more general competency in the understanding and use of medical and scientific language may result.

Key Points

Use the Key Points at the end of each chapter in the textbook to help with review for exams.

Reading Hints

When reading each chapter in the textbook, look at the subject headings to learn what each section is about. Read first for the general meaning. Then reread parts you did not understand. It may help to read those parts aloud. Carefully read the information given in each table and study each figure and its caption.

Concepts

While studying, put difficult concepts into your own words to see if you understand them. Check this understanding with another student or the instructor. Write these in your notebook.

Class Notes

When taking lecture notes in class, leave a large margin on the left side of each notebook page and write only on right-hand pages, leaving all left-hand pages blank. Look over your lecture notes soon after each class, while your memory is fresh. Fill in missing words, complete sentences and ideas, and underline key phrases, definitions, and concepts. At the top of each page, write the topic of that page. In the left margin, write the key word for that part of your notes. On the opposite left-hand page, write a summary or outline that combines material from both the textbook and the lecture. These can be your study notes for review.

Study Groups

Form a study group with some other students so you can help one another. Practice speaking and reading aloud. Ask questions about material you are not sure about. Work together to find answers.

References for Improving Study Skills

Good study skills are essential for achieving your goals in nursing. Time management, efficient use of study time, and a consistent approach to studying are all beneficial. There are various study methods for reading a textbook and for taking class notes. Some methods that have proven helpful can be found in *Saunders Student Nurse Planner: A Guide to Success in Nursing School*. This book contains helpful information on test taking and preparing for clinical experiences. It includes an example of a "time map" for planning study time and a blank form that the student can use to formulate a personal time map.

ADDITIONAL STUDY HINTS FOR ENGLISH AS SECOND-LANGUAGE (ESL) STUDENTS

Vocabulary

If you find a nontechnical word you do not know (e.g., *drowsy*), try to guess its meaning from the sentence (e.g., *With electrolyte imbalance, the patient may feel fatigued and drowsy*). If you are not sure of the meaning, or if it seems particularly important, look it up in the dictionary.

Vocabulary Notebook

Keep a small alphabetized notebook or address book in your pocket or purse. Write down new nontechnical words you read or hear along with their meanings and pronunciations. Write each word under its initial letter so you can find it easily, as in a dictionary. For words you do not know or for words that have a different meaning in nursing, write down how they are used and sound. Look up their meanings in a dictionary or ask your instructor or first-language buddy. Then write the different meanings or usages that you have found in your book, including the nursing meaning. Continue to add new words as you discover them. For example:

primary
- of most importance; main: *the primary problem or disease*
- the first one; elementary: *primary school*

secondary
- of less importance; resulting from another problem or disease: *a secondary symptom*
- the second one: *secondary school (in the United States, high school)*

First Language Buddy

ESL students should find a first-language buddy – another student who is a native speaker of English and who is willing to answer questions about word meanings, pronunciations, and culture. Maybe your buddy would like to learn about your language and culture as well. This could help in his or her nursing experience as well.

Contents

Definitions, Names, Standards, and Information Sources

Review Sheet

The QUESTION column and the ANSWER column have been offset so that you can cover the answer while reading the question, allowing you to assess your knowledge.

Question	Answer
1. Define *pharmacology*.	
2. Define *drugs*.	1. Pharmacology deals with the study of drugs and their actions on living organisms.
3. Define *medicine*.	2. Drugs are chemical substances that have an effect on living organisms.
4. What is the chemical name of a drug?	3. Therapeutic drugs are often called *medicines*; they are drugs used in the prevention and treatment of disease.
5. What is the generic or nonproprietary name of a drug?	4. The chemical name of a drug is the chemical constitution of the drug and the exact placing of its atoms or molecular groupings. This name is most meaningful to the chemist.
6. What is the official name of a drug?	5. Before a drug becomes official, it is given a generic name or common name. A generic name is simpler than the chemical name.
7. What is the trademark, brand, or proprietary name of a drug?	6. The official name of a drug is the name under which the drug is listed by the U.S. Food and Drug Administration.
8. What are some of the drug standards or official sources of American drug standards?	7. This is the name of the drug that is registered and used by the owner of the drug who is usually the manufacturer.
9. Summarize the Controlled Substances Act of 1970.	8. Refer to the text for a review of these publications.
10. Summarize the steps of new drug development in the United States.	9. This Act repealed almost 50 other laws written since 1914 that relate to the control of drugs. The new composite law was designed to improve the administration and regulation of manufacturing, distributing, and dispensing of drugs that have been found necessary to be controlled. The Drug Enforcement Administration (DEA) was organized to enforce the Act. The basic structure of the Act consists of five classifications or schedules of controlled substances. Refer to the text for a detailed explanation of these five schedules.

10. Preclinical research: Begins with discovery, synthesis, and purification of the drugs. The goal at this stage is to use laboratory studies to determine whether the experimental drug has therapeutic value and whether the drug appears to be safe in animals.

Clinical research and development: The "testing in humans" stage is subdivided into three phases. Phase 1 studies determine an experimental drug's pharmacologic properties, such as its pharmacokinetics, metabolism, and potential for toxicity at certain dosage. Phase 2 uses a smaller population of patients who have the condition the drug was designed to treat, and in phase 3 an even larger patient population is used to ensure statistical significance of the results.

New Drug Application: When sufficient data have been collected to demonstrate that the experimental drug is both safe and effective, a New Drug Application is submitted to the FDA formally requesting approval to market a new drug for human use.

Postmarketing surveillance: After the manufacturer decides to market the drug, this phase consists of an ongoing review of adverse effects of the new drug, as well as periodic inspection of the manufacturing facilities and products.

Definitions, Names, Standards, and Information Sources

Learning Activities

FILL-IN-THE-BLANK

Finish each of the following statements using the correct term.

1. Therapeutic drugs, often called _____, are those drugs used in the prevention or treatment of diseases.

2. Before a drug becomes official, it is given a(n) _____ name or common name. This name may be used in any country and by any manufacturer.

3. _____ drugs, sometimes referred to as *recreational drugs*, are drugs or chemical substances used for nontherapeutic purposes.

4. The study of drugs and the actions they have in the human body is _____.

5. The actual substance that causes the response in a living organism is a(n) _____.

MATCHING

Using the textbook and other resources, match the drug with the corresponding DEA schedule. Schedules may be used more than once.

_____ 6. Darvocet N

_____ 7. Percodan

_____ 8. Tylox capsules

_____ 9. LevoDromoran

_____ 10. Diazepam

_____ 11. Flurazepam

_____ 12. Morphine sulfate

_____ 13. Meperidine

_____ 14. Tylenol with codeine no. 2

_____ 15. Tylenol with codeine no. 3

_____ 16. Tylenol with codeine no. 4

a. Schedule I
b. Schedule II
c. Schedule III
d. Schedule IV

TRUE OR FALSE

Write "T" for true and "F" for false for each statement. Correct all false statements.

_____ 17. Drugs are chemical substances that have an effect on living organisms.

_____ 18. The Controlled Substances Act was passed by Congress in 2000.

_____ 19. The basic structure of the Controlled Substances Act consists of five classifications, or schedules, of controlled substances.

Definitions, Names, Standards, and Information Sources

Practice Questions for the NCLEX® Examination

_____ 1. Those patients who participate in "testing in humans" are part of which phase of new drug development?
1. Preclinical research and development stage
2. Clinical research and development stage
3. New drug application review
4. Postmarketing surveillance

_____ 2. Which drug name used in the United States is the one listed by the U.S. Food and Drug Administration (FDA)?
1. Chemical name
2. Generic name
3. Official name
4. Trademark name

_____ 3. Which methods are considered to be therapeutic methods for the treatment of illness? (Select all that apply.)
1. Drug therapy
2. Diet therapy
3. Physiotherapy
4. Psychological therapy
5. Occupational therapy

_____ 4. According to the Controlled Substances Act of 1970, drugs with a high potential for abuse that have no current accepted medical use in the United States and that have a lack of accepted safety for use under medical supervision are classified under which schedule?
1. Schedule I
2. Schedule II
3. Schedule III
4. Schedule IV

_____ 5. Which resources are acceptable sources of drug information when seeking information about prescription medications? (Select all that apply.)
1. _American Drug Index_
2. _Physician's Drug Reference_
3. _American Hospital Formulary Service, Drug Information_
4. _Drug Interaction Facts_
5. _Drug Facts and Comparisons_

_____ 6. When prescribing controlled substances, the prescriber includes which elements on the prescription? (Select all that apply.)
1. Health care provider's name
2. Health care provider's address
3. DEA registration number
4. Prescriber's signature
5. Patient's name
6. Patient's address
7. Date of issue

_____ 7. Information about a medication states, "In adequate, well-controlled studies in pregnant women, the drug has not shown an increased risk of fetal abnormalities." To which current category for drug use in pregnancy does this medication belong?
1. A
2. B
3. C
4. D

Principles of Drug Action and Drug Interactions

Review Sheet

Note: Understanding the vocabulary associated with the study of pharmacology is fundamental to understanding the remaining information presented in the textbook. Therefore, the first step is to define and memorize the vocabulary. The second step is to apply the vocabulary learned during the pharmacology course. The third step in learning pharmacology is to apply the vocabulary during the actual clinical practice of nursing.

The QUESTION column and the ANSWER column have been offset so you can cover the answer while reading the question, allowing you to assess your knowledge. Define the following vocabulary.

Question	Answer
1. Pharmacodynamics	
2. Receptors	1. The study of drug interactions including the drug receptors and the series of events that culminates in a pharmacologic response.
3. Agonists	2. Sites on the cells where chemical bonding of drugs occurs are receptors.
4. Antagonists	3. Drugs that stimulate a response at a receptor site are agonists.
5. Partial agonists	4. Drugs that attach to receptor sites but do NOT stimulate a response are antagonists.
6. ADME	5. Drugs that interact with a receptor to stimulate a response and concurrently inhibit other responses are partial agonists.
7. Pharmacokinetics	6. ADME is an abbreviation for the four stages of drug processing: absorption, distribution, metabolism, and excretion.
8. Absorption	7. Pharmacokinetics is the study of the mathematical relationship among the absorption, distribution, metabolism, and excretion of medicines.
9. Enteral	8. Absorption is the process by which a drug is made available to the body fluids for distribution.
10. Parenteral	9. The enteral route of drug administration is placing the drug directly into the gastrointestinal tract by oral, rectal, or nasogastric routes.
11. Percutaneous	10. Parenteral routes of drug administration are subcutaneous, intramuscular (IM), or intravenous (IV) injection.
12. Distribution	11. Percutaneous drug administration is done via inhalation, sublingual, or topical routes.

13. Drug blood level

14. Biotransformation (metabolism)

15. Excretion

16. Half-life

17. Desired action

18. Common adverse effects

19. Serious adverse effects

20. Idiosyncratic reaction

21. Allergic reactions

22. Urticaria (hives)

23. Carcinogenicity

24. Teratogen

25. Placebo
26. Tolerance

12. The term *distribution* refers to the ways in which drugs are transported by the circulating body fluids to the sites of action (receptors) for metabolism and excretion.

13. The drug blood level measures the amount of a drug present in the blood to determine if it is within the therapeutic range, below the range (subtherapeutic), or above the range (toxic).

14. *Metabolism* and *biotransformation* are defined as the process by which a drug is inactivated (broken down). The terms are used interchangeably.

15. Excretion of a drug is the elimination of the active drug or its metabolites from the body.

16. The time required for one-half, or 50%, of the drug administered to be excreted from the body.

17. Desired action is the achievement of the expected response to the drug administered.

18. Common adverse effects are predictable responses seen when a specific drug is administered. (The drug monographs throughout the textbook will give suggested nursing actions that can make these anticipated reactions more tolerable to the patient.)

19. Serious adverse effects are side effects that are more serious and require reporting to the health care provider for further orders on how to manage these reactions. These are sometimes referred to as *drug toxicity reactions*. Adverse effects are labeled "serious adverse effects" throughout this textbook. See also World Health Organization definition on p. 21.

20. Idiosyncratic reactions are reactions that are not predictable; they are unusual or abnormal responses to the drug administered.

21. An allergic reaction, also called a *hypersensitivity reaction*, occurs in an individual who has previously taken the drug and is sensitized to it. With repeated administration of the drug, antibodies formed when the drug was first given respond to the repeated exposure, producing an undesirable response such as severe itching, urticaria (hives), or in more severe cases, collapse of the respiratory and cardiovascular systems, known as *anaphylactic reaction* or *anaphylaxis*, a life-threatening situation.

22. Urticaria or hives are elevated, irregular, patchlike rashes on the skin accompanied by itching.

23. Carcinogenicity is the ability of a drug to cause living cells to be altered (mutate) and become cancerous.

24. A drug that causes birth defects is a teratogen.

25. A placebo is a drug dosage form that contains no active ingredients.

27. Drug dependence

28. Drug accumulation

29. Drug interaction

30. Unbound drug

31. Additive effect

32. Synergistic effect

33. Antagonistic effect

34. Displacement

35. Interference

36. Incompatibility

26. Tolerance occurs when higher doses of a drug are required to achieve the same effects that a lower dose once achieved.

27. Drug dependence, also called *addiction* or *habituation*, occurs when the individual is no longer able to control the ingestion of the drug.

28. Drug accumulation occurs when there is an excess amount of a drug in the body due to a number of possible physiologic variables. This can result in drug toxicity.

29. Drug interaction occurs when one drug being administered changes the action of other drugs being used at the same time.

30. Unbound or free drug is the active amount of drug available to achieve the desired physiologic response.

31. Additive effect occurs when two drugs with similar actions have an increased effect.

32. Synergistic effect occurs when the combined effect of two drugs is greater than the effect of each drug given alone.

33. Antagonistic effect occurs when one drug interferes with the action of another.

34. Displacement occurs when one drug is moved from the protein binding sites by a second drug. This usually increases the activity of the first drug because it is now unbound.

35. Interference occurs when one drug inhibits the metabolism or excretion of a second drug, causing increased activity of the second drug.

36. Incompatibility occurs when one drug is chemically incompatible with another drug, resulting in deterioration of the drug.

Principles of Drug Action and Drug Interactions

Learning Activities

FILL-IN-THE-BLANK

Finish each of the following statements using the correct term.

1. Drugs that interact with a receptor to stimulate a response are known as _____.

2. The study of the mathematical relationships among the absorption, distribution, metabolism, and excretion of individual medicines over time is called _____.

3. _____ is the process by which a drug is transferred from its site of entry into the body to the circulating fluids of the body for distribution.

4. _____ or _____ is a skin reaction to antibodies that is most commonly manifested as raised irregularly shaped patches on the skin with severe itching.

5. _____ is the ability of a drug to induce living cells to mutate and become cancerous.

6. A drug interaction that produces an increased action is known as a(n) _____ effect.

7. Two drugs with similar actions that produce an effect substantially greater than either drug administered alone are said to be _____.

8. When one drug moves the original drug administered from a binding site to produce an increased drug effect, it is known as _____.

9. Drug _____ is defined as one drug chemically destroying a second drug if mixed together prior to administration.

TRUE OR FALSE

Write "T" for true or "F" for false for each statement. Correct all false statements.

_____ 10. Drugs that attach to a receptor but do not stimulate a response are called *antagonists*.

_____ 11. In the enteral route, the drug bypasses the gastrointestinal tract.

_____ 12. Drugs that interact with a receptor to stimulate a response but inhibit other responses are called *partial agonists*.

_____ 13. A drug that induces a birth defect is known as a *teratogen*.

_____ 14. Drug dependence occurs when a person begins to require a higher dosage to produce the same effects that a lower dosage once provided.

_____ 15. Percutaneous route is the administration of drugs by subcutaneous, intramuscular, or intravenous injection.

_____ 16. Enteral route is the administration of drugs to the gastrointestinal tract.

_____ 17. Agonists stimulate a response at a receptor site on the cells.

_____ 18. Partial agonists stimulate some responses while inhibiting others at a receptor site on the cells.

_____ 19. Parenteral route is the administration of drugs by inhalation, sublingual, or topical methods.

_____ 20. Receptors are specific sites within the body where a drug acts.

_____ 21. Antagonists cause a drug response at a receptor site.

_____ 22. *Absorption* refers to the ability of a drug to be integrated into the body fluids.

_____ 23. Metabolism is the activation of a drug for use by the body.

_____ 24. Distribution is the transportation of a drug by the body fluids for utilization within the body.

_____ 25. Excretion of a drug is the elimination of a drug from the body.

_____ 26. *Biotransformation* is another term for excretion of a drug.

_____ 27. Drug blood level is a measurement of the amount of drug present in the blood at the specific time of the blood draw.

Principles of Drug Action and Drug Interactions

Practice Questions for the NCLEX® Examination

_____ 1. What are the two primary routes for drug excretion?
1. Skin and lungs
2. Gastrointestinal tract and skin
3. Renal tubules and GI tract
4. Lungs and renal tubules

_____ 2. How does drug distribution occur?
1. By decreasing body protein levels
2. By transporting in blood and lymphatic systems
3. By keeping the drug at toxic levels
4. By increasing the amount of adipose tissue

_____ 3. When a combination of two drugs will provide a greater effect than the sum of the effect of each drug if given alone, what is this called?
1. Additive effect
2. Synergistic effect
3. Antagonistic effect
4. Displacement

_____ 4. A partial agonist is a drug that does what?
1. Stimulates action at receptor sites within the circulating blood
2. Stimulates one response and inhibits another response
3. Inhibits response when attached to a receptor site
4. Stimulates a response at a receptor site

_____ 5. What is another name for an idiosyncratic reaction?
1. Allergic reaction
2. Unexpected reaction
3. Teratogenic reaction
4. Drug overresponse

_____ 6. The literature states that the half-life of a particular drug is 8 hours. This means that what percentage of the drug will have been excreted in this time period?
1. 25
2. 30
3. 50
4. 75

_____ 7. What is a _desired_ drug action?
1. The predictable/usual response to the drug
2. An unusual or idiosyncratic response to a drug
3. Capable of inducing cell mutations
4. The development of symptoms that should be reported to the prescribing physician

_____ 8. A patient now requires a higher dose of a pain medication to produce the same effect that a lower dose of the medication once provided. What does the nurse identify this phenomenon as?
1. Placebo effect
2. Tolerance
3. Drug dependence
4. Drug accumulation

_____ 9. Which term is used to describe the effect of a first drug inhibiting metabolism or excretion of a second drug, causing increased activity of the second drug?
1. Interference
2. Incompatibility
3. Displacement
4. Reaction

_____ 10. Nurses working with patients who have disease of which organ are at an increased risk of developing toxicity to the drug because most drugs are eliminated through this organ system?
1. Lungs
2. Pancreas
3. Heart
4. Kidneys

_____ 11. Which factors affect pharmacokinetics? *(Select all that apply.)*
1. Age
2. Disease
3. Dehydration
4. Psychological factors
5. Drug tolerance
6. Height

_____ 12. Which methods are considered percutaneous routes of drug administration? *(Select all that apply.)*
1. Subcutaneous
2. Inhalation
3. Sublingual
4. Rectal
5. Topical

_____ 13. If a patient is given 100 mg of a drug that has a half-life of 12 hours, how much of the drug will remain in the body after 12 hours?
1. 50 mg (50%)
2. 25 mg (25%)
3. 12.5 mg (12.5%)
4. 6.25 mg (6.25%)

_____ 14. Patients who have an anaphylactic reaction from an administered drug typically experience which signs/symptoms? *(Select all that apply.)*
1. Severe itching
2. Urticaria
3. Diarrhea
4. Respiratory distress
5. Cardiovascular collapse

Drug Action Across the Life Span

chapter

3

Review Sheet

The QUESTION column and the ANSWER column have been offset so you can cover the answer while reading the question, allowing you to assess your knowledge.

Question	Answer
1. What are common terms used to refer to individuals of different ages up to 5 years old?	
2. What is the meaning of *gender-specific medicine*?	1. Fewer than 38 weeks = premature, 0–1 months = newborn or neonate, 1–24 months = infant or baby, 1–5 years = young child.
3. What are the underlying rationales for the erratic absorption of intramuscular (IM) drugs in both the neonate and the geriatric population?	2. Gender-specific medicine is a developing science that studies the differences in the response of females and males to prescribed drugs.
4. Define *passive diffusion*. (Research other sources.)	3. The underlying rationales for the erratic absorption of IM drugs are differences in muscle mass and blood flow to muscles and muscular inactivity in the bedridden patient.
5. Define *carrier-mediated diffusion*. (Research other sources.)	4. Passive diffusion is the most common mechanism associated with drug absorption. It requires no cellular energy and involves the movement of a drug from an area of high concentration to an area of low concentration.
6. Define *active transport*. (Research other sources.)	5. Carrier-mediated diffusion, or facilitated transport or diffusion, occurs when the drug molecules combine with a carrier substance such as an enzyme or other protein. An example is glucose combining with insulin to be carried from the bloodstream into the cell, moving from an area of high concentration (the bloodstream) to an area of low concentration (the cell). In other words, the drug needs help to pass across the cell membrane and the insulin passively provides the transport. This passive process requires no cellular energy.
7. State two factors that influence drug absorption from the gastrointestinal tract.	6. Active transport involves the movement of drug molecules from an area of low concentration to an area of high concentration. This process requires cellular energy to accomplish the movement.
8. Compare the gastric pH in a premature infant, newborn, infant, adult, and older adult.	7. Passive diffusion and gastric emptying time influence the absorption of drugs in the intestinal tract. Both passive diffusion and gastric emptying time are dependent on pH.

Copyright © 2010, 2007, 2004, 2001, 1997 by Mosby, Inc., an affiliate of Elsevier Inc. All rights reserved.

13

9. Compare gastric emptying time in a premature infant, adult, and older adult.

10. Look up the term *hydrolysis* in a dictionary.

11. In the newborn, what factor affects the absorption of drugs during the process of hydrolysis?

12. If gastric emptying time increases, what happens to the speed of absorption of a drug?

13. What is the purpose of performing therapeutic drug monitoring?

14. What effect does the route of drug administration have on drug absorption?

15. List accurate methods of measuring oral liquid medications.

16. What nursing actions are appropriate when "off-label use" of medications is prescribed?

17. Why is transdermal absorption of a drug in an older adult difficult to predict?

18. What factors affect drug distribution?

19. Examine Table 3-1 on p. 29 of the text. Compare the total percentage of body water in a premature infant, a full-term infant, a 1-year-old infant, and a male adult. What conclusion(s) did you reach?

20. What effect will a higher percentage of total body water have on drug absorption?

8. The gastric pH values are:
   premature   6–8
   newborn   6–8; decreases to 2–4 in 24 hrs
   infant   1–3
   adult   1–3
   older adult   pH is increased due to decreasing number of acid-secreting cells

9. Premature infants and geriatric patients have slower gastric emptying time; therefore, the drug is in contact with the absorptive tissue longer. This may result in more absorption and a higher serum concentration of the drug in the blood.

10. Hydrolysis is the chemical alteration or decomposition of a compound with water.

11. In an infant, the absence of enzymes needed for hydrolysis of certain drugs influences the ability of the drug to be absorbed.

12. The faster the gastric emptying time, the less time the drug has to be absorbed; therefore, drug absorption is decreased.

13. Assays measure blood levels of specific drugs, providing a means to identify needed dosage adjustments.

14. In general, drug absorption is affected by: dosage form (e.g., liquid versus enteric-coated tablets); route of drug administration (e.g., oral, intramuscular, inhalation); solubility of the drug; gastrointestinal function; the condition of the absorptive surface (e.g., inflamed, open skin area versus intact skin); and blood flow to and from the site.

15. Use medicine cups, droppers provided with a specific medication, or oral syringes to measure liquid forms of oral medications accurately.

16. "Off-label use" of medications is legal; however, nurses should check reliable references or with the pharmacist for further information. In all cases, monitor the patient carefully for common and serious adverse effects whenever the medicine is administered.

17. In an older adult, there is decreased dermal thickness that may increase drug absorption; however, there may be drying, wrinkling, and decreased hair follicles that decrease absorption. There is often decreased cardiac output, which results in decreased blood flow to the tissues (decreased tissue perfusion), which results in decreased drug absorption.

18. Distribution is dependent on pH, body water concentration (intracellular, extracellular, and total body water), presence and quantity of fat tissue, protein binding, cardiac output, and regional blood flow.

19. The younger the individual, the higher the percentage of the total body water.

21. Research the meaning of *lipid-soluble* and *water-soluble*.

22. Define *protein binding*.

23. What happens to the concentration of albumin in the body after the age 40?

24. What happens to the rate of drug metabolism in older adults?

25. How functional is the renal filtration system of preterm infants and of full-term newborns when compared to that of an adult?

26. What effect do age and renal function have on drug dosages?

27. What test is used as the best predictor to estimate renal function in older adults?

28. Define *polypharmacy*.

29. Describe the safest method of initiating newly prescribed medications to a geriatric patient.

30. Identify principles of drug administration that are specifically applicable to a pregnant patient.

20. A higher percentage of total body water means drugs that are water-soluble will be more rapidly distributed and the individual may require a higher dose of these drugs. Conversely, fat-soluble drugs would be poorly absorbed.

21. Water-soluble drugs have an affinity for body fluids and are quickly absorbed and excreted through the kidneys; therefore, water-soluble drugs often have a shorter half-life. Lipid-soluble drugs have an affinity for fat tissue in the body and will often have a longer half-life.

22. Protein binding occurs when a drug binds to proteins in the body, such as albumin. When "bound," the drug is not "free" or actively available for use at the receptor sites for action.

23. Total albumin concentration decreases after age 40, while other proteins increase. This results in an increase in unbound drug making more free drug available for action and metabolism.

24. The number of functioning hepatic cells and the blood flow decreases with aging, resulting in slower drug metabolism. As drug metabolism decreases, drug doses must be reduced to prevent accumulation of the drug, producing toxicity.

25. At birth, preterm infants have approximately 15% of the renal capacity of an adult and full-term infants have approximately 35%.

26. Drug doses must be adjusted so an adequate, therapeutic serum blood concentration is maintained. Increased age and decreased renal function often require a reduced dosage.

27. The urine creatinine test is used to estimate renal function in older adults.

28. Polypharmacy is the use of multiple drugs concurrently.

29. Drug dosage should be initiated at 1/3 to 1/2 the normal adult dose and, whenever available, therapeutic drug monitoring should be completed.

30. Take a thorough drug history of all prescribed and over-the-counter medications and "street drugs" being taken. Ask specifically about any herbal remedies or nutritional supplements being taken. Ask about the use of alcohol, tobacco, and herbal products during pregnancy. Refer to Tables 3-6 and 3-7, p. 35 in the textbook.

Drug Action Across the Life Span

Learning Activities

FILL-IN-THE-BLANK

Finish each of the following statements using the correct term.

1. _____ medicine is a developing science that studies the differences in the normal function of men and women and how people of each sex perceive and experience disease.

2. At _____ year(s) of age, the child's stomach pH approximates that of an adult.

3. Drugs that are relatively insoluble are transported in the circulation by being bound to _____ proteins.

4. Certain medicines require that blood be drawn twice to assess both subtherapeutic levels and the potential for toxicity. One of the levels is drawn at 30 minutes before the next dose is to be administered to obtain the _____ or lowest blood level of medicine, and another is drawn at 20 minutes after the medicine has been administered intravenously to obtain the _____ or highest blood level.

5. _____ is the term used to describe patients requiring multiple drug therapy.

TRUE OR FALSE

Write "T" for true and "F" for false for each statement. Correct all false statements.

_____ 6. Transdermal administration of drugs to the geriatric population is often difficult to predict because dermal thickness increases with aging.

_____ 7. Medicines given intramuscularly are usually erratically absorbed in both neonates and older adults.

_____ 8. Men and women respond to medications differently.

_____ 9. Therapeutic drug monitoring is the measurement of a drug's concentration in biologic fluids to correlate the dosage administered and the level of medicine in the body with the pharmacologic response.

_____ 10. Drug metabolism is the process by which the body inactivates medicines.

_____ 11. The older adult population includes people 65 years and older.

_____ 12. Absorption of drugs administered intramuscularly is consistent and predictable.

_____ 13. Transdermal drug absorption has a predictable rate.

_____ 14. Enteric-coated and sustained-release tablets are absorbed erratically if crushed.

_____ 15. Passive diffusion requires cellular energy.

_____ 16. The gastric emptying time of an older adult and a premature infant are slow and result in increased drug absorption.

_____ 17. Hydrolysis involves the chemical breakdown of a compound, such as a drug, in water.

_____ 18. The older adult patient has a greater percentage of total body fluid than an infant.

_____ 19. Drug elimination is affected by the number of functional renal tubules.

_____ 20. Albumin is a protein to which drugs bind for transport.

_____ 21. "Unbound" drug is the active portion of the drug dose available for the desired drug action.

_____ 22. "Bound" drug is the portion of the drug causing the desired drug action.

_____ 23. The term _infant_ is used to signify babies 0–1 month of age.

_____ 24. Gender-specific medicine studies how disease differences affect normal functions of men and women.

_____ 25. The pH environment of the gastrointestinal tract affects passive diffusion and gastric emptying time.

_____ 26. Some drugs such as erythromycin, prednisolone, diazepam, and verapamil are metabolized more rapidly in men than in women.

_____ 27. Saliva assays may be used for therapeutic drug monitoring of some types of medications.

_____ 28. "Peak" and "trough" laboratory values should be communicated promptly to the prescribing health care provider.

_____ 29. Household teaspoons provide a safe, reliable measurement for drug doses.

_____ 30. Many drugs, in addition to street drugs, may be teratogenic.

Drug Action Across the Life Span

Practice Questions for the NCLEX® Examination

_____ 1. Which statement about the specific needs of pediatric patients receiving medications is correct?
1. Infants and young children have lower total body water content than adults.
2. Many medicines are not approved by the FDA for use in children.
3. Salicylates are most effective when administered to pediatric patients from infancy through their teenage years.
4. Administration of ibuprofen to children is a common cause of Reye's syndrome.

_____ 2. Which type of medication is most likely to cause an allergic reaction in a 2-year-old child?
1. Pain relievers
2. Cough suppressants
3. Antibiotics
4. Topical lotions

_____ 3. An older adult patient has just completed a teaching session with the nurse on safe medication administration. Which statement made by the patient indicates a need for further teaching?
1. "I should not start any type of pills including those from the health food store unless I first clear it with my primary health care provider."
2. "I will go to the laboratory as directed to have my blood levels of drugs measured as indicated."
3. "I will get rid of any old pills I was taking to avoid confusion with the current pills I am taking."
4. "I will take all of my pills at the same time each day to avoid having to take them throughout the day."

_____ 4. When teaching a group of pregnant patients about the use of medications during pregnancy, which statement does the nurse include?
1. "Because of the potential for injury to the developing fetus, drug therapy during pregnancy should be avoided if at all possible."
2. "It is all right to drink alcohol during pregnancy as long as you keep it to just wine."
3. "If you smoke, you should cut back to just five cigarettes a day. That way you are guaranteed to have no problems."
4. "You can use any herbal medicine you like because they are natural and will not hurt the baby."

_____ 5. The nurse is teaching a postdelivery patient about breastfeeding, including information on drug administration with breastfeeding mothers. Which statement made by the patient indicates that more teaching is needed?
1. "It is safe for me to take all of my prescription medications because my doctor would not order anything that isn't all right."
2. "If I need to take medicine, I will take it immediately after my baby has finished breastfeeding."
3. "I will discuss the use of any herbal products with my primary care provider before I take them because they can affect my baby."
4. "I know that many drugs are known to enter breast milk, so I will be sure to ask my primary care provider about any drugs before I take them."

_____ 6. Which statements about drug absorption and age considerations are true? *(Select all that apply.)*
1. Water-soluble drugs are absorbed more readily in infants.
2. Transdermal absorption in older adult patients is often difficult to predict.
3. Sublingual tablets should not be crushed.
4. Absorption of medications given intramuscularly (IM) may be affected in patients who are bedridden.
5. Dermal thickness increases with aging.

_____ 7. A mother who is nursing her young infant tells the nurse that she has been taking aspirin for stress headaches. What is the nurse's best response?
1. "An aspirin once in a while will have no effect on the baby."
2. "We really don't know the effect of aspirin on nursing babies."
3. "You cannot take any medication at all while you are nursing."
4. "Aspirin has been associated with significant adverse effects on nursing infants."

_____ 8. The prescriber orders peak and trough levels on a patient receiving gentamicin therapy at 0800, 1600, and 2400. The first dose of gentamicin was administered at 1600. At what time does the nurse obtain the trough level?
1. 1630
2. 1800
3. 2330
4. 0730

The Nursing Process and Pharmacology

Review Sheet

The QUESTION column and the ANSWER column have been offset so that you can cover the answer while reading the question, allowing you to assess your knowledge.

Question	Answer
1. Identify the purpose of nursing classification systems.	
2. Define *nursing diagnosis*.	1. Nursing classification systems provide a standardized language for recording and analysis of individualized nursing care delivery.
3. State the five steps of the nursing process.	2. A nursing diagnosis is a clinical judgment about individual, family, or community responses to actual or potential health problems/life processes.
4. Explain the purpose of the assessment phase of the nursing process.	3. The five steps of the nursing process are assessment, nursing diagnosis, planning, implementation, and evaluation.
5. What are defining characteristics?	4. Assessment is an ongoing data-gathering process that starts with the admission of the patient and continues until the patient is discharged from care. It is the problem-identifying phase of the nursing process used to identify existing (actual) patient problems and/or to identify patient problems that may be evolving.
6. How does a medical diagnosis differ from a nursing diagnosis?	5. Defining characteristics are existing signs and symptoms that help define the presence of a patient problem. They provide clinical evidence of an existing or developing patient problem.
7. What is a collaborative problem?	6. A medical diagnosis is a statement relating to a disease's or disorder's effect on the individual's physiologic functioning. A nursing diagnosis usually refers to the patient's ability to function in activities in daily living (ADLs) in relation to the impairment induced by the medical diagnosis. It identifies the individual's or group's response to the illness and defines a patient problem in which the nurse can intervene.
8. Why is a focused assessment beneficial to the nurse?	7. Collaborative problems require both medical or dental prescriptive orders and nursing interventions to monitor and evaluate the existing condition.

9. Differentiate among actual, risk/high risk, health promotion and wellness, and syndrome nursing diagnoses.

10. Explain the intent of using critical pathways.

11. What are the four phases of the planning process used to prepare to provide patient care?

12. Use Maslow's hierarchy of needs on p. 45 of the text to label and prioritize the following individual needs:
    a. need for family visitors
    b. need to avoid falls while ambulating
    c. need for basic care to prevent skin breakdown
    d. need for praise for learning about self-care

13. Which of the following are nursing actions?
    a. giving a bed bath
    b. forcing fluids
    c. taking vital signs
    d. developing a medical diagnosis statement

14. Label the following nursing actions as "D" for dependent, "I" for interdependent, and "ID" for independent:
    a. administering a tube feeding
    b. administering PRN medications
    c. positioning patient for comfort
    d. providing oral hygiene
    e. monitoring respiratory function between treatments by respiratory therapist

15. Develop a short-term goal for a patient receiving Maalox.

16. Explain why a drug history may be beneficial.

17. Label the following statements "S" for subjective data or "O" for objective data.
    a. "My medication makes me dizzy."
    b. "Yesterday the pain medication gave me good pain relief."
    c. One hour after administration of chemotherapy the nurse charts, "Patient vomited 4 ounces greenish-tinged, watery vomitus."

8. After establishing that a patient problem may or does exist, a focused assessment allows the nurse to concentrate the data collection process on a specific area that would help to define, validate, or negate the existence of a specific nursing diagnosis.

9. See definitions in textbook, p. 40.

10. Critical pathways provide a sequential, detailed plan for clinical interventions within a specified time period for a particular disease or disorder.

11. Planning encompasses: a) setting priorities, b) developing measurable goal statements, c) formulating nursing interventions, and d) developing anticipated therapeutic outcomes as a basis for evaluating the patient's status.

12. During a period of ambulation, these needs would be in the following order: b, c, a, d. The priority may vary depending on variables present.

13. a, b, and c are nursing actions.

14. Items a and b are dependent, c and d are independent, and e is interdependent. Note: d could be dependent if the oral hygiene was specifically ordered by the health care provider.

15. Multiple possible answers. One example is: The patient will be able to state the correct schedule for self-administration of Maalox on Tuesday, (date).

16. A drug history can be used to identify current drugs, OTC, and herbal products being taken or problems relating to drug therapy and to evaluate the need for medications.

18. Turn to a drug classification section in the textbook. Find the area labeled "Nursing Diagnosis." Explain the difference between indications and adverse effects when used to designate the nursing diagnoses associated with drug therapy.
19. Develop a statement for the therapeutic intent of a sedative for a patient having surgery tomorrow morning.

20. Differentiate between common and serious adverse effects.
21. List common laboratory studies used to evaluate liver (hepatic) function and those used to evaluate kidney (renal) function.

22. When are culture and sensitivity (C&S) tests taken?

23. What changes in the baseline CBC report should be reported to the health care provider?
24. Why are serum drug levels monitored?

25. What patient education should be done prior to discharge for all patients with medications prescribed?

26. List a minimum of five drugs that can be monitored by a blood draw.

17. Items a and b are subjective; c is objective.

18. Indications are nursing diagnosis statements that exist as a result of patient problems being experienced due to disruption of normal functioning by a disease process or disorder. Adverse effects are patient problems that have evolved as a result of drug therapy.
19. Therapeutic intent is to "provide rest and relaxation prior to surgery."
20. Common adverse effects are those that can generally be anticipated when the drug therapy is prescribed. It is important for the nurse to teach the patient steps he or she can take to minimize the adverse effects to make the drug therapy more tolerable. Serious adverse effects, also known as *adverse drug effects*, are those that require notification of the health care provider regarding the drug's action.
21. Hepatic function tests include AST, ALT, alkaline phosphatase, LDH, and GGT. Renal function tests include serum creatinine, creatinine clearance, blood urea nitrogen (BUN), and urinalysis.
22. C&S specimens (e.g., throat culture) are usually obtained prior to initiation of antibiotic therapy for an infection.
23. Elevated WBCs, bands, "segs," and/or lymphocytes should be reported.
24. Serum drug levels are monitored to establish whether the serum blood level of the specific drug is too low or in the nontherapeutic range, within the normal range and therapeutic, or too high and toxic to the patient.
25. Patient education before discharge should include drug name, dosage, route, and specific time(s) of administration; reason for taking the drug (therapeutic outcome or intent); common adverse effects and ways these can be minimized or eliminated; serious adverse effects; what to do if a dose is missed; and how to have the medication prescription filled.
26. Digoxin, theophylline, gentamicin, tobramycin, lithium, lidocaine, phenytoin, procainamide, quinidine, vancomycin, cyclosporine, and chloramphenicol can be monitored by a blood draw.

The Nursing Process and Pharmacology

Learning Activities

FILL-IN-THE-BLANK

Complete the following statements using the correct term.

1. A(n) _____ diagnosis is a statement of the patient's alterations in structure and function, and results in a diagnosis of a disease or disorder that impairs normal physiologic function.

2. A(n) _____ _____ and _____ nursing diagnosis is a clinical judgment about an individual, group, or community in transition from a specific level of wellness to a higher level of wellness.

3. A(n) _____ _____ _____ is a standardized care plan derived from "best practice" patterns, enabling the nurse to develop a treatment plan that sequences detailed clinical interventions to be performed over a projected amount of time for a specific case type or disease process.

4. Mary tells you she developed nausea and vomiting 4 hours after taking the first dose of her newly prescribed antibiotic. This would be an example of (subjective, objective) data.

5. The nursing instructor tells the student nurse to collect further data relating to Mary's case. The collection of patient data is known as the _____ phase of the nursing process.

6. Further inquiry reveals that Mary took the antibiotic on an empty stomach. In addition to gaining further information about the nausea and vomiting, the student nurse also asks Mary to tell her of all other medications being taken, both prescription and nonprescription. This is known as taking a(n) _____ . Mary indicates that she does not regularly take any other medicine.

7. After collecting the data, the student reviews the drug monograph on the antibiotic. It states that nausea and vomiting are common adverse effects if taken on an empty stomach. The student nurse compares the signs and symptoms present with the _____ _____ listed in a nursing diagnosis resource book to establish the actual _____ _____ .

8. Rescheduling of the time the medication is taken is an example of a nursing _____ . The student nurse suggests that Mary take the next dose of the medication with food.

9. Mary will self-administer the prescribed antibiotic with food at 6 AM, 12 noon, 6 PM, and midnight starting with the next dose. This is a(n) _____ _____ statement.

10. When a culture and sensitivity is ordered on a patient, it is important to be sure the test is performed _____ the first dose of medication is administered.

11. Nursing diagnosis statements dealing with a patient with a family history of a disease who is likely to develop the disease would be called _____ nursing diagnosis statements.

12. An example of a phase of the nursing process called _____ is the periodic review of goals/outcomes of care.

13. A nursing minimum data set is an example of a(n) _____ _____ _____ .

TRUE OR FALSE

Write "T" for true and "F" for false for each statement. Correct all false statements.

_____ 14. The nursing process is the foundation for the clinical practice of nursing.

_____ 15. Nurses should familiarize themselves with the nurse practice act in the state where they practice, to identify the educational and experiential qualifications necessary to perform physical assessment and develop nursing diagnoses.

_____ 16. A risk/high-risk nursing diagnosis is a clinical judgment that an individual, family, or community is more susceptible to the problem than others in the same or similar situation.

_____ 17. The measurable goal statements start with the specific amount of time allotted for attainment of a certain behavior followed by the nursing actions to be followed.

_____ 18. Evaluation of the expected outcomes of the patient's behavior is the final step of the nursing process.

The Nursing Process and Pharmacology

Practice Questions for the NCLEX® Examination

_____ 1. Which is the proper sequence of the nursing process?
1. Planning, intervention, evaluation, assessment
2. Nursing diagnosis statement, assessment, planning, intervention, evaluation
3. Assessment, nursing diagnoses statement, planning, intervention, evaluation
4. Planning, nursing diagnosis statement, intervention, evaluation

_____ 2. In which phase of the nursing process does the nurse set priorities, develop written outcome statements, formulate nursing interventions, formulate anticipated therapeutic outcomes, and integrate outcomes/classification system into critical pathways and/or care plans?
1. Implementation
2. Evaluation
3. Nursing diagnosis
4. Planning

_____ 3. Which is the priority ranking of Maslow's subcategory of human needs?
1. Personal growth and maturity
2. Love and affection
3. Protection from physical harm
4. Oxygen, circulation

_____ 4. When incorporating the nursing process into medication administration, the nurse follows which practices in obtaining a drug history? _(Select all that apply.)_
1. Reports any weight loss associated with use of the drug but not weight gain because this is an expected adverse effect of medication administration
2. Asks the patient about drugs currently being taken as well as those drugs which the patient has taken in the past year
3. Asks the patient about any drug allergies and the specifics about the reaction that occurs as well as treatments used for the reaction
4. Records any over-the-counter medications the patient states are being taken into the clinical record
5. Determines the presence of other disease processes

_____ 5. Which pieces of information are necessary when obtaining a medication history of a patient? _(Select all that apply.)_
1. Use of herbal medicines
2. Diet
3. Allergy to certain medications
4. Use of over-the-counter medications
5. Use of vitamins

_____ 6. Which are components of the planning phase of the nursing process? _(Select all that apply.)_
1. Set priorities
2. Formulate nursing diagnosis statements
3. Provide for patient safety
4. Formulate nursing interventions
5. Determine revisions

_____ 7. Which are nursing diagnoses approved by the North American Nursing Diagnosis Association—International (NANDA-I)? *(Select all that apply.)*
1. Congestive heart failure
2. Hypertension
3. Anxiety
4. Diarrhea
5. Powerlessness

_____ 8. Which is an example of a self-actualization need according to Maslow's subcategories of human needs?
1. Increased learning
2. Appreciation from others
3. Stability
4. Energy

_____ 9. When administering medications, which procedures does the nurse use to ensure patient safety? *(Select all that apply.)*
1. Uses the room number to identify the patient
2. Looks at the patient's name band for identity, and also requests that the patient state his or her name and birth date
3. When noncompliance is identified, collaboratively discusses reasons for not following the regimen
4. Documents development of common adverse effects
5. Identifies the patient each time a medication is to be administered

Patient Education and Health Promotion

Review Sheet

The QUESTION column and the ANSWER column have been offset so that you can cover the answer while reading the question, allowing you to assess your knowledge.

Question	Answer
1. Explain the *cognitive domain*.	
2. Explain the *affective domain*.	1. The cognitive domain is the level at which basic knowledge is learned and stored. It is the thinking portion of the learning process and incorporates a person's previous experience and perceptions.
3. Explain the *psychomotor domain*.	2. The affective domain is the most intangible portion of the learning process. Affective behavior is conduct that expresses feelings, needs, beliefs, values, and opinions.
4. When preparing to teach the patient and family health-related information, how is the process best started?	3. The psychomotor domain involves the learning of a new procedure or skill. It is often referred to as the *doing* domain.
5. What is the most effective way to ensure mastery of psychomotor skills being taught?	4. Glean what information is essential, then consider what the patient wants to know. It is best to begin with the patient's questions and proceed from there. Otherwise, you may be explaining things the patient is not interested in knowing, and the individual may not be focused on the presentation.
6. Before initiating a teaching plan, what is most important for the nurse to do first?	5. Reciprocal demonstrations are particularly useful for ensuring mastery. It helps to allow the learner to practice the task several times. Giving the person immediate feedback on skills mastered, and then giving time to practice the skills that are more difficult allows the learner to improve in manual dexterity and master the sequencing of the procedure.
7. What must the nurse take into consideration when assessing a child's readiness to learn?	6. The nurse must be certain that the patient is able to focus and concentrate on the tasks and material to be learned. The patient's basic needs such as food, oxygen, and pain relief must be met before he or she is able to focus on learning.

8. What must the nurse take into consideration when teaching the older adult?

9. How would you develop a plan to teach a patient how to take a medication?

7. Psychosocial, cognitive, and language abilities must be considered. Cognitive and motor development, as well as the learner's language usage and understanding, must be assessed. Age definitely influences the type and amount of self-care activities the child is capable of learning and executing independently.

8. The older adult needs additional assessment before health teaching is implemented. Assess vision, hearing, and short- and long-term memory. If a task is to be taught, assess fine and gross motor abilities. When teaching an older adult patient, it is prudent to slow the pace of the presentation and limit the length of each session to prevent overtiring. Older adults can learn the material, but often they process things more slowly than younger people because their short-term memory may be more limited.

9. Refer to Box 5-1 in the text.

Patient Education and Health Promotion

Learning Activities

FILL-IN-THE-BLANK

Complete the following statements using the correct term.

1. The _____ domain is the level at which basic knowledge is learned and stored.

2. The _____ domain involves the learning of a new procedure or skill; it is often referred to as the *doing* domain.

3. _____ is the assumption that one's culture provides the right way, the best way, and the only way to live.

TRUE OR FALSE

Write "T" for true and "F" for false for each statement. Correct all false statements.

_____ 4. Affective behavior is conduct that expresses feelings, needs, beliefs, values, and opinions.

_____ 5. When providing patient teaching, it is best to begin with the information that the nurse feels is most important to be taught.

_____ 6. Explaining the various self-care needs to an individual and exploring his or her prior knowledge is an example of the affective domain of learning.

_____ 7. Establishing an environment that is conducive to learning is essential to the overall learning process.

_____ 8. Deciding what to teach and how much to teach is essential to the learning process.

_____ 9. Utilizing an established teaching plan that all nurses can build on is important to the continuity of health teaching.

_____ 10. Health teaching is valued by all individuals equally.

_____ 11. Children may need adaptations in prepared learning materials based on their age, learning capabilities, and development.

_____ 12. It is best to explain all of the information needed for self-care so the teaching plan on the chart documents that all the health teaching was accomplished prior to discharge.

_____ 13. Illness may not have the same meaning for all individuals.

Patient Education and Health Promotion

chapter

5

Practice Questions for the NCLEX® Examination

_____ 1. A nurse is preparing to teach a patient the subcutaneous insulin administration process. The nurse will be working with the patient in which domain of leaning?
   1. Cognitive
   2. Psychomotor
   3. Affective
   4. Effective

_____ 2. Which is the best way for the nurse to teach a patient how to perform postoperative dressing changes at home?
   1. Show the patient a video of the correct procedure
   2. Ask the patient if he or she has any questions about the procedure
   3. Have the patient demonstrate how he or she will change the dressing
   4. Demonstrate to the patient how the procedure should be done

_____ 3. When teaching patients psychomotor skills, what is the most useful way for the nurse to ensure mastery of content taught?
   1. Written test
   2. Asking the patient if he or she understands the process
   3. Reciprocal demonstrations
   4. Verbal description of the process taught

_____ 4. Before providing teaching to a patient about the care of a colostomy, what is most important for the nurse to do?
   1. Schedule enough time to complete the teaching
   2. Plan when the next teaching session should take place
   3. Take the patient to a private room
   4. Ensure that the patient's basic needs, such as pain relief, are met before initiating a teaching plan

_____ 5. When conducting patient education using an interpreter, which techniques will the nurse be sure to use? (Select all that apply.)
   1. Looking directly at the interpreter when conversing
   2. Sometimes supplementing with pictures when interacting with the patient
   3. Using pantomime when interacting with the patient
   4. Keeping the questions brief, and asking them one at a time to the interpreter
   5. First explaining the educational session to the interpreter and the type of questions that will be asked of the patient

_____ 6. What techniques does the nurse use when teaching an older adult patient? (Select all that apply.)
   1. Slow the pace of the presentation
   2. Limit the length of each session
   3. Connect new ideas with past experiences
   4. Avoid repetition of content
   5. Evaluate mastery of psychomotor skills by paper and pencil test

_____ 7. Identify the correct sequence of the following steps that the nurse follows when teaching a patient about self-administration of an inhaled medication regimen.
1. Ask the patient to demonstrate taking the inhaled medication
2. Determine the patient's current level of knowledge and understanding of how to take the medication
3. Demonstrate the correct method of taking the medication
4. Determine mutual realistic and measurable goals or outcomes for the teaching
5. Document the teaching in the patient's chart

_____ 8. When psychomotor skills are being taught, what is most effective for the nurse to do? (*Select all that apply.*)
1. Use paper and pencil tests to ensure mastery
2. Allow the learner to practice a task several times
3. Provide immediate feedback
4. Maintain an enthusiastic attitude about the content being taught
5. Explain why a certain procedure is being done

A Review of Arithmetic

chapter

6

Learning Activities (Part 1)

EQUIVALENTS AND CONVERSION

Memorize the equivalents listed in Chapter 6, then answer the following questions.

Household Equivalents

1. 4 cups = _____ quarts

2. 1 tablespoon = _____ teaspoons

3. 8 ounces = _____ cup(s)

4. 1 pint = _____ cup(s)

Metric Equivalents

5. 1 mL = _____ cc

6. 1 liter = _____ mL

7. 1 milligram (mg) = _____ micrograms (mcg)

8. 1 gram (g) = _____ milligrams (mg)

Conversion Rules

9. To convert milligrams to grams:

STOP! IF YOU HAVE NOT MEMORIZED THE EQUIVALENTS AND THE CONVERSION RULES, YOU SHOULD NOT PROCEED UNTIL YOU HAVE DONE SO.

Copyright © 2010, 2007, 2004, 2001, 1997 by Mosby, Inc., an affiliate of Elsevier Inc. All rights reserved.

35

A Review of Arithmetic

Learning Activities (Part 2)

Roman Numerals

Convert the following Arabic numerals to Roman numerals.

1. 5 = _____

2. 7 1/2 = _____

3. 4 = _____

4. 15 = _____

5. 20 = _____

6. 24 = _____

Fractions, Decimals, and Percents

Which of the following fractions is the largest? Circle your answer.

7. 1/8 or 1/16

8. 2/3 or 3/4

9. 1/100 or 1/200

10. 1/4 or 1/3

11. 3/8 or 7/8

12. 1/150 or 1/90

Reduce the following fractions.

13. 4/16 = _____

14. 12/24 = _____

15. 4/8 = _____

16. 36/48 = _____

17. 1 12/18 = _____

18. 3 34/85 = _____

19. 1 6/8 = _____

20. 12 6/8 = _____

21. 2 30/60 = _____

22. 3/9 = _____

Write the following fractions as decimals. When applicable, carry the decimal to thousandths and round to hundredths.

23. 7/8 = _____

24. 5/6 = _____

25. 1 3/4 = _____

26. 2/3 = _____

27. 15/16 = _____

28. 1/3 = _____

29. 5/8 = _____

30. 7/9 = _____

31. 1/16 = _____

32. 1/2 = _____

Identify the numerator or denominator for each of the following fractions as indicated.

33. 1/5 numerator is _____

34. 2/3 numerator is _____

35. 3/8 numerator is _____

36. 1 1/2 denominator is _____

37. 9/10 denominator is _____

38. 2 2/5 numerator is _____

39. 6/10 denominator is _____

40. 1 1/3 denominator is _____

Multiply the following fractions. Reduce answers to lowest terms.

41. $1/3 \times 1/4 =$ _____

42. $2/3 \times 3/8 =$ _____

43. $7/8 \times 1/2 =$ _____

44. $3/4 \times 7/8 =$ _____

45. $1/2 \times 4/7 =$ _____

46. $7/8 \times 2/3 =$ _____

47. $1\,1/2 \times 3/4 =$ _____

48. $2\,2/3 \times 4/5 =$ _____

Divide the following. As appropriate, carry to hundredths and round to tenths.

49. $2/3 \div 7/8 =$ _____

50. $1/3 \div 1/2 =$ _____

51. $5/9 \div 1/4 =$ _____

52. $21.78 \div 1.23 =$ _____

53. $756 \div 12.3 =$ _____

54. $32 \div 1.78 =$ _____

55. $112 \div 0.06 =$ _____

56. $1.22 \div 0.32 =$ _____

57. $3.789 \div 0.112 =$ _____

Change the following percents to decimals and the fractions to percents. Whenever applicable, carry the decimal to the thousandths, and round to the hundredths.

58. $56\% =$ _____

59. $1/150 =$ _____%

60. $2/3 =$ _____%

61. $75\% =$ _____

62. $1/2\% =$ _____

63. $3/4 =$ _____%

64. $7/8 =$ _____%

65. $123\% =$ _____

Change the following decimals to fractions and the fractions to decimals.

66. $0.3 =$ _____

67. $0.003 =$ _____

68. $0.03 =$ _____

69. $4/10 =$ _____

70. $4/100 =$ _____

71. $4/1000 =$ _____

Change the following percents to ratios.

72. $75\% =$ _____

73. $60\% =$ _____

74. $1/2\% =$ _____

Convert the following using equivalency tables.

75. 1 quart = _____ cup(s)

76. _____ ounces = 1 pint

77. 3 teaspoons = _____ tablespoon(s)

78. 0.125 g = _____ mg

79. 250 mg = _____ g

80. 1 teaspoon = _____ mL

81. 6 lbs = _____ kg (round to hundredths)

82. 165 lbs = _____ kg

A Review of Arithmetic

Practice Questions for the NCLEX® Examination

1. Order: ibuprofen (Motrin) 0.8 g PO
   Supply: 400-mg tablets
   _____ tablet(s) are needed for each dose

2. Order: valproic acid (Depakene) 0.75 g PO
   Supply: 250 mg per 5 mL
   _____ mL are needed for each dose

3. Order: warfarin (Coumadin) 15 mg PO
   Supply: 10-mg tablets
   _____ tablet(s) are needed for each dose

4. Order: 120 mg furosemide (Lasix) IM
   Supply: 10 mg/mL
   _____ mL is administered

5. Order: haloperidol (Haldol) 4 mg IM
   Supply: 5 mg/mL
   _____ mL is administered

6. Order: Administer 1000 mL of D_5W every 8 hours IV. The drop factor is 15 gtt/mL. How many drops per minute is the IV rate?
   _____ gtt/min

7. Order: 600 mL of solution over 12 hours IV. The drop factor is 20 gtt/mL. How many gtt/min does the nurse administer? _____ gtt/min

8. A child who weighs 55 pounds weighs _____ kilogram(s).

9. A patient takes methyldopa (Aldomet), 500-mg tablets, 3 to 4 times per day. The patient is advised not to exceed a daily dose of 3 grams or _____ tablet(s).

10. A patient's temperature of 100° F converts to _____ ° C.

Principles of Medication Administration and Medication Safety

Review Sheet

The QUESTION column and the ANSWER column have been offset so you can cover the answer while reading the question, allowing you to assess your knowledge.

Question	Answer
1. What is the nurse practice act?	
2. What are the Standards of Care in relationship to nursing?	1. The nurse practice act establishes the rules and regulations for the practice of nursing at the various entry levels within a practice area in each state.
3. Can an employing agency write policies that require the nurse to exceed the standards established by the state board of nursing/nursing licensing agency?	2. Guidelines for the practice of nursing are defined by the nurse practice act of each state, by state and federal laws regulating health care facilities, The Joint Commission, as well as by professional organizations such as the American Nurses Association and other specialty nursing organizations such as the Intravenous Nurses Society, Inc.
4. What types of medications may have restrictions regarding the qualifications of an individual to administer the medicine?	3. No. Policies of the employing agency can authorize less than, but not more than, the established maximum standards.
5. What information is the nurse expected to know about a specific drug before administering it?	4. Antineoplastic medicines, magnesium sulphate, lidocaine, RhoGAM, allergy extracts, and heparin are administered in accordance with specific limitations of the employing agency. Most policies require doses of heparin and insulin to be checked by two qualified individuals. Additional policies are developed to identify guidelines within a particular clinical site for the administration of intravenous therapy.
6. What information should be recorded whenever a "PRN" medicine is to be administered?	5. See textbook, pp. 81-82.
7. What role do critical pathways have on the delivery of clinical care?	6. Before administration of any PRN medication, the patient's chart should be checked to ensure that someone else has not administered the drug, and that the specified time interval has passed since the medication was last administered. When a PRN medication is given, it should be charted immediately. Record the response to the medication.
8. Examine the sections on a medication administration record (MAR) to identify the categories used.	7. Critical pathways are a multidisciplinary plan used by all health care providers to track the individual's progress toward expected outcomes within a specified time period.

9. Where would information regarding a patient's possible allergies be found?

10. Explain the differences among the ward stock, computer-controlled ordering and dispensing system, individual prescription order, and unit dose drug distribution (acute and long-term care) systems.

11. Identify procedures for the electronic transmission of patient orders.

12. What are adverse drug events (ADEs)?

13. Referring to the controlled substance inventory form, Figure 7-12 in the textbook, list some controlled narcotic drugs routinely used in the acute care setting.

14. What information is recorded on the controlled substance inventory form when a controlled substance is administered?

15. Summarize appropriate guidelines for disposal of unused medicines.

16. Explain the differences among a stat order, standing order, PRN order, verbal order, and fax order.

17. How is a drug order verified and transcribed?

18. What are the six "rights" of drug administration?

19. What is medication reconciliation?

20. What tests are used to identify hepatic and renal function?

21. What methods are used to ensure correct identification of a patient prior to drug administration? (Discuss adults, children, and inpatient and outpatient settings.)

22. Review error-prone abbreviations, symbols, and dose designations to be avoided in written communications to prevent medication errors.

8. Medication administration records are usually divided into five sections: scheduled section, parenteral section, stat section, preoperative orders, and PRN medication section.

9. Information about a patient's allergies is recorded in the history and physical section of the chart, the Kardex, the MAR, the patient's chart holder, and on the patient's allergy bracelet.

10. See textbook pp. 91-97 under Drug Distribution Systems.

11. Faxed orders must be signed within a specified time, often 24 hours.

12. See textbook p. 100, information under Medication Safety.

13. Diazepam (Valium), meperidine (Demerol), morphine, and Tylenol with codeine.

14. The date, time, name of medicine administered, patient's name, amount wasted (if any), and the number of dosage containers (such as unit dose tablets or ampules) remaining after the drug is removed are recorded on the form. The nurse administering the medicine signs the record as well as the qualified witness if any medicine is wasted.

15. See textbook, p. 99.

16. See textbook pp. 99-100, information under Types of Medication Orders.

17. See textbook p. 102, information under Nurse's Responsibilities.

18. The six "rights" of drug administration are: right drug, right time, right dose, right patient, right route, and right documentation.

19. Medication reconciliation is the process of comparing a patient's current medication order to all of the medications that the patient is actually taking.

20. Liver function tests include aspartate aminotransferase (AST), alanine aminotransferase (ALT), alkaline phosphatase, lactic dehydrogenase (LDH), and gamma glutamyl transferase (GGT). Renal function tests include serum creatinine, creatinine clearance, blood urea nitrogen (BUN), and urinalysis.

21. See textbook p. 104, information under Right Patient.

22. See inside back cover of the textbook, ISMP's "Do Not Use" Abbreviations.

Student Name _____

Principles of Medication Administration and Medication Safety

chapter

7

Learning Activities

FILL-IN-THE-BLANK

Finish each of the following statements using the correct term.

1. A component of the patient's chart includes the _____ form which grants permission to the health care facility and physician to provide treatment.

2. A component of the patient's chart includes the _____ pathways which are standardized outcomes and timetables which require health care providers to assess the patient's progress toward the goals of discharge while maintaining quality care.

3. The MAR or _____ _____ _____ lists all medications to be administered, and provides the pharmacist and the nurse with identical medication profiles for the patient.

4. _____ _____ _____ is the drug distribution system that uses single-unit packages of drugs dispensed to fill each dose requirement as it is ordered.

5. A(n) _____ order is generally used on an emergency basis; it means that the drug is to be administered as soon as possible, but only once.

MATCHING

Match the definition with the corresponding term. Definitions may be used more than once and some may not be used.

_____ 6. PRN medications

_____ 7. physician's order form

_____ 8. MAR

_____ 9. "stat"

_____ 10. Kardex

a. Check this section of the patient chart when questioning details of a drug order on the MAR.
b. Give around the clock.
c. Give immediately.
d. Administer as required or necessary within defined limits of the drug order.
e. Record scheduled drugs administered here.
f. Section of the patient record containing the care plan.
g. Controlled substances are recorded here when administered.

TRUE OR FALSE

Write "T" for true and "F" for false for each statement. Correct all false statements.

_____ 11. Standards of care are guidelines developed for the practice of nursing that are defined by the nurse practice act of each state, by state and federal laws regulating health care facilities, by the Joint Commission, as well as by professional organizations such as the American Nurses Association and other specialty nursing organizations.

Copyright © 2010, 2007, 2004, 2001, 1997 by Mosby, Inc., an affiliate of Elsevier Inc. All rights reserved.

41

_____ 12. The graphic record is an example of manual recording of temperature, pulse, respirations, and blood pressure.

_____ 13. When a medication is ordered PRN, the nurse identifies this as meaning the patient should receive this medication every night before bedtime.

_____ 14. A standing order must be written and signed by the physician before the nurse can continue to administer the medication.

_____ 15. Medication errors can result in serious complications known as *adverse drug events*.

Principles of Medication Administration and Medication Safety

Practice Questions for the NCLEX® Examination

_____ 1. It is 0900, and the nurse is reading a patient's chart. The prescriber has written diazepam (Valium) 10 mg IV stat. How does the nurse interpret this order?
   1. The patient will receive 10 mg of diazepam IV every morning at 0900.
   2. 10 mg of diazepam IV will be administered at this time, but only once.
   3. The patient will receive the diazepam with the next group of medicines scheduled to be administered.
   4. Because the patient doesn't have an IV started, the dose of the diazepam will be doubled to 20 mg and administered orally.

_____ 2. When preparing to administer a medication to a patient, the nurse is not able to verify that the medication order is appropriate. What actions does the nurse take? *(Select all that apply.)*
   1. Documents the reasons for refusal to administer the drug in accordance with the policies of the employing institution
   2. Contacts the person who prescribed the drug
   3. If the prescriber cannot be contacted, notifies the nursing supervisor on duty
   4. Administers the medication because it went through pharmacy, and they would have caught a problem if there was one
   5. Informs the patient about the disagreement with the treatment prescribed

_____ 3. The nurse administers digoxin (Lanoxin) 0.125 mg PO and glyburide (DiaBeta) 2.5 mg PO to a patient at 0900. At 0905 the patient vomits stomach contents including the medications. What does the nurse do next?
   1. Places a nasogastric tube into the patient and administers the medications via that route
   2. Tells the patient that he or she really needs to take the medicines and administers them again
   3. Contacts the physician and discusses alternative mediation orders, since the parenteral or rectal route may be preferred
   4. Contacts the pharmacy, has the medicines sent back in rectal form, and administers via that route

_____ 4. When documenting medication administration, what does the nurse record? *(Select all that apply.)*
   1. When a drug is not administered and why
   2. Medication administration before it is administered
   3. A possible medication error
   4. Any adverse reactions concerning medication administration
   5. Patient education that took place

_____ 5. What is the most effective method the nurse uses for identifying a pediatric patient for medication administration?
   1. Asking the child his or her name
   2. Asking a family member the child's name
   3. Checking the child's identification bracelet
   4. Checking the room assignment and bed the child is in

_____ 6. What is 6 AM in military time?
   1. 0600
   2. 1200
   3. 1800
   4. 2200

_____ 7. What is 2 PM in military time?
   1. 0200
   2. 0600
   3. 1200
   4. 1400

_____ 8. At what time is the inventory control record completed?
   1. When the patient asks for a controlled substance
   2. When the controlled substance is removed
   3. When the medication is administered
   4. When the degree of pain relief is assessed

_____ 9. At what time is the PRN medication record completed?
   1. When the patient asks for a controlled substance
   2. When the controlled substance is removed
   3. Immediately after administering the drug
   4. When the degree of pain relief is assessed

_____ 10. By whom is the narcotic control count performed?
   1. Charge nurse
   2. Nurse going off duty
   3. Nurse coming on duty
   4. Two nurses; one from shift going off duty and one from shift coming on duty

_____ 11. How is a drug on a scheduled order given?
   1. As many times as needed
   2. At prescribed/designated intervals
   3. One time only
   4. Immediately

_____ 12. When a verbal order is taken, it must be co-signed and dated by the prescriber within how many days?
   1. 3
   2. 2
   3. 1
   4. 1/2

_____ 13. Which person is responsible for the transcription of a drug order?
   1. Nurse's aide
   2. Unit secretary/ward clerk
   3. Prescriber
   4. Nurse

_____ 14. When "wasting" a portion of a dose of narcotic, the nurse must have this witnessed by which person?
   1. Prescriber
   2. Charge nurse
   3. Another qualified nurse
   4. Medication aide

_____ 15. When measuring a fractional dose of a medication with a volume of less than 1 mL, what is the most accurate method to use?
   1. Medicine cup
   2. Tuberculin syringe
   3. Teaspoon
   4. Medicine dropper

_____ 16. Which is the most reliable method to calculate pediatric drug doses?
   1. Body surface area (BSA)
   2. Clark's rule
   3. A fraction of the adult dose
   4. Pyxis system of measurement

_____ 17. A patient has a new drug ordered bid. How will the drug be administered?
   1. Once daily
   2. Two times per day
   3. Three times per day
   4. Four times per day

_____ 18. To what drug dosage system does the Pyxis system refer?
   1. Narcotic inventory system
   2. Individual prescription order system
   3. Unit dose system used primarily in long-term care
   4. Electronic medication dispensing system

_____ 19. The MAR in a long-term care setting is designed to be used for how long?
1. 8 hours
2. 24 hours
3. 1 week
4. 1 month

_____ 20. Faxed medication orders are usually signed by the health care provider within how many hours?
1. 8
2. 12
3. 24
4. 48

_____ 21. Electronic database charting systems may vary, but they must comply with the guidelines/requirements of which organization while incorporating standards of care?
1. American Nurses Association
2. The Joint Commission
3. Infusion Nurses Society
4. National League of Nurses

_____ 22. Unit dose systems in a long-term care setting supply enough medication containers for what time period?
1. 8 hours
2. 24 hours
3. 48 hours
4. 1 week

_____ 23. Which are common contents of patient charts in health care facilities? _(Select all that apply.)_
1. Consent forms
2. Kardex records
3. MARs
4. Patient education records
5. Laboratory reports

Percutaneous Administration

Review Sheet

The QUESTION column and the ANSWER column have been offset so you can cover the answer while reading the question, allowing you to assess your knowledge.

Question

1. What factors affect the absorption of topical medications?

2. What is the major advantage of the percutaneous route for drug administration?

3. Explain the differences among a cream, lotion, ointment, and wet dressing, and cite the methods used to apply each.

4. What health teaching should be given to a patient using a topical form of medication?

5. What is the purpose of patch testing?

6. Describe the method used to apply allergens and read results.

7. List commonly used symbols for reading of reactions to allergen testing.

8. Describe the specific method used to apply nitroglycerin ointment and a nitroglycerin transdermal disk.

9. Why is it important for the nurse to wear gloves when applying a topical ointment or transdermal patch?

10. What types of medications are available in transdermal patch form?

Answer

1. Factors affecting the absorption of topical medications include drug concentration, the length of time the medication is in contact with the skin, size and depth of affected area, and thickness and hydration of the skin.

2. The action of the drug is primarily limited to the site of application, thereby decreasing the systemic adverse effects.

3. See textbook, pp. 108-109.

4. Patients receiving topical medications should receive the following health teaching: personal hygiene measures to treat/improve underlying condition, methods of application, ways to avoid touching affected areas, and prevention of spread of infection when present.

5. Patch testing is used to identify specific sensitivity to allergens.

6. See textbook, pp. 110-112.

7. Commonly used symbols for reading allergen patch test reactions include (see also p. 112):
   +   1+ no wheal, 3-mm flare
   ++   2+ 2–3-mm wheal with flare
   +++   3+ 3–5-mm wheal with flare
   ++++   4+ > 5-mm wheal

8. See textbook, pp. 112-113.

9. The nurse should wear gloves when administering a topical ointment or transdermal patch to avoid inadvertent absorption of the medication by the nurse through the skin.

47

11. Why is it important to discard transdermal medication patches safely after removal?

12. What schedule is used for the administration of the estrogen transdermal systems?

13. Where are sublingual and buccal forms of medication administered?

14. What is the primary advantage of the sublingual route?

15. Describe the correct techniques for administering eye drops, eye ointments, and eye disks, including patient teaching.

16. Compare the correct technique of administering an ear (otic) drug to a child and to an adult.

17. Explain the procedure for instilling nose drops/nasal sprays into an adult and a child; include health teaching.

18. Why shouldn't oily preparations be administered by inhalation?

19. Explain how to give medications by inhalation.

20. What is a metered-dose inhaler?

21. Explain how to teach a patient to administer a medication using an inhaler.

22. Explain the correct technique for inserting a vaginal suppository and proper hygiene measures used during the course of treatment.

10. Nitroglycerin, clonidine, estrogen, nicotine, scopolamine, and fentanyl are examples of some medications available in transdermal patch forms.

11. Used transdermal patches must be safely discarded because the patch may still contain some medication that could be harmful to individuals or pets for whom it is not prescribed.

12. Estrogen transdermal systems are designed to be worn continuously for 3 weeks, followed by a 1-week interval without a patch before applying the next patch.

13. Sublingual medications are administered under the tongue; buccal medications are administered in the back cheek area of the mouth.

14. In addition to being easy to access, the sublingual area provides rapid absorption and onset of action of the drug because the drug passes directly into the systemic circulation with no immediate pass through the liver, where extensive metabolism usually takes place.

15. See textbook, pp. 116-118.

16. See textbook, pp. 118-119.

17. See textbook, pp. 119-120.

18. Oily preparations should not be administered by inhaler because oil droplets would be carried to the lungs and initiate a lipid pneumonia.

19. See textbook, pp. 120-121.

20. A metered-dose inhaler is an aerosolized, pressurized inhaler that delivers a measured amount of medication with each depression of the device.

21. See textbook, pp. 121-123.

22. See textbook, pp. 123-124.

Student Name _____

Percutaneous Administration

chapter

8

Learning Activities

FILL-IN-THE-BLANK

Finish each of the following statements using the correct term.

1. _____ are semisolid emulsions containing medicinal agents for external application.

2. _____ tablets are designed to be placed under the tongue for dissolution and absorption through the vast network of blood vessels in this area, and _____ tablets are designed to be held between the cheek and molar teeth for absorption from the blood vessels of the cheek.

3. Medications that are labeled "ophthalmic" are meant for administration to the _____.

4. When administering ear drops to a child under the age of 3 years, the nurse should restrain the child, turn the head to the appropriate side, and gently pull the earlobe _____ and _____.

5. Bronchodilators and corticosteroids may be administered by oral inhalation through the mouth using an aerosolized, pressurized _____ _____ _____.

TRUE OR FALSE

Write "T" for true and "F" for false for each statement. Correct all false statements.

_____ 6. It is now recognized that a major principle in wound healing is the need for a moist environment to propagate epithelization of the wound.

_____ 7. Patch testing is a method used to identify a patient's sensitivity to contact materials.

_____ 8. After applying the prescribed amount of nitroglycerin ointment to the skin, the nurse should rub the ointment into the skin until it can no longer be seen.

_____ 9. Aerosols use a flow of air or oxygen under pressure to disperse the drug throughout the respiratory tract.

_____ 10. Douching is not recommended during pregnancy.

Copyright © 2010, 2007, 2004, 2001, 1997 by Mosby, Inc., an affiliate of Elsevier Inc. All rights reserved.

49

Percutaneous Administration

Practice Questions for the NCLEX® Examination

_____ 1. Which actions does the nurse take when applying a wet dressing to a patient?
1. Leaves about one-half of the previous dressing in place to promote epithelization and wound healing
2. Wrings out wet dressing to prevent dripping and applies the gauze in a single layer directly to the wound surface
3. Does not pack deep wounds, lightly places gauze over them
4. After the wound is dressed, pours the liquid onto the top of the dressing and leaves it open to air

_____ 2. The nurse is working in an allergy clinic. What should be taken into consideration by the nurse when administering allergy testing to patients? *(Select all that apply.)*
1. Ensuring that emergency equipment is in the immediate area in case of an anaphylactic response
2. Positioning the patient so that the surface where the test material is to be applied is horizontal
3. Administering antihistamine and anti-inflammatory agents immediately before the test
4. Cleansing the area where the allergens are to be applied with an alcohol pledget and allowing the area to dry before starting testing
5. Documenting "no reaction" at the control site on the patient's chart

_____ 3. When administering nitroglycerin percutaneously to a patient, what does the nurse do?
1. Wears gloves
2. Applies wax paper over the site of the nitroglycerin to enhance absorption of the drug
3. Ensures that the drug is on the patient 24 hours a day, 7 days a week to avoid complications
4. Always places the nitroglycerin ointment over the left chest to provide the most effective route of drug delivery to the heart

_____ 4. When administering eye drops to a patient, which practices does the nurse follow? *(Select all that apply.)*
1. Instructs the patient to look upward over the head
2. Drops the specified number of drops into the conjunctival sac
3. After instilling the drops, applies gentle pressure using a cotton ball to the outer corner of the eye for 30 seconds
4. When more than one type of eye drop is ordered for the same eye, waits 1 to 5 minutes between instillation of the different medications
5. Rubs the eye in a circular motion for 1 minute after application of the medication

_____ 5. When teaching a patient how to administer a medication for oral inhalation via a metered-dose inhaler without the use of a spacer, the nurse informs the patient to perform which actions? *(Select all that apply.)*
1. If the medication is a suspension, shake the canister before administration.
2. Close the mouth around the canister when administering the medication.
3. Activate the metered-dose inhaler and inhale deeply over 10 seconds to ensure that airways are open and that the drug is dispersed as deeply as possible.
4. If the inhaled medication is a corticosteroid, rinse the mouth with water when administration is complete.
5. Cleanse the apparatus according to the manufacturer's recommendations.

_____ 6. Eye medications may be administered by which methods? *(Select all that apply.)*
1. Irrigation
2. Drops
3. Ointment
4. Patch
5. Sub-corneal

_____ 7. When administering ear medication to an adult, in which way is the pinna pulled?
1. Up
2. Up and back
3. Down
4. Down and back

_____ 8. When administering ear medication to a child, in which way is the pinna pulled?
1. Up
2. Back and up
3. Down
4. Back and down

_____ 9. A student nurse is administering an eye ointment to a patient. Which action by the student nurse requires the supervising nurse to intervene?
1. Holding the tube between the hands for several minutes before administering the medication
2. Discarding the first centimeter of ointment when opening the tube for the first time
3. Instructing the patient to close the eyes for 1–2 minutes and roll the eyeball in all directions after the medication has been administered
4. Administering the medication under the upper lid of the eye

_____ 10. Nitroglycerin administered by which route has the longest duration of action?
1. Intravenous
2. Sublingual
3. Topical
4. Transdermal

Enteral Administration

Review Sheet

The QUESTION column and the ANSWER column have been offset so you can cover the answer while reading the question, allowing you to assess your knowledge.

Question	Answer
1. When an individual is unable to swallow or has had oral surgery, an alternative route of administration is the _____ route.	
2. A major advantage of using the rectal route for drug administration is _____.	1. Nasogastric (NG)
3. List the composition and advantages of the following dosage forms: capsules, timed-release capsules, lozenges, tablets, elixirs, emulsions, suspensions, and syrups.	2. Bypass the digestive enzymes and avoid irritation to the esophagus and stomach.
4. Why is it important to use the medicine dropper that accompanies a medication?	3. See textbook pp. 126-128, information under Dose Forms.
5. Why is an oral syringe preferred over a household teaspoon for administering a medication?	4. The dropper has been specifically made to correspond with the viscosity of the drug to deliver the correct volume of medication.
6. List the six "rights" of medication administration.	5. An oral syringe is more accurate.
7. What are the primary principles of giving a solid form and liquid form of a medication?	6. The six rights of administration are: RIGHT patient, RIGHT drug, RIGHT dosage, RIGHT time of administration, RIGHT route of administration, and RIGHT documentation.
8. Discuss the proper method(s) of checking NG tube placement prior to the administration of a drug or an enteral formula.	7. See textbook pp. 131 and 133, information under General Principles of Solid-Form Medication Administration and General Principles of Liquid-Form Oral Medication Administration.
9. Identify the color and pH values of gastric, intestinal, and pleural secretions, both with and without the administration of H_2 blockers (antagonists).	8. Verify NG location after initial placement using x-ray verification BEFORE administering any drug or enteral formula for the first time. (See textbook, pp. 134-135.)
10. Name four general categories of enteral formulas.	9. See textbook pp. 134-135, Method 1: pH and color testing of gastric contents to check for tube placement.
11. Review the procedure for NG administration of enteral formulas using bolus and continuous infusion techniques.	10. Four general types of enteral formulas are: intact (polymeric) nutrient, elemental, disease- or condition-specific, and modular nutrients.

12. State the positioning used for a patient when he or she is receiving an NG feeding using the bolus and using a continuous delivery method.

13. How are rectal suppositories inserted?

14. What position is the patient placed in to administer a disposable enema?

11. See textbook, pp. 135-137.

12. Place the patient in semi-Fowler's position with head of bed (HOB) elevated 30 degrees for 30 minutes before and at least 1 hour after a bolus feeding. Most patients with a continuous feeding are maintained at a 30- to 45-degree elevation of the HOB.

13. Apply a glove or finger cot, have suppository in a solid form, use water-soluble lubricant or plain water to moisten, then insert suppository about 1 inch past the internal sphincter in the rectum.

14. To administer a disposable enema, place the patient on the left side.

Student Name _____

Enteral Administration

chapter

9

Learning Activities

FILL-IN-THE-BLANK

Finish each of the following statements using the correct term.

1. The three routes of drug administration can be classified into the following categories: _____, _____, and _____.

2. _____ are small, cylindrical gelatin containers that hold dry powder or liquid medicinal agents.

3. _____ are dispersions of small droplets of water in oil or oil in water, and are often used to mask bitter tastes or provide better solubility to certain drugs.

4. When using the metric system, one teaspoon equals _____ mL.

5. After a patient receives a suppository, the nurse should instruct the patient to remain lying on the side for _____ to _____ minutes to allow melting and absorption of the medication.

6. Elixirs are drugs dissolved in _____ and _____.

7. Syrups are drugs dissolved in concentrated _____ with _____.

8. On the medicine cup, 1 oz (fl oz) equals _____ tbsp.

9. On the medicine cup, 1 tsp equals _____ mL.

TRUE OR FALSE

Write "T" for true and "F" for false for each statement. Correct all false statements.

_____ 10. The oral route is safe, most convenient, and relatively economical, and dose forms are readily available for most medications. The major disadvantage of this route is that it has the slowest and least dependable rate of absorption, and thus onset of action, of the commonly used routes of administration.

_____ 11. Enteric-coated tablets must not be crushed or chewed, or the active ingredients will be released prematurely and be destroyed in the stomach.

_____ 12. When a liquid medication is poured into a medicine cup, a meniscus forms in the cup. The amount of medication in the cup should be read at the lowest point of the concave curve of the meniscus.

_____ 13. Suppositories are intended only for rectal administration.

_____ 14. Patients receiving an enema should be placed in the right lateral position, unless the knee-chest position has been specified.

_____ 15. The oral dropper that accompanied a specific drug is lost. The nurse should substitute a dropper from another medication for the lost one.

_____ 16. To validate the correct placement of an NG tube prior to administering a medication or enteral feeding, it is acceptable to aspirate gastric contents and check the pH and color.

Copyright © 2010, 2007, 2004, 2001, 1997 by Mosby, Inc., an affiliate of Elsevier Inc. All rights reserved.

55

_____ 17. When flushing an NG tube, do not clamp the tube until all the solution has time to reach the stomach.

_____ 18. When documenting an enteral feeding, the amount administered is charted on the intake and output sheet and then is included in the intake total for each shift.

_____ 19. Intermittent tube feedings require that the unused formula mixed and dispensed by the pharmacy be discarded every 48 hours.

_____ 20. The HOB is elevated 30 minutes before and 30 minutes to 1 hour after administering an intermittent tube feeding.

_____ 21. Rectal suppositories are generally inserted with the patient positioned in the Sims' position.

_____ 22. A disposable enema is administered with the patient positioned on the right side.

_____ 23. When testing gastric pH for a person NOT taking an H_2 blocker such as ranitidine, the gastric contents would have a pH of 1.0–4.0.

_____ 24. When testing gastric pH for a person who is taking an H_2 blocker such as ranitidine, the gastric contents would have a pH > 4.0.

_____ 25. Aspirated intestinal fluid should be a clear- to straw-colored secretion.

_____ 26. Auscultation is an accurate method of checking NG tube placement.

Enteral Administration

Practice Questions for the NCLEX® Examination

_____ 1. When administering a liquid form of an oral medication to an infant, the nurse performs which activity?
   1. Is certain that the infant is alert
   2. Positions the infant so that the head is lowered
   3. Places the syringe or dropper at the tip of the infant's tongue
   4. Injects the medicine rapidly to facilitate swallowing of the medicine

_____ 2. When administering medications to an adult via an NG tube, what does the nurse do?
   1. Crushes timed-released capsules before administration via the nasogastric tube to prevent clogging of the tube
   2. Flushes the nasogastric tube with at least 30 mL of sterile water before and after administration of the medicine
   3. Flushes between each medication with 50 mL of water (when more than one medication is to be administered at about the same time)
   4. Checks for correct placement of the nasogastric tube after the medications are instilled

_____ 3. When checking for correct placement of an NG tube, the nurse aspirates yellow fluid from the nasogastric tube. Based on the color of the aspirate, the nurse identifies the fluid as most likely being of which type?
   1. Gastric
   2. Intestinal
   3. Pleural
   4. Tracheobronchial

_____ 4. When working with patients receiving enteral feedings via a gastrostomy tube, the nurse performs which actions? (Select all that apply.)
   1. Checks the residual volume before each feeding
   2. Checks to ensure the presence of bowel sounds
   3. Checks the position of the tube to ensure that it is still in the stomach
   4. Discards unused portions every 8 hours
   5. Changes the administration equipment every 12 hours

_____ 5. When administering an enema to an adult, what does the nurse do?
   1. Encourages the patient to hold the solution for about 5 minutes before defecating
   2. Tells the patient not to flush the toilet until you return and can see the results of the enema
   3. Inserts 1 inch of the lubricated rectal tube into the rectum
   4. Heats the enema to 101° F to ensure comfort in administration

_____ 6. When administering a solid form of medication to a patient, which procedures does the nurse apply? (Select all that apply.)
   1. Giving the most important medication first
   2. Having the patient place the medication on the front of the tongue
   3. Encouraging the patient to keep the head back while swallowing
   4. Remaining with the patient while the medication is being taken
   5. Having the patient drink a full glass of water with the medication

_____ 7. Before administering medication via an
   NG tube, the nurse checks for correct
   tube placement. Which findings indicate
   that the tube is in the correct location?
   (Select all that apply.)
   1. Aspiration of clear fluid from the na-
      sogastric tube
   2. Recent x-ray verification of tube
      placement
   3. Gastric pH result of 3.0
   4. Auscultation of air over the right up-
      per quadrant of the abdomen
   5. Palpation of the tube in the stomach

8. A patient is ordered 2/3 strength Sustacal 360
   mL to be administered over 4 hours via a gastrostomy tube. Sustacal is available in 10 fluid
   ounce cans. How many cans of Sustacal will the
   patient require? _____ can(s)

9. An order reads 2/3 strength Ensure 90 mL
   every hour for 5 hours via NG tube. Ensure is
   available in 8 fluid ounce cans. How many mL
   of water will the nurse use to dilute 300 mL of
   Ensure to the appropriate strength? _____ mL

10. A baby is ordered 3/8 strength Enfamil. The
    baby needs 32 fluid ounces of the 3/8 strength
    Enfamil for one feeding. Enfamil is available
    in 6 fluid ounce bottles. How many bottles of
    Enfamil will the baby need for one feeding?
    _____ bottle(s)

Parenteral Administration: Safe Preparation of Parenteral Medications

Review Sheet

The QUESTION column and the ANSWER column have been offset so that you can cover the answer while reading the question, allowing you to assess your knowledge.

Question	Answer
1. Define *parenteral*.	1. Parenteral medication administration routes are intradermal, intramuscular (IM), and intravenous (IV) injections.
2. What are the major advantages of parenteral medication administration?	
3. Cite specific nursing actions required during medication administration to provide for accurate, safe drug delivery to the patient.	2. See textbook, p. 141.
4. Discuss established policies and procedures used for checking and transcribing medication orders and for preparing, administering, recording, and monitoring of therapeutic responses to drug therapy in clinical sites where assigned.	3. 1) Knowledge of individual drugs ordered, prepared, and administered; 2) awareness of symptoms for which the drug is prescribed as well as baseline evaluation of desired therapeutic outcomes; 3) understanding of nursing assessments needed to detect, prevent, or ameliorate adverse events; and 4) the nurse must exercise clinical judgment when drug orders are changed, new drugs are ordered, drug doses are missed, or when substitution of therapeutically equivalent medicines are made by the pharmacy.
5. List the parts of a syringe and the method of reading the measuring scale on the tuberculin, 3 mL, and insulin syringes.	4. Instructor needs to assist the student to identify policies developed by the school and by individual clinical sites relative to this question.
6. What volume can safely be injected at one site for intradermal, subcutaneous, IM, and IV medications?	5. See Figures 10-1, 10-2, 10-5, and 10-8.
7. Identify the types of tips found on syringes.	6. See Table 10-1, p. 147.
8. Examine calibrations found on different types of syringes.	7. See Figure 10-4 A, B.
9. What are common manufacturers' names for prefilled syringes?	8. See Figure 10-2, 10-5, and 10-8.
10. Name the parts of an "insulin pen."	9. Tubex, Carpuject, insulin pen
11. What medication is contained in an Epi-Pen® and what is the intended use for this device?	10. See Figure 10-10.
12. The inner diameter of a needle is known as _____.	11. Epinephrine, p. 145. It is used in emergencies caused by allergy to insect stings, foods, or drugs. See Figure 10-11.

13. Why are different length needles available for intramuscular and subcutaneous injections?

14. What do the terms *package integrity* or *package continuity* mean?

15. What are the provisions of the Needlestick Safety and Prevention Act of 2000?

16. What is the purpose of a filter needle?

17. Research safety devices developed for syringes and needles.

18. Identify the location of the OSHA-approved sharps containers on the clinical unit where assigned.

19. Differentiate between an ampule, a vial, and a Mix-O-Vial. Read the section on removal of medications from these containers.

20. Practice the procedures involved in the removal of a drug from an ampule, vial, and Mix-O-Vial.

12. Gauge: the larger the number, the smaller the diameter.

13. Different length needles provide a means of depositing the prescribed medication into the correct location/depth for maximum drug response in individuals of different build and age.

14. The terms *package integrity* or *package continuity* mean inspecting the container to ensure sterility of the contents has been retained.

15. The Act requires OSHA to develop and revise standards for blood-borne pathogens, monitoring and reporting of needlestick injuries, and the development of safety equipment to protect health care providers.

16. A filter needle is used to screen out glass particles that may have inadvertently fallen into the ampule during removal of its top. Note: After medication is removed from the ampule, remove filter needle, apply appropriate gauge and length needle for drug administration, and measure the amount of drug prescribed.

17. Under new OSHA regulations, needleless systems are required for the collection of body fluids, or the withdrawal of body fluids after initial venous or arterial access is established, the administration of medication or fluids, and any other procedure involving the potential for occupational exposure to blood-borne pathogens as a result of percutaneous injuries from contaminated sharps. Another new delivery system under development is a jet injection system that delivers subcutaneous injections of liquid medications such as insulin and vaccine through the skin without use of a needle. See information on blunt access devices.

18. Ask your instructor.

19. See Figures 10-20, 10-21, and 10-22.

20. See Figures 10-23, 10-24, and 10-25.

Parenteral Administration: Safe Preparation of Parenteral Medications

chapter
10

Learning Activities

FILL-IN-THE-BLANK

Finish each of the following statements using the correct term.

1. The Occupational Safety and Health Administration reports that more than 5 million workers in the health care industry and related occupations are at risk for occupational exposure to blood-borne pathogens, including such devastating diseases as _____ _____ virus, _____ virus, and _____ virus.

2. The syringe has three parts: the _____ is the outer portion on which the calibrations for the measurements of drug volume are located, the _____ is the inner cylindrical portion that fits snugly into the barrel, and the _____ is the portion that holds the needle.

3. The needle _____ is the diameter of the hole through the needle.

4. The proper gauge for an intradermal injection is _____ to _____ g, and the appropriate length of the needle is _____ to _____ inch.

5. The proper needle gauge for blood administration is _____ to _____ g.

In the blanks provided, write the volume of a drug that can be injected at one site by the following methods.

6. Intradermal: _____ mL

7. Subcutaneous: _____ mL

8. Intramuscular: _____ mL
   Divided dose is: _____ mL

9. Intravenous fluid: _____ mL

LABELING

Label the syringe below.

10.

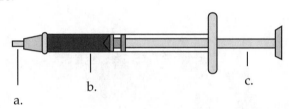

a.   b.   c.

Read the following syringes.

11. _____

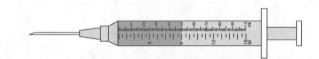

12. _____

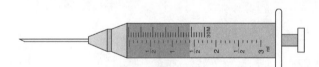

13. _____

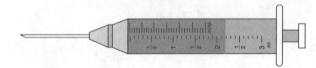

14. _____

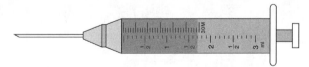

15. _____

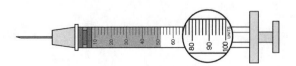

16. _____

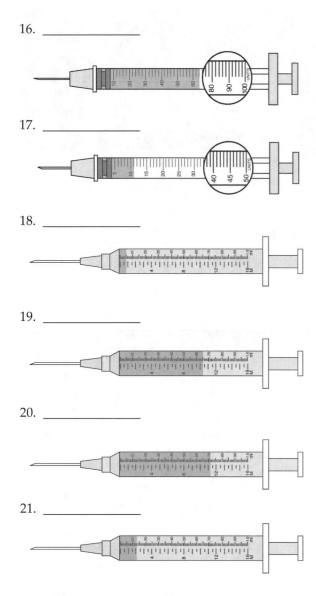

17. _____

18. _____

19. _____

20. _____

21. _____

Label the parts of a needle.

22.

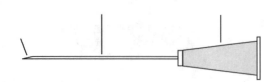

Label the following.

23. This is known as a(n) _____.

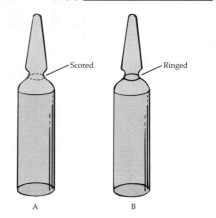

Explain how to withdraw fluid from this receptacle.

24. This is known as a(n) _____.

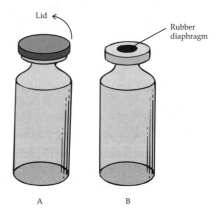

Explain how to withdraw fluid from this receptacle.

25. This is known as a(n) _____.

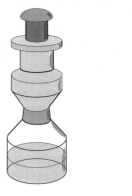

Explain how to withdraw fluid from this receptacle.

TRUE OR FALSE

Write "T" for true and "F" for false for each statement. Correct all false statements.

_____ 26. When drugs are given parenterally rather than orally, the onset of drug action is generally more rapid but of shorter duration.

_____ 27. Injection of drugs requires skill and special care because of the trauma at the site of needle puncture, possibility of infection, chance of allergic reaction, and that once medication is injected, the drug is irretrievable.

_____ 28. Insulin is now manufactured in U-50 concentration in the United States.

_____ 29. Low-dose insulin syringes are used for patients receiving 80 units or less of U-100 insulin.

_____ 30. Ampules are glass containers that usually contain a single dose of medication.

Parenteral Administration: Safe Preparation of Parenteral Medications

chapter
10

Practice Questions for the NCLEX® Examination

_____ 1. When preparing to administer a medication from an ampule, what does the nurse do?
1. Moves all of the solution to the top of the ampule
2. Covers the ampule neck with a sterile gauze pledget or antiseptic swab while breaking the top off
3. Uses a 23-gauge needle to withdraw the medication from the ampule
4. Keeps the needle straight and turns the ampule to the side so that all of the medication is removed

_____ 2. When reconstituting a sterile powder from a vial in preparation for parenteral administration, the nurse performs which actions? *(Select all that apply.)*
1. Pulls back on the plunger of the syringe to fill with an amount of air equal to the volume of solution to be withdrawn
2. Withdraws the measured volume of diluent required for reconstitution of the powdered drug
3. Inserts the needle in the diaphragm of the bottle with the powder and injects the diluent into the powder
4. Mixes the diluent and powder thoroughly
5. Withdraws the appropriate amount of reconstituted sterile powder and immediately administers the drug to the patient with the same needle

_____ 3. When administering medications in the operating room, what procedures does the nurse follow? *(Select all that apply.)*
1. Saves unused portions of medications for use in other surgical procedures
2. Tells the surgeon the name and dosage or concentration of the medication or solution handed to him or her
3. Repeats the entire medication order back to the surgeon at the time the request is made to verify all aspects of the order
4. Checks the accuracy of the drug order against the medication being prepared at least three times during the preparation phase
5. Documents the medication administration

_____ 4. When administering NPH and regular insulin together in the same syringe, what does the nurse do?
1. Discards NPH insulin if it is cloudy
2. First, injects the amount of air equal to the amount of insulin to be withdrawn into the regular insulin
3. First, draws up the NPH insulin to be administered
4. Is careful not to inject any of the first type of insulin already in the syringe into the vial

_____ 5. An obese adult is in need of an intramuscular injection. Which needle length does the nurse use?
1. 4 inches
2. 3 inches
3. 2 inches
4. 1 inch

_____ 6. When preparing to administer blood to a patient, which needle gauges does the nurse consider using? *(Select all that apply.)*
1. 18
2. 20
3. 22
4. 24

_____ 7. Which volumes of medication are acceptable for intramuscular administration at one site to an older infant? *(Select all that apply.)*
1. 0.5 mL
2. 1.0 mL
3. 1.5 mL
4. 2.0 mL
5. 2.5 mL

_____ 8. Which statements about insulin syringes are true? *(Select all that apply.)*
1. If an insulin syringe is not available, a tuberculin syringe may be substituted for insulin administration, as they both hold about 1 mL.
2. The U-100 insulin syringe holds 100 units of insulin per mL.
3. Low-dose insulin syringes may be used for patients receiving 50 units or less of U-100 insulin.
4. The small lines on the insulin syringe represent volume of the insulin as measured in minims.
5. Use of U-40 insulin requires the use of a U-40 insulin syringe.

_____ 9. A patient is ordered Novulin NPH U-100 insulin 20 units subcutaneously before breakfast. Novulin NPH U-100 insulin is available with standard 100 units and Lo-Dose 50 units U-100 insulin syringes. Which syringe does the nurse use to administer the insulin?
1. 1 cc
2. Tuberculin
3. Standard U-100
4. Lo-Dose 50 unit U-100

10. A patient's blood glucose reading taken before dinner is 399. Using the medication order and insulin sliding scale below, how many units of insulin must be administered to the patient?
_____ units

Order: Humulin regular U-100 insulin subcutaneously before meals per sliding scale

Insulin Dose	Glucose Reading
No coverage	Glucose less than 160
2 units	160–220
4 units	221–280
6 units	281–340
8 units	341–400
	Glucose greater than 400; hold insulin; call primary care provider stat

Parenteral Administration: Intradermal, Subcutaneous, and Intramuscular Routes

Review Sheet

The QUESTION column and the ANSWER column have been offset so you can cover the answer while reading the question, allowing you to assess your knowledge.

Question

1. Identify the layer of skin in which an intradermal injection is deposited.
2. Name the common intradermal injection sites.
3. Before allergy sensitivity testing begins, what medications should be stopped for 24 to 48 hours?
4. What volume can safely be injected at one site for intradermal, subcutaneous, IM, and IV medications?
5. What is the angle of the needle inserted for an intradermal injection?
6. How do you "read" a skin test?
7. List the terms associated with intradermal administration and reading of the reactions.
8. Describe patient education that should be done in advance and at the time of performing intradermal testing.
9. What types of subcutaneous injections do NOT require aspiration before injection of the medication?
10. List the injection sites used for IM injections.
11. Why is the gluteal area NOT used for IM injections in children under 3 years of age?
12. When is the Z-track method of IM injection used?
13. What is the purpose of performing a premedication assessment?

Answer

1. Intradermal injections are made into the dermal layer of skin below the epidermis.
2. Upper chest, scapular area of back, inner aspect of forearm.
3. Antihistamines, anti-inflammatory agents, certain sleep medications, and immunosuppressants. (Always check with physician before discontinuing medications.)
4. Review Table 10-1 in Chapter 10.
5. A 15-degree angle with the needle bevel upward.
6. Positive reactions are measured, both the wheal and erythema, and by palpation and measurement of the size of any induration present.
7. See textbook, pp. 157-159.
8. See textbook, pp. 157-159.
9. Heparin and insulin do not require aspiration prior to injection.
10. See textbook, pp. 162-163.
11. The gluteal muscle is not adequately developed.
12. The Z-track method is used with medications that are particularly irritating or that will stain the skin (e.g., injectable iron).
13. Premedication assessment is performed to prevent the administration of a medication to a patient whose diagnosis, symptoms, or other data indicate the medication should not be administered.

Parenteral Administration: Intradermal, Subcutaneous, and Intramuscular Routes

chapter
11

Learning Activities

FILL-IN-THE-BLANK

Finish each of the following statements using the correct term.

1. _____ injections are made by penetrating a needle through the dermis and subcutaneous tissue into the muscle layer.

2. Intramuscular injections should be made at a(n) _____-degree angle.

3. When a drug that is irritating needs to be administered intramuscularly, the _____ method is commonly used.

4. To use the _____ area for intramuscular injection, the patient should be placed in the prone position on a flat surface.

5. When administering _____ and _____ subcutaneously, the nurse should not aspirate after the needle has been inserted.

LABELING

Label the following syringes.

6. _____

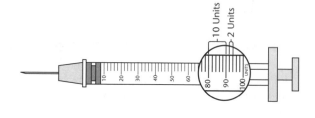

7. _____

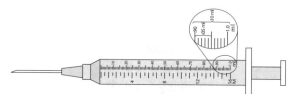

8. _____

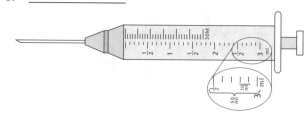

Read the following syringes.

9. _____

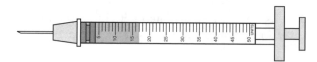

10. _____

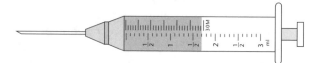

11. _____

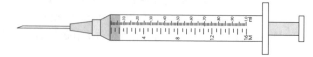

12. _____

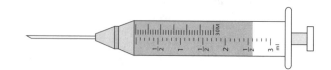

13. _____

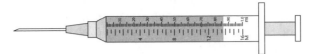

14. _____

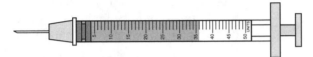

15. Label the figure below with the injection sites used for subcutaneous drug administration.

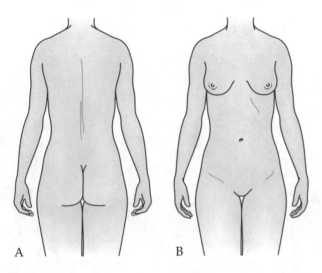

A   B

16. Label the pictures below with the sites for intramuscular injection in a child and an adult.

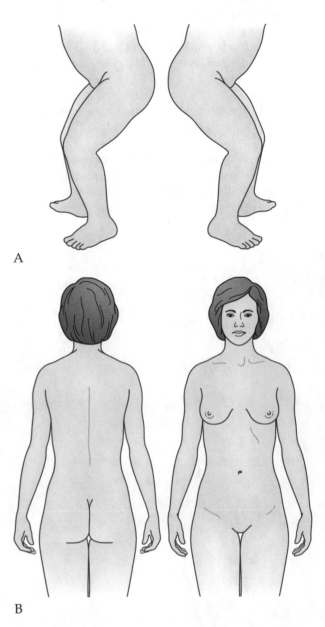

A

B

TRUE OR FALSE

Write "T" for true and "F" for false for each statement. Correct all false statements.

_____ 17. Intradermal injections are made into the dermal layer of skin just below the epidermis.

_____ 18. The usual amount of volume injected subcutaneously is 2–5 mL.

_____ 19. When administering heparin subcutaneously, insert the needle quickly at a 45-degree angle, do not aspirate, and slowly inject the medication.

_____ 20. The gluteal area must not be used for intramuscular injection of medication in children under 3 years of age because the muscle is not yet well-developed from walking.

_____ 21. When using the deltoid muscle for intramuscular drug administration in adults, the volume should be limited to 2 mL or less, and the substance must not cause irritation.

Student Name _____

Parenteral Administration: Intradermal, Subcutaneous, and Intramuscular Routes

Practice Questions for the NCLEX® Examination

_____ 1. When preparing to provide allergy testing to a patient using the intradermal injection technique, what does the nurse do?
   1. Inserts the needle at a 90-degree angle with the needle bevel facing down
   2. Recaps the needle used before disposing of it in a puncture-resistant container
   3. Wears gloves
   4. Deposits the solution being injected into the subcutaneous tissue under the skin

_____ 2. The nurse is preparing to administer an intramuscular injection in the dorsogluteal area. What does the nurse do first?
   1. Positions the patient prone with the toes pointed inward
   2. Has the patient flex the dorsogluteal muscles to minimize pain from the injection
   3. Identifies the site by forming a "V" on the greater trochanter of the femur
   4. Holds the syringe at a 30-degree angle to the surface of the patient's skin

_____ 3. How many mL of medication is the usual amount administered via the intramuscular route to adults?
   1. 2
   2. 3
   3. 4
   4. 5

_____ 4. The nurse is teaching a patient about the importance of rotating subcutaneous insulin injection sites. Which statement made by the patient indicates a need for additional teaching?
   1. "Common subcutaneous sites for administering insulin include upper arms, anterior thighs, and the abdomen."
   2. "The fastest site of absorption is when I inject into the abdomen."
   3. "I need to rotate injection sites to prevent lipohypertrophy or lipoatrophy which will slow insulin absorption."
   4. "Exercise will not affect the rate of insulin absorption."

5. What is the upper volume of medication that can be delivered to a patient via the subcutaneous route? _____ mL

6. What is the upper volume of medication that can be delivered into a muscle? _____ mL

_____ 7. The most common site for the administration of intradermal medication is the inner aspect of which body part?
   1. Thigh
   2. Forearm
   3. Upper arm
   4. Shin

8. A patient is ordered heparin 3,500 units subcutaneously every 12 hours. Heparin is available in a bottle labeled 5,000 units/mL. How many mL of the medication does the nurse administer? _____ mL

9. A patient is ordered digoxin (Lanoxin) 600 mcg IV stat. The label on the bottle reads "digoxin 0.5 mg in 2 mL." How many mL of the medication does the nurse administer? _____ mL

_____ 10. When administering intradermal allergy testing for a patient, which steps does the nurse perform? *(Select all that apply.)*
   1. Asks the patient if he or she has taken any antihistamine or anti-inflammatory agents for 24–48 hours before the test
   2. Uses an antiseptic pledget to clean the skin
   3. Injects the volume ordered, usually 0.01 to 0.05 mL, into the subcutaneous tissue
   4. Aspirates for blood once the needle has been inserted
   5. Wipes the site with alcohol after injection

Parenteral Administration: Intravenous Route

Review Sheet

The QUESTION column and the ANSWER column have been offset so that you can cover the answer while reading the question, allowing you to assess your knowledge.

Question	Answer
1. What does the term *intravenous* mean?	
2. Nurses having certification for IV therapy can use the initials ____ in their title.	1. *Intravenous* means "in the vein." In the context of this chapter, it means administration of fluids directly into the bloodstream.
3. Name two agencies that are recommended resources for establishing standards relating to IV therapy.	2. CRNI
4. What types of IV administration sets are available?	3. Infusion Nurses Society (INS) and Centers for Disease Control and Prevention (CDC)
5. What types of controller clamps are commonly used on IV administration sets?	4. See textbook, p. 169.
6. Differentiate between nonvolumetric and volumetric IV infusion controllers.	5. Roller and slide clamps. *Note*: A dial-style controller is also available for use.
7. Differentiate among peripheral access devices, midline catheters, central devices, and implantable venous infusion ports. Identify their uses, sites of insertion, and what vessel the catheter tip should be in when placement is complete.	6. Nonvolumetric infusion devices only monitor the gravity-induced flow by counting drops that pass through the drip chamber; volumetric IV controllers apply external pressure to pump the IV fluid at a specified rate.
8. How frequently should peripheral catheters be changed?	7. See textbook, pp. 171-173.
9. Describe the flushing of Hickman, Broviac, and Groshong catheters.	8. 72 to 96 hours (check policy manual where assigned)
10. What types of needles are used to access an implanted port?	9. See textbook, p. 173.
11. What does it mean when an IV solution is *isotonic, hypotonic,* or *hypertonic*?	10. All ports are accessed using a Huber needle.
12. What criteria are used to select an isotonic, hypotonic, or hypertonic IV solution for administration to a patient?	11. See textbook, p. 174.
13. Compare the preparation for administration of IV solutions delivered in glass bottles with those in plastic bags.	12. See textbook, pp. 174-175.
14. When setting up an IV fluid or medication for administration as an IV piggyback, how should the piggyback bag be positioned?	13. See Figure 12-1.

15. Compare common peripheral access devices and the intended use of each.

16. Describe vein selection for the initiation of an IV in the hand or forearm.

17. Identify common veins used for initiating IV therapy in infants and children.

18. What are the most common veins used for central venous catheter access?

19. Study and practice IV-related procedures found throughout this chapter in the laboratory setting (e.g., venipuncture, spiking and hanging an IV, adding an IV piggyback to a primary line, giving IV drugs by bolus method, preparing an ADD-Vantage or similar prepackaged system of medication for administration IV, and operating syringe pumps and volumetric and nonvolumetric infusion control devices). Check with the instructor for details.

20. Obtain copies of procedures used at the clinical site where you are assigned for:
    — frequency of changing IV tubing.
    — IV peripheral sites.
    — length of time IV solutions can remain hanging.
    — recording of IV fluids and IV medications on the MAR.
    — procedures for flushing and dressing of heparin, saline, or medlock.
    — central venous catheters and PICC lines.

21. Explain the SASH procedure used for IV therapy.

22. Which type of IV central catheter does not require flushing with heparin?

23. What is a commonly accepted rate for a TKO (to keep open) IV order?

24. What is the purpose of a premedication assessment?

25. What is the formula used to calculate an IV drip rate?

26. Describe the correct method of monitoring an infusing IV solution and site.

27. Describe how to assess for infiltration at an IV site.

14. See Figure 12-8.

15. See Figures 12-3, 12-4, and textbook pp. 171-172.

16. See Figures 12-9 and 12-10.

17. See Figure 12-11.

18. The subclavian and jugular veins are most commonly used for central IV access.

19. Consult with your instructor to obtain detailed instructions for practicing and being "checked off" on procedures relating to IV medication administration.

20. See general guidelines, textbook pp. 177-179. Guidelines of individual practice settings should always be consulted.

21. S = Saline
    A = Administer drug
    S = Saline
    H = Heparin (Not all types of vascular access devices require the use of heparin; check facility policy.)

22. Groshong

23. A commonly accepted rate for TKO IV is 10 mL/hr.

24. Premedication assessment is performed to prevent the administration of a medication to a patient whose diagnosis, symptoms, or other data indicate the medication should not be administered.

25. $$\frac{\text{mL of solution} \times \text{number of drops/mL}}{\text{hrs of administration} \times 60 \text{ min/hr}} = \text{drops/min}$$

26. Check the ordered IV solution, total amount infused, drip rate, IV tubing for kinks or air in the line, date and time the IV solution was hung, and check for IV site infiltration.

28. If you see air in the tubing of a running IV, what should you do?

29. What are the signs and symptoms of circulatory overload and pulmonary edema?

30. How is a suspected pulmonary embolism verified?

31. Differentiate between the terms *infiltration* and *extravasation*.

27. Check for limb's color, size, or skin integrity; compare with the opposite limb. See textbook for guidelines to follow and for the infiltration scale, Figure 12-19.

28. Clamp the tubing; use a syringe to withdraw the air bubble.

29. Symptoms of circulatory overload include engorged neck veins; dyspnea; reduced urine output; edema; bounding pulse; and shallow, rapid respirations. Symptoms of pulmonary edema include dyspnea, cough, anxiety, rales, rhonchi, possible cardiac dysrhythmias, thready pulse, frothy sputum, and elevation or drop in blood pressure depending on the severity.

30. A lung scan is done as well as drawing ABGs and baseline prothrombin times.

31. Infiltration is leakage of IV solution into the tissue surrounding the vein; extravasation is leakage of an irritant chemical into the tissue surrounding the vein.

Parenteral Administration: Intravenous Route

Learning Activities

FILL-IN-THE-BLANK

Finish each of the following statements using the correct term.

1. Macrodrip intravenous chambers provide ____, ____, or ____ drops/mL, whereas microdrip chambers deliver ____ drops/mL.

2. If the IV solution and the blood have approximately the same osmolality, the solution is said to be _____; if the solution has fewer dissolved particles than the blood, it is known as being _____, and those with higher concentrations of dissolved particles are considered to be _____ solutions.

3. The most commonly used veins for IV administration in infants and children are in the _____ region of the scalp, _____ of the hand, and _____ of the foot.

4. Two types of solutions are used to maintain patency of vascular access devices: _____ is used to prevent clot formation and _____ is used to clean the interior diameter of the device of blood or particles of medication.

5. Some complications of intravenous therapy include _____, which is leakage of an intravenous solution into the tissue surrounding the vein, and _____, which is the leakage of an irritant chemical into the tissue surrounding the vein.

6. The usual time interval between tube changes on lipid solutions is ____ hours.

7. Based on drop volume, an IV administration set that delivers 20 gtt/mL is called a(n) _____ set.

8. A type of IV device that holds a prefilled syringe is called a(n) _____ _____.

9. A(n) _____-the-needle catheter is commonly inserted peripherally for routine peripheral infusion therapy.

10. This type of IV infusion device is designed for use over a 2- to 4-week period. It is known as a(n) _____ _____ _____.

11. A type of central venous catheter that a qualified nurse can insert is known as a(n) _____ catheter.

12. A type of tunneled venous catheter that does not require flushing with heparin is known as a(n) _____ catheter.

13. Name three types of vessels that comprise the intravascular compartment:
    1) _____,
    2) _____, and
    3) _____.

14. Isotonic solutions have an osmolality range of ____ to ____ mOsm/L.

15. Hypertonic solutions (e.g., parenteral nutrition solutions) are administered through central infusion lines directly into the _____ _____ _____.

16. Name the agency that is recognized as a recommended resource to be consulted when establishing guidelines relating to infectious diseases. _____

LABELING

Label the following.

17. What type of drip chamber is this?

_____

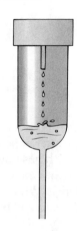

18. Figure A is a(n): _____

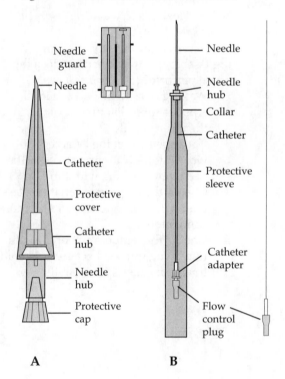

A   B

TRUE OR FALSE

Write "T" for true and "F" for false for each statement. Correct all false statements.

_____ 19. Intravenous administration is the most rapid of all parenteral routes because it bypasses all barriers to drug absorption.

_____ 20. Topical antibiotics or creams should not be used on peripheral intravenous catheters because they have the potential to promote fungal infections and antimicrobial resistance.

_____ 21. Bacteriostatic water or saline containing the benzyl preservative to reconstitute or dilute medications or to flush IV catheters of newborns should not be used because the preservative is toxic to these patients.

_____ 22. Thrombophlebitis is the inflammation of a vein, and phlebitis is inflammation of the vein with the formation of a thrombus in the area of inflammation.

_____ 23. Flushing the IV line by speeding the IV solution is not recommended because the medication still in the line would be administered too rapidly.

Parenteral Administration: Intravenous Route

Practice Questions for the NCLEX® Examination

_____ 1. A patient has been ordered a peripherally inserted central venous catheter (PICC) for the administration of medications. The nurse has taught the patient about the insertion procedure, use, and care of the PICC line. Which statement made by the patient indicates a need for further teaching?
   1. "I will be placed under general anesthesia to have this intravenous line inserted."
   2. "I will be able to go home with a PICC."
   3. "My PICC line can last up to a year if it is properly cared for."
   4. "The PICC line should be flushed with a saline-heparin solution after every use, or daily if not used."

_____ 2. Which statements about implantable infusion ports are correct? (Select all that apply.)
   1. Blood products can be administered through an implantable infusion port.
   2. One port of a two-port system may be reserved for drawing blood samples.
   3. An implanted central venous access catheter may remain in place for over a year and only requires a saline-heparin solution flush after every access or once monthly.
   4. The CDC recommends that central venous catheters be routinely replaced to prevent catheter-related infection.
   5. The infusion port can accommodate up to 100 punctures before it needs to be changed.

_____ 3. A patient has been admitted to the health care facility after experiencing a GI bleed at home which has now resolved. The patient now has an intravascular fluid volume deficit. Which IV fluid does the nurse anticipate will be ordered for the patient?
   1. 0.9% sodium chloride
   2. 0.2% sodium chloride
   3. 0.45% sodium chloride
   4. 5% dextrose in water

_____ 4. When providing care to a patient receiving IV therapy, which actions does the nurse perform? (Select all that apply.)
   1. Wears gloves to inspect the IV site
   2. Applies topical antibiotic ointment to the insertion site
   3. If it appears that the IV access device is clotted, attempts to clear the needle by flushing with fluid
   4. Checks the drip chamber; if it is less than half full, squeezes it to fill more completely
   5. Checks the temperature of the solution being infused because cold solutions can cause spasms in the vein

_____ 5. Which practices does the nurse follow when administering a medication by a heparin/saline/medlock? *(Select all that apply.)*
   1. Selects a syringe several milliliters larger than that required by the volume of the drug
   2. When a blood return is established, injects saline for flush followed by the medication at the rate specified by the manufacturer
   3. After the medication is administered, inserts another syringe containing 10 mL of normal saline to flush the remaining drug from the catheter
   4. Maintains constant pressure on the plunger of the syringe used to flush the line after the medication has been administered while simultaneously withdrawing the needle from the diaphragm to prevent backflow of blood
   5. Verifies the heparin dose with another qualified nurse

_____ 6. Which needle gauges are appropriate for the administration of blood? *(Select all that apply.)*
   1. 26
   2. 25
   3. 20
   4. 16
   5. 18

_____ 7. In calculating IV fluid rates, microdrip chambers form how many drops per milliliter?
   1. 10
   2. 15
   3. 20
   4. 60

_____ 8. Which statements about PICCs are correct? *(Select all that apply.)*
   1. They are not available for pediatric use.
   2. PICC line insertion is only attempted in the operating room.
   3. PICC lines are easier to maintain than short peripheral catheters because there is less frequent infiltration and phlebitis.
   4. They should not be used for long-term administration of total parenteral nutrition.
   5. It is necessary to flush the PICC line with a saline-heparin solution after every use, or daily if not used.

_____ 9. A patient has been ordered cefazolin (Ancef) 0.5 g in 100 mL of D_5W IV piggyback to run over 30 minutes. The drop factor of the IV tubing is 20 gtt/mL. The nurse regulates the flow rate on the IV to how many gtt/min? _____ gtt/min

_____ 10. A patient is ordered 1 L of D_5W to run at 125 mL/h. The nurse hangs the bag at 0800. The bag will need to be replaced at what time?
   1. 0200
   2. 1400
   3. 1600
   4. 1800

_____ 11. A student nurse is administering a medication by saline lock to a patient. Which action by the student nurse causes the supervising nurse to intervene?
   1. Accesses the injection portal with a syringe containing flush solution and gently pulls back on the plunger for a blood return
   2. When blood return is established, injects the medication followed by the saline for flush
   3. Observes the IV site at the catheter tip for swelling and monitors for reports of discomfort
   4. Documents the date, time, drug, dosage, rate of administration, assessment data, and how well the procedure was tolerated

Drugs Affecting the Autonomic Nervous System

Review Sheet

The QUESTION column and the ANSWER column have been offset so that you can cover the answer while reading the question, allowing you to assess your knowledge.

Question	Answer
1. What is the central nervous system composed of?	
2. The autonomic nervous system relays information from the central nervous system to _____?	1. The central nervous system (CNS) is composed of the brain and spinal cord.
3. The autonomic nervous system controls the functions of what types of tissue?	2. The autonomic nervous system (ANS) relays information from the CNS to the whole body.
4. What primary function is controlled by the motor nervous system?	3. The ANS controls the functions of all tissue except striated muscle.
5. What neurotransmitter is liberated by cholinergic fibers?	4. Skeletal muscle contractions are controlled by the motor nervous system.
6. What neurotransmitter is liberated by adrenergic fibers?	5. The cholinergic fibers secrete acetylcholine.
7. What three major types of receptors are found in the autonomic nervous system?	6. The adrenergic fibers secrete norepinephrine.
8. Stimulation of alpha$_1$ receptors causes what action on blood vessels?	7. The three major types of receptors found in the ANS are alpha-, beta-, and dopaminergic receptors.
9. Stimulation of beta$_1$ receptors produces what type of effect on the heart rate?	8. Stimulation of alpha$_1$ receptors causes vasoconstriction. This results in a rise in blood pressure; therefore, before giving alpha$_1$-type medications, the blood pressure should be checked. This action makes these drugs useful in the treatment of hypotension and shock.
10. Stimulation of beta$_2$ receptors produces what effects?	9. Stimulation of beta$_1$ receptors increases the heart rate. If excessive doses of a beta$_1$ agonist are administered, the patient may experience tachycardia and dysrhythmias.
11. Define *adrenergic agent*.	10. Stimulation of beta$_2$ receptors relaxes the smooth muscle of the bronchi, uterus, and peripheral blood vessels. These actions make these drugs useful as bronchodilators and inhibitors of preterm labor.
12. When beta-adrenergic agents are administered, what effects will be seen on blood vessels, bronchi, heart rate, blood pressure, respiration, lungs, gastric motility and tone, and blood glucose?	11. An adrenergic agent produces or mimics the effects of stimulation of the sympathetic nervous system. Therefore, these drugs are also known as "sympathomimetic" agents.

13. What premedication assessments should be completed prior to administering an adrenergic agent?

14. Giving an excessive dose of an adrenergic agent results in what adverse effects?

15. List the primary actions of alpha-adrenergic blocking agents and beta-adrenergic blocking agents.

16. Why/when are alpha- and beta-adrenergic blocking agents prescribed?

17. State the possible effects of administering beta blockers to a patient with a known respiratory disease such as asthma or emphysema.

18. Which portion of the autonomic nervous system do cholinergic agents affect?

19. What effect do beta blockers have on a patient with diabetes mellitus?

20. What pharmacologic effect may be expected when indomethacin and beta blocker therapy are combined?

21. What drug is a specific antidote for cholinergic agents?

22. Under what types of clinical conditions are cholinergic agents used?

23. What adverse effects can be anticipated when an anticholinergic agent is administered?

24. What actions of anticholinergic agents make them useful in the clinical treatment of gastrointestinal disorders?

12. When adrenergic agents are administered, blood vessels dilate, bronchi dilate, heart rate increases, blood pressure may drop, GI peristalsis decreases, relaxation of the gastric smooth muscle occurs, and blood glucose increases.

13. Before administering an adrenergic agent, the following assessments should be completed: baseline vital signs (e.g., heart rate, blood pressure), screen for respiratory tract disease, and ascertain if the patient uses bronchodilators or decongestants.

14. Excessive doses of an adrenergic agent may result in dysrhythmias, hypertension, nervousness, anxiety, and insomnia due to stimulation of the sympathetic nervous system.

15. Alpha-adrenergic blocking agents act by plugging the alpha receptors, preventing vasoconstriction of arterioles. Beta-adrenergic blocking agents act by plugging the beta-adrenergic receptors, preventing beta stimulation, especially from norepinephrine and epinephrine.

16. Alpha-adrenergic blocking agents are used to treat diseases with vasoconstriction (e.g., peripheral vascular disease, Buerger's disease, and Raynaud's disease). Beta blocking agents are used to treat hypertension, angina pectoris, cardiac dysrhythmias, and hyperthyroidism.

17. Administering a beta blocker to a person with a known respiratory disease may cause bronchoconstriction and make the person experience respiratory distress.

18. Cholinergic agents affect the parasympathetic portion of the nervous system.

19. Beta blockers induce hypoglycemia; they decrease the release of insulin in response to hypoglycemia and mask the symptoms normally associated with hypoglycemia.

20. The combination of indomethacin and beta blocker therapy may cause loss of hypertensive control. The dosage of the beta blocker may need to be increased.

21. Atropine sulfate, an anticholinergic agent, is a specific antidote for cholinergic agents.

22. Cholinergic agents can be used to treat glaucoma, urinary retention, myasthenia gravis, as a muscle relaxant to reverse nondepolarizing agents, and for gastrointestinal disorders such as paralytic ileus.

23. Anticholinergic agents produce the following adverse effects: dryness of mouth and tongue, blurring of vision, mild nausea, and nervousness. Other adverse effects include constipation, urinary hesitancy or retention, tachycardia, palpitations, mydriasis, muscle cramping, and mild transient postural hypotension.

25. Before administering any anticholinergic agent, the patient's history should be checked for the presence of what type of eye disorder?

26. Atropine is an example of an anticholinergic agent frequently used preoperatively. Which of the drug's anticholinergic properties make this drug useful preoperatively?

27. What premedication assessments should be completed before administering an anticholinergic agent?

28. The postoperative patient who has been given atropine sulfate needs to be monitored for _____?

29. Describe the action(s) and adverse effects of the following drug classifications and/or drugs: adrenergic agents, alpha-adrenergic agents, beta-adrenergic agents, cholinergic agents, anticholinergic agents, beta-adrenergic blocking agents, physostigmine, epinephrine, and atropine.

24. Anticholinergic (also known as *antispasmodic*) agents' actions include decreased secretion of saliva, hydrochloric acid, pepsin, bile, and other enzymatic fluids necessary for digestion, along with relaxation of the sphincter muscles and decreased spasm, which allows peristalsis to move the contents of the stomach and bowel through the gastrointestinal tract.

25. All patients' charts should be screened for the presence of angle-closure glaucoma before any anticholinergic agent is administered.

26. Atropine sulfate is given preoperatively to dry secretions of the mouth, nose, throat, and bronchi, and decrease secretions during surgery. It also prevents vagal stimulation and bradycardia during the placement of the endotracheal tube.

27. Check for a history of angle-closure glaucoma or history of enlarged prostate and urinary hesitancy or retention before administering an anticholinergic agent.

28. The postoperative patient who received atropine sulfate needs to be monitored frequently for urinary retention. There may also be postoperative constipation.

29. See textbook, pp. 200-209. Examine drug monographs and drug classification explanations.

Drugs Affecting the Autonomic Nervous System

Learning Activities

FILL-IN-THE-BLANK

Finish each of the following statements using the correct term.

1. The efferent and afferent nerves are known collectively as the _____.

2. The junction between one neuron and the next is called a(n) _____.

3. The two major neurotransmitters of the autonomic nervous system are _____ and _____.

4. The nerve endings that liberate acetylcholine are called _____, and those that secrete norepinephrine are called _____.

5. Catecholamines that are secreted naturally in the body are _____, _____, and _____.

6. Dopamine is secreted at what three primary sites in the body? _____, _____, _____

7. The three types of sympathetic autonomic nervous system receptors are _____, _____, and _____.

8. Cholinergic agents are also known as _____.

9. Stimulation of the adrenergic receptors causes smooth muscle _____ of the bronchial muscles, which causes _____ of the airway.

10. Stimulation of the cholinergic receptors causes smooth muscle _____ of the bronchial muscles, which causes _____ of the airway.

11. The generic names of all $beta_1$ blocking agents end in "-_____."

MATCHING

Match the generic drug name with its corresponding brand name. Each option will be used only once.

_____ 12. propantheline

_____ 13. carvedilol

_____ 14. neostigmine

_____ 15. isoproterenol

_____ 16. terbutaline

_____ 17. pyridostigmine

_____ 18. timolol

a. Isuprel
b. Pro-Banthine
c. Brethine
d. Coreg
e. Prostigmin
f. Mestinon
g. Blocadren

TRUE OR FALSE

Write "T" for true and "F" for false for each statement. Correct all false statements.

_____ 19. The brain and spinal cord make up the central nervous system.

_____ 20. The central nervous system receives signals from afferent nerves throughout the body that are transmitted to the spinal cord and brain.

_____ 21. The transmission of nerve signals or impulses occurs because of the activity of chemical substances called *neurotransmitters*.

_____ 22. Anticholinergic agents are safe to use in patients with closed-angle glaucoma.

_____ 23. Cholinergic drugs are also known as *parasympathetic agents*.

_____ 24. All beta blockers mask most of the signs and symptoms of acute hypoglycemia.

Drugs Affecting the Autonomic Nervous System

Practice Questions for the NCLEX® Examination

_____ 1. Stimulation of beta$_2$ receptors in a patient results in which assessment findings? *(Select all that apply.)*
  1. Bronchoconstriction
  2. Uterine relaxation
  3. Vasoconstriction
  4. Tachycardia
  5. Orthostatic hypotension

_____ 2. Patients with which condition would most likely benefit from the dopaminergic effects of adrenergic agents?
  1. Parkinson's disease
  2. Guillain-Barré syndrome
  3. Amyotrophic lateral sclerosis
  4. Multiple sclerosis

_____ 3. Which adrenergic agent is most useful in the treatment of digitalis toxicity?
  1. Epinephrine (Adrenalin)
  2. Metaraminol (Aramine)
  3. Isoproterenol (Isuprel)
  4. Phenylephrine (Neo-Synephrine)

_____ 4. Which medication is the preferred treatment for a patient with asthma in need of treatment with a beta blocker?
  1. Propranolol
  2. Timolol
  3. Nadolol
  4. Atenolol

_____ 5. Before administering a beta blocker to a patient, it is most important for the nurse to assess the patient for a history of which disorder?
  1. Hypertension
  2. Angina pectoris
  3. Diabetes mellitus
  4. Cardiac dysrhythmias

_____ 6. A patient experiences orthostatic hypotension as a result of taking an adrenergic blocking agent for treatment of hypertension. Which measures does the nurse incorporate into this patient's plan of care? *(Select all that apply.)*
  1. Monitors blood pressure in the standing position daily
  2. Monitors blood pressure daily in the supine position
  3. Teaches the patient to rise slowly from a supine or sitting position
  4. Encourages the patient to sit down if feeling faint
  5. Discontinues the adrenergic blocking agent

_____ 7. What are serious adverse effects of beta-adrenergic blocking agent therapy? *(Select all that apply.)*
  1. Bradycardia
  2. Wheezing
  3. Orthopnea
  4. Hypoglycemia
  5. Nausea

8. A patient is ordered albuterol (Proventil) syrup 2 mg. The medication is available as 2 mg/5 mL. How many mL of the medication does the nurse administer? _____ mL

9. A patient is ordered carvedilol (Coreg) 6.25 mg twice daily. The medication is available as 3.125 mg per tablet. How many tablets will the patient receive in a 24-hour period? _____ tablet(s)

_____ 10. A patient is ordered metoprolol (Lopressor) 300 mg PO daily. The medication is available as 25-mg, 50-mg, and 100-mg tablets. How many tablets does the nurse administer?
1. Twelve 25-mg tablets
2. Ten 25-mg tablets and one 100-mg tablet
3. Four 50-mg tablets and one 100-mg tablet
4. Three 100-mg tablets

Sedative-Hypnotics

Review Sheet

The QUESTION column and the ANSWER column have been offset so that you can cover the answer while reading the questions, allowing you to assess your knowledge.

Question	Answer
1. What are the four stages of sleep?	
2. What is another name for paradoxic sleep?	1. Sleep stages I-IV are explained in the textbook, pp. 210-211.
3. What is insomnia?	2. Rapid eye movement (REM) sleep is also called paradoxic sleep.
4. What premedication assessments should be performed prior to administering any sedative-hypnotic agent?	3. Insomnia is the inability to sleep.
5. Differentiate between the actions of a sedative and a hypnotic.	4. Before administering a sedative-hypnotic agent, assess for level of alertness, orientation, and ability to perform motor functions, as well as current blood pressure, pulse, respirations, sleep pattern, anxiety level, and environmental and nutritional factors that might impede sleep.
6. What should a nursing history relating to a patient's complaints of insomnia include?	5. Hypnotics produce sleep. Sedatives relax the patient.
7. Name two classes of drugs used as sedative-hypnotics. What ending appears on the generic drug names?	6. A nursing history related to a patient's complaints of insomnia should include usual pattern of sleep, anxiety level, environmental factors, nutritional habits, and medications or actions tried before seeking current treatment.
	7. Two classes of sedative-hypnotics are barbiturates (all end in "-tal") and benzodiazepines (all end in "-am," except chlordiazepoxide [Librium]).
8. State the effect of hypnotics on respiratory function.	8. Hypnotics produce mild to marked respiratory depression, depending on dosage and pulmonary function.
9. What changes in REM sleep occur with the administration of barbiturates?	9. Barbiturates initially decrease REM sleep; however, as tolerance builds, REM sleep returns to normal.
10. What is a rebound effect associated with discontinuing barbiturates?	10. A rebound effect associated with discontinuing barbiturates is increase in REM; it may take several weeks following barbiturate therapy for this to resolve.
11. What is meant by *morning hangover* associated with barbiturates, benzodiazepines, and miscellaneous agents used as sedative-hypnotics? State the associated health teaching that needs to be initiated.	

12. What is a paradoxical response to hypnotics and what nursing actions are required if this response occurs?

13. What laboratory studies are recommended with continued use of barbiturates and benzodiazepines?

14. List the generic and brand names of commonly prescribed barbiturates, benzodiazepines, and miscellaneous sedative-hypnotic agents as assigned by the instructor.

15. In addition to their use as sedative-hypnotics, for what other clinical uses are barbiturates prescribed?

16. What effect can the regular use of barbiturates have on oral contraceptive therapy?

17. What is the blood-brain barrier?

18. What adverse effects can be expected from the administration of sedative-hypnotics?

19. What are serious adverse effects when taking sedative-hypnotics?

20. What premedication assessments should be performed before administration of a benzodiazepine?

11. Morning hangover from sedative-hypnotics includes blurred vision, mental dullness, and mild hypotension. Health teaching about this effect should include directions to consult the health care provider if these symptoms become too bothersome; instructions to rise slowly to sitting position, equilibrate, then stand; and a caution regarding use of machinery, etc.

12. Paradoxical response is a period of excitement prior to sedation induced by use of barbiturates and other sedative-hypnotics not usually associated with benzodiazepine therapy. Appropriate nursing actions include protecting the patient from harm providing for channeling of energy.

13. RBC, WBC, and differential count lab studies should be done with continued use of barbiturates and benzodiazepines. Also immediately report sore throat, fever, progressive weakness, purpura, or jaundice.

14. Consult Tables 14-1, 14-2, and 14-3.

15. Specific agents are used as anticonvulsants and induction anesthetics.

16. The patient may need to use an alternative form of contraceptive therapy, particularly if spotting or breakthrough bleeding occurs.

17. The blood-brain barrier is a membrane that controls the passage of drugs into the central nervous system to the receptor sites on the cells within the central nervous system.

18. Adverse effects of sedative-hypnotics include hangover, sedation, lethargy, diminished alertness, blurred vision, and transient hypotension on arising.

19. Serious adverse effects of sedative-hypnotics are excessive use or abuse, paradoxical response, pruritus, rash, high fever, sore throat, purpura, and jaundice.

20. Before administering a benzodiazepine, record baseline vital signs, (blood pressure, pulse, respirations); measure blood pressure in sitting and lying positions. Check for history of blood dyscrasias or hepatic disease or whether the patient is in the first trimester of pregnancy and assess the patient's level of pain.

Sedative-Hypnotics

Learning Activities

FILL-IN-THE-BLANK

Finish each of the following statements using the correct term.

1. _____ is the most common sleep disorder known.

2. A(n) _____ is a drug that produces sleep; a(n) _____ quiets the patient and gives a feeling of relaxation and rest, not necessarily accompanied by sleep.

3. The long-acting barbiturate, phenobarbital, is also used as a(n) _____.

4. The _____ are the most commonly used sedative-hypnotics.

5. To enhance sleep, patients should be offered foods high in _____ and _____ products at a specific time before sleep.

Choose from the following vocabulary words to complete the statements: sedative, hypnotic, rebound sleep, paradoxic excitement, initial insomnia, intermittent insomnia, terminal insomnia. Not all words will be used.

Steve has difficulty falling asleep, and the health care provider he consults tells him this is known as (6.) _____. While at the sleep disorder clinic, Steve tells another patient, Walt, about his difficulty sleeping. Walt quickly explains this isn't the same as his problem. He falls asleep, but awakens about 4 AM and can't get back to sleep. Walt's insomnia pattern is called (7.) _____.

Prior to surgery, the health care provider prescribes a(n) (8.) _____ to help James to sleep. The next morning, a(n) (9.) _____ is ordered for 8 AM (0800) for the purpose of providing relaxation and rest while awaiting scheduled surgery

at 10:30 AM (1030). Two days after surgery, James asks the nurse if it would be OK to ask the provider for a prescription for the "wonderful medication" he took before surgery because he had the best sleep that day. The nurse asks him about his sleep pattern. He describes that he generally has difficulty sleeping all night at home. He sleeps a while, awakens, and sleeps in cycles several times nightly. The nurse tells him this is known as (10.) _____ .

MATCHING

Match the generic drug name with its corresponding brand name. Each option will be used only once.

_____ 11. triazolam

_____ 12. midazolam

_____ 13. flurazepam

_____ 14. phenobarbital

_____ 15. amobarbital

_____ 16. dexmedetomidine

_____ 17. zolpidem

_____ 18. ramelteon

a. Versed
b. Amytal
c. Dalmane
d. Halcion
e. Luminal
f. Precedex
g. Ambien
h. Rozerem

TRUE OR FALSE

Write "T" for true and "F" for false for each statement. Correct all false statements.

_____ 19. Insomnia is not a disease but a symptom of physical or mental stress.

_____ 20. A common adverse effect of barbiturate therapy is daytime sedation.

_____ 21. Most cases of insomnia are short-lived and can be effectively treated by non-pharmacologic methods.

_____ 22. Habitual use of benzodiazepines does not ever result in physical dependence.

_____ 23. Smoking enhances the metabolism of benzodiazepines.

Sedative-Hypnotics

chapter

14

Practice Questions for the NCLEX® Examination

_____ 1. Which statements does the nurse include when teaching a patient about zolpidem (Ambien) therapy?
  1. "Daytime drowsiness is generally not a problem with this medication."
  2. "If you have difficulty sleeping, increase the dose by one-half."
  3. "No physical dependency will develop with use of this drug."
  4. "Take the medication about 3 hours before you plan on going to sleep."

_____ 2. Barbiturates are known to reduce the effects of which medications? *(Select all that apply.)*
  1. Estrogen (Menest)
  2. Warfarin (Coumadin)
  3. Metronidazole (Flagyl)
  4. Lorazepam (Ativan)
  5. Doxycycline (Vibramycin)

_____ 3. A patient is admitted to the unit because of rapid discontinuation of barbiturate therapy. The nurse expects the patient to exhibit which signs/symptoms? *(Select all that apply.)*
  1. Anxiety
  2. Delirium
  3. Grand mal seizures
  4. Drowsiness
  5. Diarrhea
  6. Weakness

_____ 4. A patient is ordered 7.5 mg of tempazepam (Restoril) PO at bedtime PRN. What does the nurse do next?
  1. Administers the medication to ensure the patient has a good night's sleep
  2. Does not administer the medication unless the patient is having difficulty sleeping, and other measures to meet comfort and psychological needs have failed to produce the desired effect
  3. Leaves the medication at the patient's bedside and instructs the patient to take it if he or she has difficulty falling asleep
  4. Tells the patient that he or she should not take the medication because of a risk of addiction

_____ 5. Upon assessing a patient in REM sleep, which signs does the nurse expects to observe?
  1. Bradycardia
  2. Irregular breathing
  3. Flaccid muscles
  4. Hypothermia

_____ 6. While teaching patients about nonpharmacologic methods to enhance sleep, which statement does the nurse include?
  1. "Do not go to bed at the same time each night; go to bed when you feel the most tired."
  2. "Eat your heaviest meal of the day about 45 minutes before you plan to go to bed."
  3. "Exercise during the day, not near bedtime."
  4. "Avoid drinking milk before going to bed."

_____ 7. Which medications and/or substances
        does the nurse identify as potentially in-
        ducing or aggravating insomnia? *(Select
        all that apply.)*
        1. Corticosteroids
        2. SSRI antidepressants
        3. Caffeine
        4. Nicotine
        5. Alcohol

8. A patient is ordered triazolam (Halcion) 0.25
    mg PO at bedtime. The medication is available
    in 0.125-mg tablets. How many tablets does the
    nurse administer? _____ tablet(s)

_____ 9. A patient is ordered phenobarbital
        (Luminal) 60 mg. The medication is
        available as phenobarbital elixir 20 mg/
        5 mL. How many mL of the elixir does
        the nurse administer?
        1. 5 mL
        2. 10 mL
        3. 15 mL
        4. 20 mL

_____ 10. After receiving secobarbital (Seconal) 100
        mg PO at bedtime, an older adult patient
        experiences a paradoxical response to
        the medication. Which actions does the
        nurse take? *(Select all that apply.)*
        1. Provides supportive physical care
        2. Provides for patient safety
        3. Places the patient in restraints
        4. Provides for physical channeling
           such as walking
        5. Seeks a change in the medication or-
           der

Drugs Used for Parkinson's Disease

Review Sheet

The QUESTION column and the ANSWER column have been offset so that you can cover the answer while reading the question, allowing you to assess your knowledge.

Question

1. Prepare a list of signs and symptoms of parkinsonism.
2. Summarize the purpose of giving medications to treat Parkinson's disease.

3. Identify the basic components of a baseline assessment of a patient's neurologic function.

4. What are the monitoring parameters found on the Unified Parkinson's Disease Rating Scale (UPDRS)?

5. How is a rating scale such as the UPDRS used to assess the severity of Parkinson's disease based on the degree of disability exhibited by the patient?
6. What are the meanings of the terms: *tremors; dyskinesia; propulsive, uncontrolled movement; bradykinesia;* and *akinesia*?
7. Because of the many adverse effects known to occur with medications used to treat parkinsonism, what health teaching should be initiated?

Answer

1. Signs and symptoms of parkinsonism are expressionlessness; masklike face; tremors of hands, lips, tongue, and jaw; "pill-rolling" movements of fingers; excessive salivation; and dyskinesia.
2. Medications are given to treat Parkinson's disease to provide maximum relief of symptoms and to optimize independence of movement and activity. See also Drug Therapy for Parkinson's Disease, textbook p. 225.
3. Baseline neurologic assessment includes orientation to name, date, time, and place; degree of alertness; ability to comprehend and follow instructions; and degree of involvement in activities of daily life.
4. See textbook, p. 225.

5. See textbook p. 225.

6. Tremors occur primarily at rest, but are more noticeable during emotional turmoil or periods of increased concentration. A "pill rolling" motion in the fingers and thumbs is characteristic. Tremors are usually reduced with voluntary movement. Dyskinesia: inability to perform voluntary movements. Propulsive, uncontrolled movement: quick, short steps forward or backward that cannot be controlled. Bradykinesia is the extremely slow body movements that may eventually progress to akinesia: lack of movement.

8. Summarize the action of the monoamine oxidase-B inhibitors.

9. Summarize the adverse effects associated with medication therapy used in the treatment of parkinsonism. State nursing actions that could be used to alleviate and/or prevent the adverse effects.

10. What type of glaucoma prohibits the use of levodopa?

11. What effect does pyridoxine (vitamin B$_6$) have on levodopa (Larodopa) therapy?

12. List three drugs used to treat parkinsonism.

13. What drugs may be combined with levodopa to improve its effectiveness?

14. People taking levodopa (Larodopa) for several months may develop what type of central nervous system adverse effects?

15. Why should a baseline neurologic assessment be done prior to and periodically during the administration of commonly prescribed drugs for treatment of Parkinson's disease?

16. What is the primary mechanism of action of anticholinergic agents?

17. What are the therapeutic outcomes desired when an anticholinergic agent is prescribed for a Parkinson's patient?

18. When the ability to perform motor functions is impaired, what nursing diagnosis statement could be made?

7. Prepare a list of symptoms the patient has before starting therapy and involve the patient in keeping track of alterations (as the individual's abilities permit). Explain the need for continuing therapy for a period sufficient for the effectiveness of medications to be evaluated. Have the patient report effects that are particularly bothersome; work cooperatively to plan approaches to alleviate the problems.

8. Selegiline and rasagiline are potent monoamine oxidase-type B inhibitors that reduce the metabolism of dopamine in the brain, allowing greater dopaminergic activity.

9. See p. 233 (levodopa), p. 237 (entacapone), and pp. 237-238 (anticholinergic agents).

10. Angle-closure glaucoma prohibits the use of levodopa.

11. Pyridoxine (vitamin B$_6$) in oral doses of 5 to 10 mg reverses the therapeutic and toxic effects of levodopa (Larodopa). Normal diets contain less than 1 mg of pyridoxine, so dietary restrictions are not necessary. However, the ingredients of multiple vitamins should be considered.

12. Drugs used to treat parkinsonism include levodopa (Larodopa), carbidopa (Sinemet), and ropinirole (Requip).

13. Carbidopa, an enzyme inhibitor that reduces the metabolism of levodopa, allowing a greater portion of the administered levodopa to reach the receptor sites in the basal ganglia. Entacapone inhibits the metabolism of dopamine, resulting in a more constant dopaminergic stimulation in the brain.

14. Long-term use of levodopa can cause abnormal movements (e.g., rocking, facial grimacing, chewing motions, head and neck bobbing).

15. Several of the drugs used to treat Parkinson's disease can cause adverse effects such as confusion and hallucinations. It is important to know which is a progression of the disease and which is due to an adverse effect of drug therapy.

16. The primary mechanism of action of anticholinergic agents is to reduce overstimulation caused by the excess of acetylcholine, a cholinergic neurotransmitter.

17. The desired effects are reduction in drooling, sweating, tremors, and depression.

18. Risk for injury related to Parkinson's disease; manifested by propulsive gait, unsteadiness, and progressive inability to walk unassisted.

Student Name _____

Drugs Used for Parkinson's Disease

Learning Activities

FILL-IN-THE-BLANK

Finish each of the following statements using the correct term.

1. Selegiline (Eldepryl) may be used to slow the course of Parkinson's disease by possibly slowing the progression of deterioration of _____ nerve cells.

2. _____ is the impairment of the individual's ability to perform voluntary movements.

3. _____ is extremely slow body movement, which may eventually progress to _____, or lack of movement.

4. Patients taking levodopa (Larodopa) therapy should be warned that the metabolites of levodopa react with toilet-bowl cleaners to turn the urine _____ to _____ in color.

5. _____ is an antibiotic which inhibits the metabolism of ropinirole hydrochloride (Requip).

6. Anticholinergics reduce the severity of the _____ and drooling associated with parkinsonism.

7. The goal of treatment of parkinsonism is to restore dopamine neurotransmitter function as close to normal as possible, and relieve symptoms caused by _____ acetylcholine.

8. With Parkinson's disease, the neurotransmitter _____ is deficient, leaving a relative excess of the neurotransmitter _____.

9. To help reduce an excess amount of acetylcholine, _____ agents are prescribed.

10. The major action of the drug carbidopa (Sinemet) is to reduce metabolism of _____.

11. The major action of the drug levodopa (Larodopa) is to cross into the brain and be metabolized to _____.

12. The major action of the drug entacapone (Comtan) is to reduce destruction of _____ in peripheral tissue.

13. The term used for the lack of ability to move is _____.

MATCHING

Match the generic drug name with its corresponding brand name. Each option will be used only once.

_____ 14. apomorphine

_____ 15. diphenhydramine hydrochloride

_____ 16. carbidopa

_____ 17. benztropine mesylate

_____ 18. pramipexole

a. Sinemet
b. Apokyn
c. Cogentin
d. Mirapex
e. Benadryl

TRUE OR FALSE

Write "T" for true and "F" for false for each statement. Correct all false statements.

_____ 19. The symptoms associated with parkinsonism are caused by a dopamine deficiency in the extrapyramidal system within the basal ganglia of the brain.

_____ 20. In most cases of drug-induced parkinsonism, there is no recovery if the chemical is discontinued.

_____ 21. There is no cure for parkinsonism.

_____ 22. Orthostatic hypotension is a rare adverse effect with most of the medicines used to treat Parkinson's disease.

_____ 23. Carbidopa (Sinemet) is used to reduce the dose of levodopa (Larodopa) required by approximately 75%.

_____ 24. Carbidopa (Sinemet) has no effect when used alone; it must be used in combination with levodopa (Larodopa)

_____ 25. Dopamine does not enter the brain when administered orally.

Drugs Used for Parkinson's Disease

Practice Questions for the NCLEX® Examination

_____ 1. Constipation resulting from drug therapy for Parkinson's disease is best treated by which method?
1. Limiting fluid intake to four six-ounce glasses of water daily
2. Adding bulk-forming laxatives to the daily regimen
3. Decreasing bulk in the diet
4. Eliminating fruits from the diet

_____ 2. Which statement about tremors associated with Parkinson's disease is true?
1. They are usually a "pill rolling" motion in the fingers and thumbs.
2. They are usually increased with voluntary movement.
3. They occur primarily with motion.
4. They start with rapid movement of the arms and hands.

_____ 3. When performing an admission assessment on a patient with Parkinson's disease, what does the nurse expect to find?
1. A spine that is erect and shoulders that are parallel to the hips
2. Eyes that are bulging
3. Increased salivation
4. Muscle relaxation and weakness

_____ 4. When teaching a patient about diet therapy and levodopa (Larodopa), which information does the nurse include?
1. Vitamin C will decrease the effects of levodopa (Larodopa).
2. Pyridoxine (vitamin B_6) will reduce the therapeutic effect of levodopa.
3. A low-protein diet is recommended for patients with parkinsonism.
4. Patients taking levodopa therapy should be weighed every other month.

_____ 5. Which statements does the nurse include when teaching a patient about Parkinson's disease? _(Select all that apply.)_
1. "Parkinson's disease is curable."
2. "Diarrhea is a frequent problem in patients with Parkinson's disease."
3. "The goal of treatment of parkinsonism is minimizing symptoms."
4. "The motor symptoms of parkinsonism start insidiously."
5. "The cause of parkinsonism is not known."

_____ 6. Before administering levodopa (Larodopa) therapy, the nurse must assess the patient for a history of which condition?
1. Hypertension
2. Allergy to penicillin
3. Asthma
4. Acute angle-closure glaucoma

_____ 7. Which drug is contraindicated for patients receiving selegiline (Eldepryl)?
1. Morphine
2. Meperidine (Demerol)
3. Acetaminophen (Tylenol)
4. Aspirin

_____ 8. Which foods or beverages are high in tyramine content? _(Select all that apply.)_
1. Chianti wine
2. Chicken
3. Fava beans
4. Cheeses
5. Almonds

_____ 9. Which statement does the nurse include when teaching a patient with Parkinson's disease about the drug apomorphine (Apokyn)?
1. It is chemically related to morphine, but does not have any opioid activity.
2. It is used to treat hypermobility associated with the "weaning off" of dopamine agonists.
3. It is administered intravenously.
4. It commonly causes hypertension in patients who initially start therapy with this drug.

_____ 10. Which medication used in treating patients with Parkinson's disease reduces the destruction of dopamine in the peripheral tissues, allowing significantly more dopamine to reach the brain to eliminate the symptoms of parkinsonism?
1. Entacapone (Comtan)
2. Ropinirole (Requip)
3. Apomorphine (Apokyn)
4. Selegiline (Eldepryl)

_____ 11. Which signs or symptoms does the nurse expect to find in a patient who has had Parkinson's disease for 12 years? *(Select all that apply.)*
1. Tremors
2. Dyskinesia
3. Obesity
4. Dry mouth
5. Masklike face

_____ 12. Which statements about Parkinson's disease and its treatment are true? *(Select all that apply.)*
1. Parkinson's disease is a progressive neurologic disorder.
2. The symptoms associated with Parkinson's disease develop because of a relative excess of dopamine in the brain.
3. Selegiline (Eldepryl) therapy is often started first to slow the development of symptoms.
4. Nonpharmacologic treatment of Parkinson's disease is equally important in maintaining the long-term well-being of the patient.
5. Pyridoxine (vitamin B_6) has been found to enhance the therapeutic and toxic effects of levodopa.

_____ 13. Which statements about the use of apomorphine (Apokyn) in the treatment of Parkinson's disease are true? *(Select all that apply.)*
1. Apomorphine is chemically related to morphine and has twice as much opioid activity as morphine.
2. Apomorphine is used to treat the muscular rigidity associated with Parkinson's disease.
3. Emesis is one of the pharmacologic actions of apomorphine.
4. Apomorphine should not be administered intravenously.
5. Ondansetron (Zofran) is the treatment of choice for nausea associated with apomorphine therapy.

_____ 14. Which statements about the proper administration of selegiline (Eldepryl) orally disintegrating tablets does the nurse include in a patient's teaching plan? *(Select all that apply.)*
1. "Do not ingest food or liquids for 5 minutes before and after taking selegiline."
2. "Take the tablets before bedtime."
3. "Be sure your hands are dry when handling the tablets."
4. "Remove the tablets from the packaging by pushing them through the foil backing."
5. "Place the tablet under your tongue."

_____ 15. Which are nursing considerations for patients on apomorphine (Apokyn) therapy? *(Select all that apply.)*
1. Administer prochlorperazine (Compazine) for nausea associated with apomorphine therapy.
2. Assess patients on apomorphine therapy for orthostatic hypotension.
3. Calculate apomorphine dose based on milligrams.
4. Do not administer apomorphine intravenously.
5. Assess patients receiving apomorphine therapy for sudden sleep attacks.

_____ 16. A prescriber's order reads benztropine mesylate (Cogentin) 5.5 mg PO at bedtime. Cogentin comes in strengths of 0.5-mg, 1-mg, and 2-mg tablets. Which dosage does the nurse select?
  1. Four 1-mg tablets and one 0.5-mg tablet
  2. One 2-mg tablet and one 0.5-mg tablet
  3. Two 2-mg tablets, one 1-mg tablet, and one 0.5-mg tablet
  4. Two 2-mg tablets and one-half of a 1-mg tablet

17. A patient is scheduled to receive 60 mg of orphenadrine citrate (Banflex) intramuscularly. Banflex is available as 30 mg/mL in a 10-mL vial. How many mL of medication does the nurse administer? _____ mL

Drugs Used for Anxiety Disorders

chapter

16

Review Sheet

The QUESTION column and the ANSWER column have been offset so that you can cover the answers while reading the questions, allowing you to assess your knowledge.

Question	Answer
1. Define *generalized anxiety disorder*.	
2. What is a phobia?	1. Generalized anxiety disorder is described as excessive and unrealistic worry about two or more life circumstances for 6 months or more. (See textbook, p. 240.)
3. What is panic disorder?	2. Phobias are irrational fears of a specific object, activity, or situation. The patient recognizes the fear as exaggerated or unrealistic. The fear persists, however, and the patient seeks to avoid the situation.
4 What is obsessive-compulsive disorder?	3. Panic disorder begins as a series of acute or unprovoked anxiety (panic) attacks involving an intense, terrifying fear. The attacks do not occur on exposure to an anxiety-causing situation as phobias do.
5. State another common name for tranquilizers.	4. An obsession is an unwanted thought, idea, image, or urge that a patient recognizes as time-consuming and senseless but that repeatedly intrudes into the consciousness despite attempts to ignore, prevent, or counteract it. A compulsion is a repetitive, intentional, purposeful behavior performed to decrease the anxiety associated with an obsession.
6. Summarize nursing assessments and interventions that are used for the patient displaying anxiety.	5. Tranquilizers are also called *anxiolytic agents* or *antianxiety medications*.
7. State the action of benzodiazepines.	6. See textbook, pp. 242-244.
8. What is the ending spelling of all generic drug names of benzodiazepines except chlordiazepoxide?	7. Benzodiazepines stimulate an inhibitory neurotransmitter gamma-aminobutyric acid (GABA).
9. Name three benzodiazepines that are relatively short-acting and therefore most appropriate for an older adult or an individual with reduced hepatic function.	8. All generic drug names of benzodiazepines end in "-am."

10. What premedication assessments should be performed prior to administering a benzodiazepine?

11. State the desired therapeutic outcome for any drug prescribed for an anxiety disorder.

12. Why is the use of benzodiazepines avoided during the first trimester of pregnancy?

13. Describe common adverse effects of buspirone (BuSpar), hydroxyzine (Vistaril, Atarax), and meprobamate (Miltown).

14. Based on the adverse effects of the drugs listed in question 13, what nursing diagnosis could be developed?

15. When you read a drug monograph that lists possible orthostatic hypotension as an adverse effect, what nursing actions would be appropriate, in addition to teaching the patient to rise slowly from a supine to sitting position?

16. What are additive effects associated with concurrent CNS system depressants?

17. What are symptoms of hepatotoxicity?

18. What are the common adverse effects of hydroxyzine (Vistaril, Atarax)?

19. What is the major advantage of buspirone (BuSpar), an azaspirone agent, over other antianxiety agents?

20. What is the action of fluvoxamine (Luvox), an SSRI agent?

21. When used as a preoperative medication, what are the desired actions of hydroxyzine (Vistaril, Atarax)?

9. Alprazolam (Xanax), lorazepam (Ativan), oxazepam (Serax) are appropriate benzodiazepines for older adults or individuals with reduced hepatic function.

10. Before administering a benzodiazepine, assess for level of anxiety present; vital signs, especially blood pressure in sitting and supine positions; blood dyscrasias; hepatic disease; and whether the patient is in the first trimester of pregnancy or breastfeeding.

11. The desired outcome of drug therapy for anxiety disorders is a decreased level of anxiety so that the individual can function normally in life's daily activities.

12. Use of benzodiazepines in the first trimester of pregnancy is associated with increased incidence of birth defects.

13. Common adverse effects include sedation and lethargy with buspirone; blurred vision, constipation, dryness of mucous membranes, and sedation with hydroxyzine; and sedation, slurred speech, and dizziness with meprobamate.

14. A possible nursing diagnosis is: Injury, high risk for, related to antianxiety drug therapy (meprobamate, buspirone, hydroxyzine) manifested by lethargy, sedation, blurred vision, dizziness.

15. Monitor blood pressure in supine and standing positions every shift and provide for patient safety.

16. Combining more than one drug that depresses the CNS will cause exaggeration of the depressant effects and could reach potentially fatal levels.

17. Symptoms of hepatotoxicity include anorexia, jaundice, nausea, vomiting, hepatomegaly, splenomegaly, and abnormal liver function tests (elevated bilirubin, AST, ALT, GGT, alkaline phosphatase, and prothrombin time).

18. Common adverse effects of hydroxyzine include blurred vision, constipation, dry mucosa (thirst), and sedation.

19. There is lower incidence of sedation with buspirone.

20. Fluvoxamine inhibits serotonin reuptake at the nerve endings, prolonging the serotonin activity. It is used to assist patients with obsessive-compulsive disorder to gain better control over obsessive actions.

21. Used preoperatively, hydroxyzine causes sedation, acts as an antiemetic, and reduces the narcotic dose needed for analgesia.

Drugs Used for Anxiety Disorders

Learning Activities

FILL-IN-THE-BLANK

Finish each of the following statements using the correct term.

1. _____ is an unpleasant feeling of apprehension or nervousness caused by the perception of potential or actual danger that threatens a person's security.

2. A(n) _____ is an unwanted thought, idea, image, or urge that the patient recognizes as time-consuming and senseless but repeatedly intrudes into the consciousness, despite attempts to ignore, prevent, or counteract it.

3. The most common drug class used for the treatment of anxiety disorders are the _____.

4. A patient is admitted to the emergency department from his place of employment after he started to breathe fast and feel anxious when a butterfly entered his office space. The patient states, "I am so afraid of butterflies. I know they will kill me, and I can't stop thinking that that butterfly was in my office. I am terrified of them." The nurse understands that the patient most likely is exhibiting evidence of a(n) _____.

5. The _____ are the most commonly used drugs for the treatment of anxiety disorders because they are more consistently effective, less likely to interact with other drugs, less likely to cause overdose, and have less potential for abuse than other antianxiety agents.

MATCHING

Match the generic drug name with its corresponding brand name. Each option will be used only once.

_____ 6. alprazolam

_____ 7. diazepam

_____ 8. lorazepam

_____ 9. oxazepam

a. Serax
b. Ativan
c. Valium
d. Xanax

TRUE OR FALSE

Write "T" for true and "F" for false for each statement. Correct all false statements.

_____ 10. Anxiety disorders are the most commonly encountered mental disorder in clinical practice.

_____ 11. Panic attacks occur on exposure to an anxiety-causing situation.

_____ 12. Patients generally respond to benzodiazepine therapy in one week.

_____ 13. It is recommended that benzodiazepines not be administered during at least the first trimester of pregnancy.

_____ 14. Larger doses of benzodiazepines may be necessary to maintain anxiolytic effects in patients who smoke.

Drugs Used for Anxiety Disorders

Practice Questions for the NCLEX® Examination

_____ 1. Which statement about buspirone (BuSpar) is true?
1. It is a controlled substance.
2. It has a high potential for abuse.
3. It is sometimes called a *midbrain modulator*.
4. It requires 2–3 days of treatment before initial signs of improvement are evident.

_____ 2. Which drug used for anxiety disorders is also used routinely as a preoperative or postoperative sedative to control vomiting, diminish anxiety, and reduce the amount of narcotics needed for anesthesia?
1. Meprobamate (Miltown)
2. Hydroxyzine (Vistaril)
3. Buspirone (BuSpar)
4. Fluvoxamine (Luvox)

_____ 3. Which intervention by the nurse is the most effective in dealing with a patient who has orthostatic hypotension caused by meprobamate (Miltown) therapy?
1. Asking the patient to rise from a sitting position rapidly
2. Encouraging the patient to sit down if feeling faint
3. Encouraging the patient to sleep in a chair at night; do not lie down
4. Informing the patient to reduce the dose of meprobamate by half

_____ 4. What is the most common adverse effect of buspirone (BuSpar)?
1. Constipation
2. Dry mouth
3. CNS disturbances
4. Hepatotoxicity

_____ 5. Anxiety is a component of many medical illnesses involving which systems? *(Select all that apply.)*
1. Cardiovascular
2. Pulmonary
3. Digestive
4. Endocrine
5. Sensory

_____ 6. When a patient is withdrawn from long-term use of benzodiazepines, the nurse assesses for which signs/symptoms? *(Select all that apply.)*
1. Restlessness
2. Worsening of anxiety
3. Tremor
4. Muscle tension
5. Auditory hypersensitivity

7. A patient is prescribed hydroxyzine (Vistaril) 10 mg PO qid. The medication is available as 25 mg/5 mL. There is 120 mL in the container. How much medication does the nurse administer? _____ mL

_____ 8. A patient is prescribed alprazolam (Xanax) 5 mg three times daily. What does the nurse do next?
1. Plans to administer the medication at breakfast, lunch, and dinner
2. Administers the medication when the patient has an empty stomach
3. Assesses the patient for allergy to shrimp before administering the medication
4. Questions the dose of medication ordered

_____ 9. When assessing a patient before administering buspirone (BuSpar), which finding is of most concern to the nurse?
1. Slurred speech
2. Insomnia
3. Nervousness
4. Dizziness

Drugs Used for Mood Disorders

Review Sheet

The QUESTION column and the ANSWER column have been offset so that you can cover the answers while reading the questions, allowing you to assess your knowledge.

Question	Answer
1. Define *mood disorders*.	
2. Which neurotransmitters are affected by depression?	1. Mood disorders are also known as *affective disorders*. The person's ability to function is impaired for a prolonged period of time going beyond brief periods of emotional upset from negative life experiences. Mood disorders are characterized by abnormal feelings of euphoria and/or depression.
3. What are characteristic symptoms found in a person experiencing depression?	2. Norepinephrine, serotonin, and dopamine are the neurotransmitters affected by depression.
4. Define *bipolar disorder*.	3. Characteristic symptoms of depression are persistent, reduced ability to experience pleasure in life's usual activities, sometimes accompanied by personality change and sadness.
5. Define *flight of ideas*.	4. Bipolar disorder is characterized by distinct episodes of mania (euphoria) and depression separated by intervals without mood disturbances.
6. Cite the incidence of attempted suicide in individuals with mood disorders.	5. Quick thoughts that rapidly change from one topic to another are called *flight of ideas*.
7. Cite the three stages that patients with mood disorders experience as they strive for achievement of full functioning status.	6. The frequency of suicide attempts in individuals with mood disorders is 15%, 30 times higher than general population.
8. Give two examples of cognitive symptoms and psychomotor symptoms.	7. The stages one goes through during treatment of a mood disorder are: acute, continuation, and maintenance. See textbook p. 252 for definitions of each.
9. Define *labile moods*.	8. Cognitive symptoms involve the ability to concentrate and altered clarity of thought (e.g., confusion, poor short-term memory). Psychomotor symptoms include slowed or retarded movements, pacing, and outbursts of shouting.
10. Define *grandiose thinking*.	9. Labile moods are rapid shifts in mood. A person may be happy, then rapidly switch to anger and irritability.
11. List the drug classifications used in the treatment of depression.	10. Grandiose thinking is overestimation of oneself and one's abilities or importance.

12. Describe basic components of assessment for an individual with a mood disorder.

13. In general, what is the decision-making capacity of an individual with a mood disorder?

14. What are the basic actions of medicines used to treat depression?

15. Why is it necessary to closely monitor patients taking antidepressants?

16. What is the anticipated therapeutic outcome for antidepressant therapy?

17. Discuss premedication assessments needed for an individual who is to receive 1) MAOIs; 2) SSRIs; 3) tricyclic antidepressants; or 4) miscellaneous agents, including bupropion hydrochloride (Wellbutrin, Zyban), mirtazapine (Remeron), nefazodone, and trazodone hydrochloride.

18. State appropriate nursing diagnoses as indicators of antidepressant therapy.

19. Name the drug used to treat manic episodes. List the important premedication assessments as well as assessments needed for long-term therapy.

20. List the normal serum level for lithium carbonate.

21. Describe teaching that should be completed about sodium intake while receiving lithium therapy.

11. Drugs used in the treatment of depression include MAOIs, SSRIs, SNRIs, tricyclic antidepressants, and a miscellaneous group of agents.

12. Basic components of assessment for mood disorders include history of mood disorders, basic mental status, interpersonal relationships, mood/affect, clarity of thought, thoughts of death, psychomotor function, sleep pattern, and dietary history.

13. The decision-making capacity of an individual with a mood disorder is highly variable. The nurse must evaluate the individual's abilities and need to be protected from self-harm.

14. All antidepressants have varying degrees of effect on norepinephrine, dopamine, and serotonin by blocking reuptake and reducing destruction of these neurotransmitters, thereby prolonging their action.

15. Patients taking antidepressants may be suicidal. When drug therapy is initiated, it may take 1–4 weeks before a therapeutic response is evident. An early improvement in mood or other symptoms should not be used as an indicator that the depression is no longer present. Individuals may require 4–6 weeks to reach a full therapeutic level of the medicine.

16. The anticipated therapeutic outcome for individuals taking antidepressants is improvement of mood with a concurrent reduction in the feelings of depression.

17. MAOIs, textbook p. 257; SSRIs, textbook p. 261; tricyclic antidepressants, textbook p. 263; miscellaneous agents, textbook pp. 265-268.

18. Risk for self-directed violence (indication); Hopelessness (indication); Dysfunctional grieving (indication); Ineffective coping (indication); Social isolation (indication); Disturbed sensory perception, visual or auditory (indication).

19. Lithium carbonate (Eskalith, Lithane) is used to treat manic episodes. Before beginning lithium therapy, stress importance of the need for adequate hydration and sodium intake. Teach the patient the signs of lithium toxicity (e.g., nausea, vomiting, abdominal pain, diarrhea, lethargy, speech difficulty, mild dizziness, muscle twitching, and tremors).

20. Normal serum lithium range is 0.4–1.5 mEq/L.

22. Why is behavioral monitoring during anti-depressant therapy done?

21. During lithium therapy, normal daily intake of sodium is essential, as is adequate hydration. Stress using salt in cooking and at the table. The person should also drink 10–12 8-oz glasses of water daily.

22. Behavioral monitoring during antidepressant therapy is done to detect development of extrapyramidal symptoms and to monitor for degree of therapeutic response to therapy.

Drugs Used for Mood Disorders

Learning Activities

FILL-IN-THE-BLANK

Finish each of the following statements using the correct term.

1. Bipolar disorder was formerly known as
   _____ _____ .

2. The most common gastrointestinal adverse effect when taking tricyclic antidepressants is
   _____ .

3. St. John's wort may _____ toxic effects of antidepressant medicines.

4. _____ is used to treat acute mania and for the prophylaxis of recurrent manic and depressive episodes in bipolar disorder.

5. Periods of elation or euphoria are known as
   _____ .

6. People taking MAOIs must omit foods containing _____ .

MATCHING

Match the generic drug name with its corresponding brand name. Each option will be used only once.

_____ 7. sertraline

_____ 8. paroxetine

_____ 9. fluvoxamine

_____ 10. fluoxetine

_____ 11. citalopram

_____ 12. imipramine

_____ 13. clomipramine

_____ 14. duloxetine

a. Cymbalta
b. Anafranil
c. Tofranil
d. Celexa
e. Luvox
f. Paxil
g. Zoloft
h. Prozac

TRUE OR FALSE

Write "T" for true and "F" for false for each statement. Correct all false statements.

_____ 15. Major depression currently ranks as the second leading cause of disease burden in the United States.

_____ 16. Anxiety symptoms are present in almost 90% of depressed patients.

_____ 17. All patients with depression should be assessed for suicidal thoughts.

_____ 18. For most antidepressants, the lag time between initiation of therapy and therapeutic response is one week.

_____ 19. Electroconvulsive therapy is contraindicated in the treatment of patients with cardiovascular disease.

_____ 20. Dosages of fluvoxamine (Luvox) may need to be decreased for full therapeutic response in patients who smoke.

Drugs Used for Mood Disorders

Practice Questions for the NCLEX® Examination

_____ 1. What is the highest priority of care for a patient with severe mood disorders?
1. Monitoring serum drug levels
2. The provision of patient safety and supervision at intervals consistent with severity of the suicidal threat
3. Maintaining a calm environment
4. Maintenance of physical restraints

_____ 2. Patients with severe mood disorders would most likely benefit from which type of diet?
1. High protein
2. High sodium
3. High fat
4. Low calorie

_____ 3. When foods with high tyramine content are ingested by a patient taking monoamine oxidase inhibitors (MAOIs), what is the most common adverse effect?
1. Allergic reaction
2. Renal failure
3. Hypertensive crisis
4. Respiratory depression

_____ 4. Which drug for pain is contraindicated for use in a patient who is receiving MAOI therapy?
1. Meperidine
2. Morphine
3. Acetaminophen
4. Codeine

_____ 5. For a patient on bupropion hydrochloride (Wellbutrin) therapy, the concurrent use of nicotine patches may cause which sign?
1. Development of a rash
2. Low heart rate
3. Chronic cough
4. High blood pressure

_____ 6. The fluid and electrolyte status of a patient taking lithium carbonate (Eskalith) must be closely monitored by the nurse, because lithium may do what?
1. Deplete potassium stores
2. Enhance sodium depletion
3. Cause calcium toxicity
4. Result in acidosis

_____ 7. The nurse is teaching a patient about lithium carbonate (Lithane) therapy. Which statement does the nurse include in the teaching plan?
1. "If nausea should occur, discontinue therapy immediately."
2. "Continue with the usual dose of lithium if weakness should develop."
3. "Maintain a normal dietary intake of sodium with adequate maintenance fluids."
4. "Lithium will cause a metallic taste in your mouth that you will get used to."

_____ 8. Which approach does the nurse use when interacting with a patient who is in the manic phase?
1. Allow the patient to make decisions if capable.
2. Maintain flexibility with unit rules.
3. Isolate the patient if he or she is highly agitated.
4. Medicate the patient immediately.

_____ 9. Tricyclic antidepressants are can be used to treat which conditions? *(Select all that apply.)*
1. Phantom limb pain
2. Peripheral neuropathy
3. Premenstrual symptoms
4. Obstructive sleep apnea
5. Parkinson's disease

_____ 10. A patient is diagnosed with serotonin syndrome. Which manifestations of the disease will the nurse assess for? (Select all that apply.)
1. Mental status changes
2. Hypertension
3. Sweating
4. Hyperpyrexia
5. Tremors

_____ 11. What is the most widely used drug class of antidepressant medications?
1. SSRIs
2. MAOIs
3. Tricyclic antidepressants
4. Miscellaneous agents

12. A patient is ordered duloxetine (Cymbalta) 120 mg PO daily. The medication is available in 30-mg capsules. How many capsules does the nurse administer? _____ capsule(s)

13. A patient is ordered escitalopram (Lexapro) oral solution 10 mg PO once daily. The medication is available as 5 mg/5 mL. How many mL of the medication does the nurse administer? _____ mL

_____ 14. The nurse is teaching a patient diagnosed with depression about tricyclic antidepressant therapy. Which statement by the patient indicates the nurse's instruction has been successful?
1. "I can expect to feel better in about 10 days."
2. "I may experience sweating while taking this drug."
3. "I will double the dose of St. John's wort while taking this medication."
4. "I may continue to drink alcohol while taking this medication."

_____ 15. A patient has been prescribed bupropion hydrochloride (Zyban) for smoking cessation. Which statement by the patient indicates a need for further teaching on the use of this drug?
1. "I will need to stop smoking first, then start to take the medication."
2. "I can expect to be on the medication for about 7 to 12 weeks."
3. "It takes 6 weeks for the medication to become effective."
4. "I don't need to taper the medication dose when I no longer need to take it."

Drugs Used for Psychoses

Review Sheet

The QUESTION column and the ANSWER column have been offset so that you can cover the answer while reading the questions, allowing you to assess your knowledge.

Question	Answer
1. Define *psychosis*.	
2. Differentiate among delusions, hallucinations, and disorganized thinking.	1. Psychosis does not have a single definition, but is a clinical descriptor that means that a person is out of touch with reality.
3. What is change in affect?	2. Delusions are false, irrational beliefs unchanged in the presence of data to the contrary. Hallucinations are false sensory perceptions experienced by an individual without external stimulus. Disorganized thinking is recognized when an individual switches rapidly from one idea or thought to another unrelated topic.
4. What is meant by *target symptoms*?	3. Change in affect is characterized by diminished emotional expression, reduced spontaneous movement, and poor eye contact. The individual withdraws from effective functioning in interpersonal relations, work, education, and self-care.
5. What rating scales have been developed for objective measurement of target symptoms due to psychotherapy and pharmacology?	4. Target symptoms are those symptoms to be assessed to evaluate therapeutic response to drug therapy and nonpharmacologic interventions.
6. What is another name for an antipsychotic agent?	5. Brief Psychiatric Rating Scale (BPRS), the Positive and Negative Scale for Schizophrenia (PANSS), the Clinical Global Impression (CGI) scale, and the Rating of Aggression Against People and/or Property (RAAPP) Scale are recently developed scales in use for objective measurement of target symptoms. Adverse effects scales include GDS, TWSTRS for dystonias, DISCUS or AIMS for extrapyramidal symptoms. (Note: Students can benefit from further online research of the scales listed.)
7. Differentiate between the terms *low-potency* and *high-potency* antipsychotic agents.	6. Neuroleptic agent—usually reserved for the typical antipsychotic agents.
8. What are typical and atypical antipsychotic agents?	7. These terms refer ONLY to the milligram doses and not to the difference in effectiveness of antipsychotic agents.
9. Cite the desired therapeutic outcome(s) from antipsychotic therapy.	8. Typical and atypical antipsychotic agents are listed in Table 18-1.

10. Define *extrapyramidal symptoms*, including dystonia, pseudoparkinsonian symptoms, akathisia, and tardive dyskinesia.

11. What causes pseudoparkinsonian symptoms?

12. What monitoring scales are used to rate dystonia?

13. What are the DISCUS or AIMS scales?

14. Describe common adverse effects associated with antipsychotic therapy.

15. What is neuroleptic malignant syndrome? What are the symptoms, and how is it treated?

16. Summarize nursing implementations and patient education used for patients being treated for psychoses.

17. Memorize the generic and brand names of these commonly prescribed antipsychotic agents: haloperidol, molindone, aripiprazole, clozapine, olanzapine, quetiapine, and risperidone.

9. Calmed the individual, reduced psychomotor agitation and insomnia, reduced thought disorders so the individual is able to function with minimal exacerbation of psychotic symptoms.

10. Dystonia is spasmodic movements of muscle groups (e.g., tongue protrusion, rolling back of the eyes). Pseudoparkinsonian symptoms are tremors, muscular rigidity, masklike expression, shuffling gait, and loss or weakness of motor function. Akathisia is a feeling of anxiety, restlessness, pacing, rocking, and inability to sit still. Tardive dyskinesia is progressive symptoms of involuntary, hyperkinetic, abnormal movements.

11. Pseudoparkinsonian symptoms are caused by a relative deficiency of dopamine and an excess of acetylcholine, caused by antipsychotic agents.

12. Toronto Western Spasmodic Torticollis Rating Scale (TWSTRS), Global Dystonia Scale (GDS), Unified Dystonia Scale (UDRS), and the Fahn-Marsden Scale. (See also related websites on documentation of dystonia.)

13. Both the DISCUS and AIMS scales are involuntary movement scales for rating dyskinetic movements. (See Appendix F [DISCUS] on the text's Companion CD or the Evolve website at http://evolve.elsevier.com/Clayton.)

14. Adverse effects of antipsychotic therapy include sedation, drowsiness, appetite stimulation, postural hypotension, reflex tachycardia, lowering of seizure threshold, and development of symptoms of tardive dyskinesia.

15. See textbook, p. 277. Symptoms of neuroleptic malignant syndrome include fever, extrapyramidal symptoms, and lead-pipe rigidity, probably due to excessive dopamine depletion. It is treated with bromocriptine or amantadine as dopamine agonists and dantrolene, a muscle relaxant. Fever is treated with cooling blankets, adequate hydration, and antipyretics.

16. See textbook, pp. 280-281.

17. The generic and brand names of commonly prescribed antipsychotic agents are: haloperidol (Haldol), molindone (Moban), aripiprazole (Abilify), clozapine (Clozaril), olanzapine (Zyprexa), quetiapine (Seroquel), and risperidone (Risperdal).

Drugs Used for Psychoses

Learning Activities

FILL-IN-THE-BLANK

Finish each of the following statements using the correct term.

1. _____ does not have a single definition but is a clinical descriptor that means being out of touch with reality.

2. A(n) _____ is a false or irrational belief that is firmly held despite obvious evidence to the contrary.

3. The typical antipsychotic agents antagonize the neurotransmitter _____ in the central nervous system.

4. With the use of antipsychotic therapy, reduction in hallucinations, delusions, and thought disorder often requires _____ to _____ weeks of therapy for full therapeutic effect.

5. _____ _____ syndrome is a potentially fatal adverse effect of antipsychotic therapy in which the patient displays extrapyramidal manifestations as part of the symptoms of the disorder.

6. _____ is a syndrome consisting of subjective feelings of anxiety and restlessness and objective signs of pacing, rocking, and inability to sit or stand in one place for extended periods.

7. A(n) _____ is a false sensory perception that is experienced without an external stimulus but that nevertheless seems real to the patient.

8. Persistent and involuntary hyperkinetic abnormal movements in a patient taking antipsychotic drugs is called _____ _____ .

MATCHING

Match the generic drug name with its corresponding brand name. Each option will be used only once.

_____ 9. risperidone

_____ 10. haloperidol

_____ 11. aripiprazole

_____ 12. prochlorperazine

_____ 13. olanzepine

a. Haldol
b. Risperdal
c. Abilify
d. Zyprexa
e. Compazine

Select the definition that best describes the term(s) listed. Not all definitions will be used.

_____ 14. hallucinations

_____ 15. delusions

_____ 16. akathisia

_____ 17. tardive dyskinesia

_____ 18. dystonia

a. Syndrome demonstrated by anxiety, restlessness, pacing, and rocking
b. Alternating feelings of danger and elation
c. Involuntary hyperkinetic abnormal movements
d. False sensory perceptions experienced without external stimulus
e. Prolonged spasmodic movements of muscle groups
f. A false, irrational belief that a patient embraces despite evidence to the contrary

TRUE OR FALSE

Write "T" for true and "F" for false for each statement. Correct all false statements.

_____ 19. In some instances, it is necessary to use injection of long-acting medicines to overcome the nonadherence problem in selected patients with psychotic symptoms.

_____ 20. Rapid increases in dosages of antipsychotic medication will reduce the antipsychotic response time and decrease the frequency of adverse effects.

_____ 21. Extrapyramidal effects are the most troublesome adverse effects and the most common cause of nonadherence associated with antipsychotic therapy.

_____ 22. Acute dystonia has the latest onset of all the extrapyramidal symptoms.

_____ 23. Neuroleptic malignant syndrome (NMS) typically occurs after 3–9 days of treatment with antipsychotic agents and is not related to dosage or previous drug exposure.

_____ 24. It is hypothesized that the cause of the symptoms seen in neuroleptic malignant syndrome is excessive dopamine depletion.

_____ 25. Patients taking clozapine (Clozaril) are particularly susceptible to developing agranulocytosis.

Drugs Used for Psychoses

chapter
18

Practice Questions for the NCLEX® Examination

_____ 1. Which statement does the nurse include when teaching patients taking antipsychotic agents about acute dystonia?
1. "Acute dystonia reactions occur most often in the first 72 hours of therapy."
2. "Dystonic reactions occur most often in females."
3. "There are no treatments for dystonic reactions."
4. "Dystonic reactions usually last for 1 week."

_____ 2. When working with diabetic or prediabetic patients who are taking antipsychotic drugs, what is most important for the nurse to do?
1. Monitor the patient for the development of hyperglycemia, particularly during the early weeks of therapy.
2. Reduce the amount of oral hypoglycemic agents by one-half.
3. Increase the amount of insulin by one unit per milligram of antipsychotic agent taken.4. Discontinue blood glucose monitoring.

_____ 3. Which statement does the nurse include when teaching patients about drug therapy for psychoses?
1. "Expect a rash to develop and continue taking the medication."
2. "If fine tremors of the tongue or lip smacking develop, discontinue use of the antipsychotic drug immediately."
3. "Avoid prolonged exposure to sunlight and ultraviolet light."
4. "Hypertension is a common adverse effect from the use of these drugs."

_____ 4. Patients experiencing neuroleptic malignant syndrome typically manifest which signs and symptoms? _(Select all that apply.)_
1. Lead-pipe rigidity
2. Tachycardia
3. Labile hypertension
4. Hypothermia
5. Diaphoresis

_____ 5. Which is the best treatment approach to tardive dyskinesia for patients receiving antipsychotic therapy?
1. Reducing the antipsychotic drug dose
2. Discontinuing the antipsychotic drug
3. Administering dopamine agonists
4. Assessing for early signs of tardive dyskinesia, at least semiannually and preferably quarterly

_____ 6. Which statement about tardive dyskinesia is true?
1. Symptoms improve when the antipsychotic dosage is decreased.
2. It typically appears after antipsychotic disease reduction or discontinuation takes place.
3. It improves with administration of anticholinergic agents.
4. It rapidly goes away after antipsychotic medications are discontinued.

_____ 7. A patient receiving antipsychotic therapy develops pseudoparkinsonian symptoms. The patient's spouse wants to know what to expect now that these symptoms have developed. What information does the nurse give to the patient's spouse?
1. "The antipsychotic medication will need to be discontinued due to this complication."
2. "These symptoms are an adverse effect of the antipsychotic drug therapy and no treatment is effective."
3. "The patient has now developed parkinsonism and there is no treatment."
4. "These symptoms are well-controlled by anticholinergic antiparkinsonian agents."

_____ 8. What is the most common cause of nonadherence associated with antipsychotic therapy?
1. The high cost of these medications
2. Extrapyramidal effects
3. Drowsiness
4. Hypertension

_____ 9. A patient in the emergency department tells the nurse that he is the creator of the universe. What does the nurse suspect that this patient is experiencing?
1. Disorganized thinking
2. Change of affect
3. Hallucinations
4. Delusions

_____ 10. Patients taking antipsychotic drug therapy are most likely to experience which adverse effects? (_Select all that apply._)
1. Pseudoparkinsonism
2. Weight loss
3. Hypoglycemia
4. Akathisia
5. Seizures

_____ 11. Patients taking antipsychotic medications may experience which adverse effects as a result of the anticholinergic effects produced by these agents? (_Select all that apply._)
1. Diarrhea
2. Chronic fatigue
3. Dry mouth
4. Blurred vision
5. Urinary retention

12. A patient is prescribed aripiprazole (Abilify) 30 mg. Aripiprazole is available in 10-mg tablets. How many tablets does the nurse administer? _____ tablet(s)

_____ 13. A patient is diagnosed with neuroleptic malignant syndrome. The nurse anticipates that the patient's medication regimen will include which drug?
1. Dantrolene (Dantrium)
2. Chlorpromazine (Largactil)
3. Molindone (Moban)
4. Clozapine (Clozaril)

_____ 14. A patient has been started on clozapine (Clozatril) therapy. For the first 6 months of therapy, which lab result is most important for the nurse to monitor?
1. Red blood cell counts
2. White blood cell counts
3. Blood glucose
4. Serum potassium

Drugs Used for Seizure Disorders

Review Sheet

The QUESTION column and the ANSWER column have been offset so that you can cover the answer while reading the question, allowing you to assess your knowledge.

Question	Answer
Question	**Answer**

1. Define *seizures*.
2. Describe *epilepsy*.

1. Seizures are symptoms of an abnormality in nerve centers of the brain. They are brief periods of abnormal electrical activity in these nerve centers. Seizures may be convulsive (accompanied by violent, involuntary muscle contractions) or nonconvulsive.

3. Describe tonic-clonic (grand mal) seizures, atonic or akinetic seizures, myoclonic seizures, generalized nonconvulsive seizures, and partial (localized) seizures.

2. Epilepsy is the most common of all neurologic disorders. It is not a single disease but several different disorders that have one common characteristic; a sudden discharge of excessive electrical energy from nerve cells in the brain.

4. What is status epilepticus?

3. Tonic-clonic (grand mal) seizures are the most common type of seizure. In the tonic phase, patients suddenly develop intense muscular contractions that cause them to fall to the ground, lose consciousness, and lie rigid. The back may arch, arms may flex, legs extend, and the teeth clench. Air is forced up the larynx, extruding saliva as foam and producing audible sound like a cry. Respirations stop and the patient may become cyanotic. This phase usually lasts 20–60 seconds before diffuse trembling sets in. The clonic phase is manifested by bilaterally symmetric jerks alternating with relaxation of the extremities. The clonic phase starts slightly and gradually becomes more violent, involving the whole body. Patients often bite their tongues and become incontinent of urine or feces. This phase usually lasts 60 seconds.
   Atonic or akinetic seizures manifest as a sudden loss of muscle tone. They are also referred to as a *drop attack*. This may be described as a head drop, the dropping of a limb, or slumping to the ground. A sudden loss of muscle tone results in a dramatic fall. Patients usually remain conscious. The attacks are short, but frequent injury occurs from the un-

controlled falls. These patients often wear protective headgear to minimize the trauma.

Myoclonic seizures involve lightening-like repetitive contractions of the voluntary muscles of the face, trunk, and extremities.

Absence (petit mal) seizures are attacks that consist of paroxysmal episodes of altered consciousness lasting for 5–20 seconds. Patients appear to be staring into space and may exhibit a few rhythmic movements of the eyes, or head, lip smacking, mumbling, chewing, or swallowing movements.

Partial (localized) seizures are subdivided into partial simple motor seizures (jacksonian) seizures which involve localized convulsions of voluntary muscles and partial seizures with complex symptoms (psychomotor seizures). The person experiencing this type of seizure may appear normal, but they may wander aimlessly and have unusual and repeated chewing, lip smacking, or swallowing movements.

5. Describe the postictal state.

6. Describe the terms *treatment responsive* and *treatment resistant*.

7. Describe nonpharmacologic treatment of seizures.

8. What is the relationship between use of antiepileptic drugs and suicide? What are the indications for health care professionals?

9. When a child is on anticonvulsant therapy, what information should be discussed with the health care provider, family, and teachers?

4. Status epilepticus is a rapidly recurring generalized seizure that does not allow the individual to regain normal function between seizures. It a medical emergency that requires prompt treatment to minimize permanent nerve damage and death.

5. After the clonic phase of a tonic-clonic (grand mal) seizure, the patient proceeds to a resting, recovery phase of flaccid paralysis and sleep lasting 2–3 hours called the *postictal state*. The patient has no recollection of the attack upon awakening.

6. Patients with newly diagnosed epilepsy who respond to treatment are referred to as "treatment responsive." Patients who do not respond to first-line agents are referred to as "treatment resistant."

7. Nonpharmacologic treatment of refractory seizures includes surgical intervention with use of an implantable vagus nerve stimulator for children 12 and older, and a ketogenic diet. The ketogenic diet is used in children, and includes restriction of carbohydrates and protein intake; fat is the primary fuel to produce acidosis and ketosis.

8. In January 2008, the FDA released a report that revealed patients receiving antiepileptic drugs had approximately twice the risk of suicidal behavior or ideation (0.43%) compared to patients receiving placebo (0.22%). Health care professionals should closely monitor all patients currently receiving antiepileptic drugs for notable changes in behavior that could indicate the emergence or worsening of suicidal thoughts or behavior, or depression.

10. In general, how should anticonvulsant therapy start?

11. What is the general action of anticonvulsant therapy?

12. What assessments should the nurse make during seizure activity?

13. Describe the treatment of a patient in status epilepticus.

14. What action should a patient who takes drug therapy for seizure disorder take if pregnancy is suspected?

15. What actions do benzodiazepines have on seizure activity?

16. What symptoms would be seen if benzodiazepines are suddenly stopped?

17. What time period should be used for the gradual withdrawal of benzodiazepines?

18. What precaution should be used when administering diazepam or phenytoin intravenously?

9. In children, anticonvulsant therapy may cause a change in personality and possible indifference to school activities and family activities. Behavioral differences must be discussed with the health care provider, family, and teachers. The school nurse must be informed or medications prescribed.

10. Anticonvulsant therapy should start with use of a single agent selected from a group of first-line agents based on the type of seizure. (See Table 19-1.)

11. Anticonvulsants increase the seizure threshold and regulate neuronal firing by either inhibiting excitatory processes or enhancing inhibitory processes. These medications can also prevent seizures from spreading to adjacent neurons.

12. During seizure activity, the nurse should note a description of the seizure, including onset, duration, body parts involved, any progression of symptoms, state of consciousness, respiratory pattern, salivation, pupil size and eye movement, as well as incontinence.

13. Status epilepticus treatment is found on textbook p. 289.

14. If pregnancy is suspected, the patient should consult an obstetrician as soon as possible. The health care provider should be informed of the seizure medications. The patient should not discontinue medications unless told to do so by the health care provider.

15. The mechanism of action for benzodiazepines is not fully understood, but it is thought that the benzodiazepines inhibit neurotransmission by enhancing the effects of GABA in postsynaptic clefts between nerve cells.

16. Rapid withdrawal of benzodiazepines can result in symptoms similar to those seen with alcohol withdrawal. These may vary from weakness and anxiety to delirium and generalized tonic-clonic seizures.

17. Benzodiazepines require a 2- to 4-week period of gradual withdrawal.

19. Name the drugs known as *hydantoins*.

20. What nursing action should be taken when a patient with diabetes is receiving phenytoin?

21. Describe the oral hygiene measures needed for patients taking hydantoin therapy.

22. What is the therapeutic range of a blood serum level for phenytoin?

23. What is a brand name of phenytoin?

24. The succinimides are used to treat which type of seizures?

25. What are the uses of carbamazepine (Tegretol)?

26. What premedication assessments should be completed before carbamazepine (Tegretol) therapy is initiated?

27. Describe the action and use of gabapentin (Neurontin).

18. Do not mix parenteral diazepam or phenytoin in the same syringe, and do not add either medication to other IV solutions because of precipitate formation. Always check for IV incompatibility before administering either medicine through an established IV line and use the SAS technique. Administer diazepam slowly at a rate of 5 mg per minute. Administer phenytoin slowly at a rate of 25–50 mg per minute. During administration of either medication it is recommended that an ECG monitor be used to closely observe for bradycardia. Should bradycardia occur, stop the bolus infusion until the heart rate returns to normal. Observe the patient during administration for respiratory depression and hypotension.

19. Hydantoins include phenytoin, ethotoin, and fosphenytoin. (Note that these drug names all end in "-toin.")

20. Hydantoins may elevate blood glucose levels, especially if higher doses are used; patients with diabetes mellitus are more susceptible to hyperglycemia. Particularly during the early weeks of therapy, diabetic or prediabetic patients must be monitored for the development of hyperglycemia.

21. The frequency of gingival hyperplasia (gum overgrowth) associated with phenytoin therapy may be reduced by good oral hygiene, including gum massage, frequent brushing, and proper dental care.

22. The therapeutic blood levels for phenytoin are 10 to 20 mg/L.

23. Dilantin is the brand name of phenytoin.

24. The succinimides are used to control absence (petit mal) seizures.

25. Carbamazepine (Tegretol) is an anticonvulsant often used in combination with other anticonvulsants to control generalized tonic-clonic and partial seizures. It has also been used successfully to treat the pain associated with trigeminal neuralgia. It may also be used to treat manic-depressive disorders when lithium therapy has not been optimal.

26. As a result of serious adverse reactions, CBC, LFT, urinalysis, BUN, serum creatinine and ophthalmic examinations should be performed to obtain baseline status of the patient. The patient's history should be reviewed to exclude Asian ancestry. A dangerous and possibly fatal skin reaction may occur with the use of carbamazepine in this particular patient population.

28. What is the action of lamotrigine (Lamictal)?

29. Why is it necessary to check on whether a patient is already taking valproic acid before initiating therapy with lamotrigine (Lamictal)?

30. What is the therapeutic blood level for phenobarbital (Luminal)?

31. What are the therapeutic uses of the drug pregabalin (Lyrica)?

32. Describe the action of primidone (Mysoline).

33. Why is the hydration status of a patient of particular concern if topiramate (Topamax) is used?

34. What considerations must be considered when a patient with diabetes mellitus is prescribed valproic acid (Depakene) therapy?

27. The exact mechanism of action of gabapentin (Neurontin) is unknown. It does not appear to enhance GABA. It is an anticonvulsant usually used in combination with other anticonvulsants to control partial seizures. Gabapentin (Neurontin) is also approved for use in postherpetic neuralgia, a complication of acute herpes zoster infection often described as unbearable itching, electric shock-like pain, or burning.

28. Lamotrigine (Lamictal) is a newer anticonvulsant of the phenyltriazine class, unrelated to other antiepileptic medicines currently available. It is thought to act by blocking voltage-sensitive sodium channels in neuronal membranes. This stabilizes the neuronal membranes and inhibits the release of excitatory neurotransmitters such as glutamate that may induce seizure activity.

29. Valproic acid reduces the metabolism of lamotrigine (Lamictal) by as much as 50%. Significant lamotrigine dosage reductions may be required.

30. The therapeutic blood levels for phenobarbital are 15 to 45 mg/L.

31. Pregabalin (Lyrica) is an anticonvulsant used in combination with other anticonvulsants to control partial seizures. Pregabalin is also approved for the treatment of pain associated with fibromyalgia, diabetic neuropathy, and postherpetic neuralgia.

32. Primidone (Mysline) is structurally related to the barbiturates. It is metabolized into phenobarbital and phenylethylmalonamide (PEMA), both of which are active anticonvulsants. The exact mechanism of anticonvulsant action is unknown.

33. Decreased sweating and overheating have been reported with the use of topiramate (Topamax), primarily in children. Most cases occurred in association with exposure to elevated environmental temperatures and/or vigorous activity. Proper hydration before and during activities such as exercise or exposure to warm temperatures is recommended.

34. One of the metabolites of valproic aid is a ketone. It is excreted in the urine and may produce a false-positive test for urine ketones.

Drugs Used for Seizure Disorders

Learning Activities

FILL-IN-THE-BLANK

Finish each of the following statements using the correct term.

1. A patient having seizures that are chronic and recurrent is diagnosed as having _____.

2. _____ _____ is a rapidly recurring generalized seizure that does not allow the individual to regain normal function between seizures.

3. The period of time immediately after the seizure is complete is referred to as the _____ period.

4. In describing seizures, a sudden loss of muscle tone is known as a(n) _____ seizure or drop attack.

5. _____ is by far the most commonly used anticonvulsant of the hydantoins.

6. Diazepam (Valium) should be administered at a slow rate of _____ mg/min when given intravenously.

7. Serious adverse effects of valproic acid (Depakene) affecting the gastrointestinal system include _____ and _____.

8. The benzodiazepines can cause _____ in a patient with diabetes mellitus.

9. Drug treatment for status epilepticus includes intravenous administration of _____, _____, _____, _____.

10. Along with the treatment of seizure disorders, pregabalin (Lyrica) is also approved for the treatment of pain associated with _____, diabetic neuropathy, and _____ _____.

MATCHING

Match the generic drug name with its corresponding brand name. Each option will be used only once.

_____ 11. phenytoin

_____ 12. lorazepam

_____ 13. diazepam

_____ 14. clonazepam

_____ 15. fosphenytoin

_____ 16. methsuximide

_____ 17. clorazepate

_____ 18. ethotoin

a. Klonopin
b. Valium
c. Dilantin
d. Ativan
e. Tranxene
f. Peganone
g. Cerebyx
h. Celontin

TRUE OR FALSE

Write "T" for true and "F" for false for each statement. Correct all false statements.

_____ 19. *Generalized seizures* refer to those that affect both hemispheres of the brain, are accompanied by loss of consciousness, and may be subdivided into convulsive and nonconvulsive types.

_____ 20. Epilepsy is treated almost exclusively with medications known as *anticonvulsants*.

_____ 21. In children, anticonvulsant therapy may cause a change in personality and possible indifference to school and family activities.

_____ 22. Individuals who are having a seizure should be restrained to protect them from further injury.

_____ 23. Smaller doses of benzodiazepines may be necessary to maintain effects in patients who smoke.

_____ 24. The mechanism of action of the hydantoins is unknown.

_____ 25. Hypoglycemia may be caused by hydantoin therapy in patients with diabetes.

_____ 26. Carbamazepine is not effective in controlling myoclonic or absence seizures.

Drugs Used for Seizure Disorders

Practice Questions for the NCLEX® Examination

_____ 1. When administering diazepam (Valium) intravenously, what does the nurse do?
1. Administers slowly at a rate of 25 to 50 mg over at least one minute
2. Uses the SAS technique
3. Assesses the patient for the development of tachycardia
4. Piggybacks the diazepam to the maintenance IV

_____ 2. Patients taking which group of anticonvulsants are most at risk for the development of gingival hyperplasia?
1. Barbiturates
2. Benzodiazepines
3. Hydantoins
4. Succinimides

_____ 3. Patients receiving zonisamide (Zonegran) for the treatment of seizure disorder should be assessed for an allergy to which drug class?
1. Penicillins
2. Loop diuretics
3. Sulfonamides
4. Digitalis glycosides

_____ 4. A patient who has been taking lamotrigine (Lamictal) for treatment of a seizure disorder develops a skin rash in the second week of therapy. What does the nurse do?
1. Discontinues the lamotrigine
2. Promptly notifies the health care provider of development of the rash
3. Administers diphenhydramine hydrochloride (Benadryl) to the patient
4. Packs the area of the skin rash in ice

_____ 5. Before starting treatment with valproic acid (Depakene), the nurse ensures which baseline studies are completed? *(Select all that apply.)*
1. Electrocardiogram
2. Liver function tests
3. Bleeding time determination
4. Platelet count
5. Urinalysis

_____ 6. The nurse is teaching a female patient about the use of topiramate (Topamax) for seizure control. What does the nurse tell the patient about also taking oral contraceptives with this medication?
1. "You will not be able to become pregnant because of the topiramate therapy."
2. "Topiramate therapy should be stopped if you experience spotting or bleeding."
3. "An alternative form of birth control should be used when taking topiramate with oral contraceptives."
4. "There are no contraindications for using these two drugs together."

_____ 7. A patient taking oxcarbazepine (Trileptal) for the treatment of a seizure disorder develops nausea, malaise, headache, lethargy, and is confused. The patient is most likely experiencing symptoms of which disorder?
1. Hyponatremia
2. Hypokalemia
3. Hypocalcemia
4. Hypomagnesemia

_____ 8. The nurse is teaching a patient about the use of gabapentin (Neurontin). What does the nurse tell the patient to do if sedation, drowsiness, dizziness, or blurred vision develop?
1. Discontinue use of the gabapentin.
2. Reduce the dose of the gabapentin by half.
3. Consult the health care provider.
4. Take the gabapentin before going to sleep.

_____ 9. Which action does the nurse take when working with a patient experiencing a seizure?
1. Restrains the patient
2. Places a tongue blade in the patient's mouth
3. Once the patient enters into the relaxation stage, turns him or her slightly onto the side to allow secretions to drain from the mouth.
4. Medicates the patient immediately

10. A patient is ordered 100 mg of carbamazepine (Tegretol) PO, qid. The medication is available as a suspension, 100 mg/5 mL. How many mL of the medication does the nurse administer? _____ mL

11. A patient is ordered pregabalin (Lyrica) 300 mg PO bid. The medication is available in 150-mg tablets. How many tablets will the patient receive in a 24-hour period? _____ tablets

12. A patient is ordered lorazepam (Ativan) 8 mg IV. The medication is available as 4 mg/mL. How many mL of the medication does the nurse administer? _____ mL

Drugs Used for Pain Management

Review Sheet

The QUESTION column and the ANSWER column have been offset so that you can cover the answer while reading the questions, allowing you to assess your knowledge.

Question

1. Define *pain perception, pain threshold,* and *pain tolerance.*
2. Compare nociceptive pain, somatic pain, visceral pain, neuropathic pain, and idiopathic pain.

3. Define *analgesic.*

4. Name the classes of analgesics.
5. What neurotransmitters are known to stimulate nociceptors?

6. What are the four types of opiate receptors?

7. What drug is usually prescribed for severe, chronic pain?
8. Summarize the nursing process for pain management.

9. Discuss the World Health Organization's stepwise approach to pain management.
10. What are the primary therapeutic outcomes appropriate for pain management therapy?
11. Read the Pain Care Bill of Rights.
12. Obtain a copy of the pain assessment tools used in local clinical sites and discuss the appropriate assessments and recording of pain events using the tools assembled.

Answer

1. Pain perception is awareness of the pain sensation. Pain threshold is the point at which pain is felt. Pain tolerance is an individual's ability to withstand the pain experience.
2. Nociceptive pain is a result of stimulus to pain receptors (dull, aching); somatic pain originates in the skin, bone, or muscle; visceral pain originates in the organs of the thorax or abdomen; neuropathic pain results from injury to the peripheral or central nervous systems; and idiopathic pain is of unknown origin.
3. Analgesics are drugs that relieve pain.
4. Opiate agonists, opiate partial agonists, opiate antagonists, anti-inflammatory, nonsteroidal anti-inflammatory, and miscellaneous agents
5. The neurotransmitters bradykinin, prostaglandins, leukotrienes, histamines, and serotonin sensitize nociceptors.
6. The four types of opiate receptors are mu, delta, kappa, and sigma receptors.
7. Morphine sulfate is usually prescribed for severe, chronic pain. It may also be combined with other drugs such as antidepressants.
8. See textbook, pp. 310-318.

9. See textbook, pp. 309-310.

10. See textbook, p. 310.
11. See Box 20-1, p. 311.

13. What is the most effective route for administering an analgesic when immediate relief is needed?
14. Explain the benefits of patient-controlled analgesia (PCA).
15. What is meant by "on demand" in relation to the use of a PCA pump?

16. Differentiate among addiction, physical dependence, and tolerance.

17. Define *agonists, antagonists,* and *partial agonists.*
18. Opiate agonists are subdivided into what four groups?

19. Identify pain assessment data needed to establish a baseline for monitoring therapy before initiating treatment for pain.

20. For what type(s) of pain are opiate agonists used?

21. What premedication assessments should be performed before administering an opiate agonist?
22. Will naloxone (Narcan) reverse CNS depression caused by sedative/hypnotics or tranquilizers?
23. When is naloxone (Narcan) effective?

24. What three drugs are antidotes for opiate agonists and opiate partial agonists?
25. Do opiate partial agonists relieve pain effectively in people who have recently taken opiate agonists?
26. Give an example of an opiate partial agonist.

12. Individualize to local clinical facilities.

13. The intravenous route gives the most immediate pain relief.
14. With PCA, the patient can initiate the administration of analgesics, allowing pain relief to be obtained rapidly. Most important is the sense of control a patient feels toward the pain and scheduling daily activities. The PCA system monitors the total dose(s) administered and limits can be set on the total amount that can be self-administered during a specified period.
15. "On demand" means the patient can self-administer a dosage of pain medication when needed. There is a "lock-out" safety device that limits the number of administrations over a specific period of time.
16. Research on the Internet definitions of *addiction, physical dependence,* and *tolerance.*
17. Agonists interact with receptors to stimulate response. Antagonists attach to a receptor but do not stimulate a response or block a response. Partial agonists are drugs that interact with a receptor to stimulate a response, but may inhibit other responses.
18. Opiate agonists are divided into four groups: morphinelike derivatives, meperidinelike derivatives, methadonelike derivatives, and other opiate agonists.
19. Baseline vital signs, neurologic exam, prior analgesics administered, and degree of pain control; voiding and bowel pattern.
20. Opiate agonists are used for moderate to severe pain.
21. Baseline vital signs, neurologic exam, prior analgesics administered, degree of pain control; voiding and bowel pattern.
22. Naloxone will not reverse CNS depression caused by sedative/hypnotics or tranquilizers.
23. Naloxone reverses the CNS depressant effects of the opiate agonists.
24. Naloxone (Narcan) and naltrexone (ReVia) are antidotes for opiate agonists and opiate partial agonists.
25. Opiate partial agonists usually do not alleviate pain in people who have recently taken opiate agonists.

27. What are the most common analgesics used for relief slight to moderate pain?

28. What three pharmacologic effects are associated with the salicylates?

29. Describe uses for the salicylates. When should they not be used?

30. What is salicylism?

31. What is the antidote for salicylism?

32. What are premedication assessments to perform before administering nonsteroidal anti-inflammatory drugs (NSAIDs)?

33. What are NSAIDs?

34. How do NSAIDs act?

35. What are the primary therapeutic outcomes expected from the NSAIDs?

36. What is the major adverse effect of NSAIDs?

37. Name five commonly used NSAIDs.

38. What are the therapeutic outcomes for acetaminophen (Tylenol)?

39. How do the therapeutic outcomes of NSAIDs and acetaminophen (Tylenol) compare?

26. See Table 20-2, p. 323.

27. The salicylates are the most common analgesics used to relieve of slight to moderate pain.

28. Three pharmacologic effects of salicylates are analgesic, antipyretic, and anti-inflammatory.

29. The salicylates are the drugs of choice for symptomatic relief of discomfort, pain, inflammation, or fever associated with bacterial or viral infections, headache, muscle aches, and rheumatoid arthritis. Because of its antiplatelet activity, aspirin is indicated for reducing the risk of recurrent TIA or stroke in men. Aspirin is also used to reduce the risk of myocardial infarction (MI) in patients with previous MI or unstable angina pectoris. Salicylates should not be used in children because of the associated risk of Reye's syndrome.

30. Salicylism is seen with high doses of salicylates. Symptoms include tinnitus, impaired hearing, sweating, dizziness, mental confusion, and nausea and vomiting.

31. There is no antidote for salicylism. Use gastric lavage, force IV fluids, and alkalization of urine with IV sodium bicarbonate; stop salicylates.

32. See textbook, p. 331.

33. NSAIDs or nonsteroidal anti-inflammatory drugs are also known as "aspirinlike" drugs. They are chemically unrelated to the salicylates but are prostaglandin inhibitors and share many of the same therapeutic actions and adverse effects.

34. NSAIDs act by blocking cyclooxygenase (COX-1 and COX-2).

35. The primary therapeutic outcomes expected from the NSAIDs are reduced pain, reduced inflammation, and elimination of fever.

36. The major adverse effect of NSAID therapy is increased risk of potentially fatal cardiovascular adverse effects including heart attack and stroke, gastric irritation, gastric bleeding, constipation, dizziness, drowsiness, confusion, hives, pruritus, rash, nephrotoxicity, hepatotoxicity, and blood dyscrasias.

37. See Table 20-3, pp. 327-329.

38. The primary therapeutic outcomes expected from acetaminophen (Tylenol) are reduced pain and fever.

40. What are early indications of acetaminophen (Tylenol) toxicity?

41. What premedication assessments are required for each classification of drug used to treat pain?

42. What effect does aspirin have on phenytoin (Dilantin), valproic acid, and oral hypoglycemic agents?

39. Acetaminophen has no anti-inflammatory effect. However, it is a very good antipyretic and analgesic. NSAIDs are used for their anti-inflammatory, antipyretic, and analgesic effects.

40. Early indications of acetaminophen toxicity include nausea, anorexia, vomiting, and jaundice accompanied by an elevation in liver function tests.

41. This information can be found in sections listed as Premedication Assessments in the drug monographs throughout Chapter 20.

42. When taken with aspirin, phenytoin levels are increased, causing toxicity: nystagmus, lethargy, sedation. Dosage adjustment may be required. Valproic acid levels are increased when taken with aspirin; dose adjustment may be needed. With oral hypoglycemics, aspirin increases potential for hypoglycemia.

Drugs Used for Pain Management

Learning Activities

FILL-IN-THE-BLANK

Finish each of the following statements using the correct term.

1. The three terms used in relationship to the pain experience are pain _____, pain _____, and pain _____.

2. _____ pain is a nonspecific pain of unknown origin.

3. _____ are drugs that relieve pain without producing loss of consciousness or reflex activity.

4. Antidotes for opiate antagonists include _____, _____, and naltrexone (ReVia).

5. Opiate partial agonist drugs should be held and the health care provider notified if the patient's respirations are below _____.

6. NSAID is an abbreviation for _____ _____.

7. The primary therapeutic outcomes expected from acetaminophen (Tylenol) are reduced _____ and _____.

8. The NSAIDs exert their therapeutic effect by blocking _____ and _____.

MATCHING

Match the generic drug name with its corresponding brand name. Each option will be used only once.

_____ 9. butorphanol

_____ 10. buprenorphine

_____ 11. nalbuphine

_____ 12. oxaprozin

_____ 13. naproxen

_____ 14. meloxicam

a. Daypro
b. Aleve
c. Mobic
d. Stadol
e. Buprenex
f. Nubain

TRUE OR FALSE

Write "T" for true and "F" for false for each statement. Correct all false statements.

_____ 15. The sympathetic nervous system is activated when a person experiences acute pain.

_____ 16. Chronic pain has a slower onset and lasts longer than 2 months beyond the healing process.

_____ 17. The first step leading to the sensation of pain is the stimulation of receptors known as *nociceptors*.

_____ 18. Pain is expected with aging.

_____ 19. Patients should be taught to request pain medication before the pain escalates and becomes severe for optimal effectiveness.

_____ 20. The word *narcotic* should be abandoned in exchange for *opiate agonists* and *opiate partial agonists*.

_____ 21. Symptoms of withdrawal from opiate agonists reach a peak at 12 hours after discontinuation of the medication and disappear over the next 24 hours.

_____ 22. Meperidine (Demerol), once a commonly prescribed opioid agonist for the management of pain, is less frequently prescribed due to the adverse effects associated with its active metabolite, normeperidine.

_____ 23. Urinary retention can occur with the use of opiate agonists.

_____ 24. A unique property of aspirin when compared with other salicylates is inhibition of platelet aggregation and enhancement of bleeding time.

_____ 25. Although considered acceptable at one time, placebo therapy should never be used with pain management.

_____ 26. The rating of pain has been designated "the fifth vital sign."

Drugs Used for Pain Management

Practice Questions for the NCLEX® Examination

_____ 1. Patients experiencing acute pain would be most likely to exhibit which sign?
   1. Bradypnea
   2. Bradycardia
   3. Constricted pupils
   4. Hypertension

_____ 2. Which type of pain originates from the abdominal and thoracic organs?
   1. Nociceptive
   2. Somatic
   3. Visceral
   4. Neuropathic

_____ 3. Which statement about the use of the transdermal opioid analgesic fentanyl (Duragesic) is true?
   1. Fentanyl is commonly used for acute pain.
   2. It takes approximately 2 hours for the initial patch of medication to reach a steady blood level.
   3. The patch provides relief for up to 72 hours.
   4. No other analgesics may be used with fentanyl.

_____ 4. A patient is receiving drugs for pain. Which statement about nutritional aspects of care for this patient is correct?
   1. Constipation is a common effect from opiate use.
   2. Caffeine should be encouraged to counteract the sedating effects of other medications.
   3. Limit fluid intake to four 8-ounce glasses daily.
   4. The diet should be low fiber.

_____ 5. A patient prescribed opiates is suspected of being addicted to opiate agonists. What is the best course of action for this patient's care?
   1. Treat the addiction after the patient experiences the symptoms of withdrawal.
   2. Abruptly reduce the patient's daily opiate doses.
   3. Give the patient methadone if withdrawal symptoms become severe.
   4. Withhold tranquilizers and sedatives while the patient withdraws from opiate agonist addiction.

_____ 6. If an opiate partial agonist is administered to a patient who is addicted to opiate agonists, what must the nurse assess for?
   1. Withdrawal symptoms from the opiate agonist
   2. Constipation
   3. Hypotension
   4. Hypothermia

_____ 7. A patient has been taking an oral hypoglycemic agent, and is now ordered salicylate therapy for pain management. What does the nurse anticipate will happen when these two types of drugs are taken together?
   1. The patient will need to switch to subcutaneous insulin therapy for the duration of the salicylate therapy.
   2. Urine glucose determinations with Clinitest will be required for blood glucose measurements.
   3. The dose of the oral hypoglycemic agent will be doubled while the patient is on salicylate therapy.
   4. Salicylates may enhance the hypoglycemic effects of oral hypoglycemic agents; therefore, the patient will be monitored for hypoglycemia.

_____ 8. Which statement about opiate partial agonists is true?
1. Constipation does not occur with use of these drugs.
2. These drugs have no effect on the respiratory center of the brain.
3. Addiction is not an issue with use of these drugs.
4. The potency with the first few weeks of therapy is similar to that of morphine; however, after prolonged use, tolerance may develop.

_____ 9. Visceral pain usually originates from which parts of the body? (Select all that apply.)
1. Skin
2. Bones
3. Abdominal organs
4. Joints
5. Thoracic organs

_____ 10. What nonpharmacologic comfort measures may the nurse provide for a patient with pain? (Select all that apply.)
1. Backrubs
2. Cold applications
3. Exercise
4. Transcutaneous electrical nerve stimulation (TENS)
5. Hot baths

_____ 11. A patient is receiving opiate agonists for pain control. Which adverse effects does the nurse report to the health care provider? (Select all that apply.)
1. Patient reports feeling lightheaded
2. Respiratory rate of 7
3. Orthostatic hypotension
4. Urinary retention
5. Constipation

_____ 12. While assessing a patient who has overdosed on acetaminophen (Tylenol), it is most important for the nurse to assess which body system?
1. Cardiovascular
2. Hepatic
3. Central nervous
4. Reproductive

13. A patient is ordered acetaminophen (Tylenol) #3, 1 grain PO every 4 hours PRN. The medication is available as 30 mg per tablet. How many tablets does the nurse administer?
_____ tablet(s)

14. A patient is ordered acetaminophen (Tylenol), 0.325 g PO every 4 hours PRN for pain. The medication is available as 325 mg/5 mL. How many teaspoons does the nurse administer?
_____ teaspoon(s)

15. A patient is ordered codeine 1/4 grain PO daily. The medication is available as 30 mg per tablet. How many tablets does the nurse administer?
_____ tablet(s)

Introduction to Cardiovascular Disease and Metabolic Syndrome

Review Sheet

The QUESTION column and the ANSWER column have been offset so that you can cover the answer while reading the question, allowing you to assess your knowledge.

Question	Answer
1. Define *cardiovascular disease*.	1. *Cardiovascular disease* is a collective term used to refer to disorders of the circulatory system.
2. What are the characteristics of metabolic syndrome?	2. The presence of type 2 diabetes mellitus, abdominal obesity, hypertriglyceridemia, low high-density lipoproteins (HDL), and hypertension.
3. What are the risk factors for the development of metabolic syndrome?	3. Poor diet, sedentary lifestyle, and genetic predisposition.
4. In addition to type 2 diabetes and heart disease, what other consequences are associated with metabolic syndrome?	4. Renal disease, obstructive sleep apnea, polycystic ovary syndrome, cognitive decline in older adults, and dementia in older adults.
5. Summarize the overall treatment goals for metabolic syndrome.	5. Refer to Box 21-2, p. 338.
6. What is the drug therapy for hypertension associated with metabolic syndrome?	6. A combination of a thiazide diuretic plus an angiotensin-converting enzyme inhibitor or a beta blocker.
7. What is the treatment for dyslipidemia associated with metabolic syndrome?	7. Treatment of dyslipidemia is generally to lower the triglycerides and LDL cholesterol and raise the HDL cholesterol. After lifestyle changes, medicines most commonly used are the 3-hydroxy-methyl-glutaryl coenzyme A reductase inhibitors, fibrinic acid derivatives, and niacin.
8. What is the mechanism of action of the thiazolidinediones in the treatment of type 2 diabetes mellitus in metabolic syndrome?	8. The thiazolidinediones reduce insulin resistance in peripheral tissues.
9. What is the mechanism of action of metformin (Glucophage) in the treatment of type 2 diabetes mellitus in metabolic syndrome?	9. Metformin decreases production of glucose by the liver and to a lesser extent, reduces insulin resistance in peripheral tissues.
10. What is mechanism of action of the alpha-glycosidase inhibitors in the treatment of type 2 diabetes mellitus in metabolic syndrome?	10. The alpha-glycosidase inhibitors reduce the absorption of glucose from the intestine, reducing postprandial hyperglycemia.
11. What is the mechanism of action of the sulfonylureas and meglitinides in the treatment of type 2 diabetes mellitus in metabolic syndrome?	11. The sulfonylureas and meglitinides stimulate the beta cells of the pancreas to release more insulin.

Introduction to Cardiovascular Disease and Metabolic Syndrome

chapter

21

Learning Activities

FILL-IN-THE-BLANK

Finish each of the following statements using the correct term.

1. _____ _____ _____ is the term pertaining to narrowing or obstruction of the arteries of the heart which leads to angina pectoris and myocardial infarction.

2. _____ has been recognized as the greatest contributor to the development of cardiovascular disease.

3. Weight in proportion to height is referred to as _____ _____ _____.

4. _____ diseases are a major cause of premature death in the United States.

TRUE OR FALSE

Write "T" for true and "F" for false for each statement. Correct all false statements.

_____ 5. The treatment of dyslipidemia is generally to lower triglycerides and HDL cholesterol and raise LDL cholesterol.

_____ 6. Insulin injections are used in the treatment of patients with metabolic syndrome who do not secrete adequate amounts of insulin.

_____ 7. The reductase inhibitors used to treat dyslipidemias are also known as "statins."

_____ 8. A weight loss of 10–15 pounds can improve hypertension and hyperglycemia associated with metabolic syndrome.

_____ 9. A hemoglobin A_{1c} of 10% is considered as meeting the general treatment goals for patients with metabolic syndrome.

Introduction to Cardiovascular Disease and Metabolic Syndrome

chapter

21

Practice Questions for the NCLEX® Examination

_____ 1. When teaching a group of patients about metabolic syndrome, which information does the nurse include? *(Select all that apply.)*
1. Type 1 diabetes mellitus is a common characteristic of metabolic syndrome.
2. Mexican-American women have the highest rate of metabolic syndrome in the U.S. within ethnic groups.
3. Patients with metabolic syndrome commonly have low high-density lipoproteins.
4. Hypertension is commonly found in patients with metabolic syndrome.
5. Hypertriglyceridemia is commonly found in patients with metabolic syndrome.

_____ 2. Which lab values indicate that the general treatment goals for patients with metabolic syndrome are being met? *(Select all that apply.)*
1. Blood pressure of 139/91 mm Hg
2. High-density lipoproteins of 45 mg/dL
3. Triglycerides of 140 mg/dL
4. Hemoglobin A_{1c} of 5%
5. Fasting plasma glucose of 118 mg/dL

_____ 3. Which drug class used in the treatment of type 2 diabetes mellitus reduces insulin resistance in peripheral tissues?
1. Meglitinides
2. Alpha-glycosidase inhibitors
3. Sulfonylureas
4. Thiazolidinediones

_____ 4. When teaching a group of patients with metabolic syndrome the importance of weight loss and healthy diet, which statement does the nurse include?
1. "Restrict the total amount of fat you consume each day to approximately 45% of your total calories."
2. "You must limit the amount of protein you eat to 2 ounces once a day."
3. "Most of the dietary fat you consume should be saturated."
4. "Olive oil is an example of the type of 'good' fat you may eat."

_____ 5. Which drugs and/or drug classes used to treat type 2 diabetes mellitus associated with metabolic syndrome stimulate the beta cells of the pancreas to release more insulin? *(Select all that apply.)*
1. Sulfonylureas
2. Metformin (Glucophage)
3. Alpha-glycosidase (Acarbose)
4. Meglitinides
5. Thiazolidinediones

_____ 6. Which factors does the nurse encourage when teaching health promotion to patients with metabolic syndrome? *(Select all that apply.)*
1. Smoking cessation
2. Weight reduction
3. Vigorous exercise
4. Stress reduction
5. Dietary modification

7. A patient is prescribed chlorpropamide (Diabinese) 125 mg PO daily. The supply available is 100-mg or 250-mg tablets. Which tablets and how many of them does the nurse administer?

_____-mg tablet

_____ tablet(s)

8. A patient is prescribed gemfibrozil (Lopid) 0.6 g PO bid. The medication is available in 600-mg tablets. How many tablets does the nurse administer? _____ tablet(s)

_____ 9. A patient with diabetes mellitus is admitted for coronary artery bypass surgery. The patient informs the nurse that he takes metformin (Glucophage) 500 mg PO bid to control diabetes. What change does the nurse expect in the patient's treatment of diabetes mellitus?
1. No change in therapy
2. Administration of half of the metformin therapy while hospitalized
3. Administration of insulin glargine (Lantus) bid
4. A transfer to insulin therapy

Drugs Used to Treat Dyslipidemias

Review Sheet

The QUESTION column and the ANSWER column have been offset so that you can cover the answer while reading the questions, allowing you to assess your knowledge.

Question	Answer
1. Define *atherosclerosis, hyperlipidemia, dyslipidemia, chylomicrons, triglycerides,* and *lipoproteins.*	
2. What lifestyle changes should be used to treat hyperlipidemia before starting drug therapy?	1. See textbook, p. 341.
3. What are the primary drugs for lowering serum cholesterol levels?	2. Lifestyle changes should be attempted for treatment of hyperlipidemia before starting drug therapy, including dietary changes (e.g., fat intake less than 30% of calories, decreased cholesterol and saturated fat intake, increased polyunsaturated and monounsaturated fats), weight reduction, and regular exercise.
4. Why aren't fibric acid agents used as first-line drugs for the treatment of hyperlipidemias?	3. Bile acid resins, niacin, and HMG-CoA reductase inhibitors (statins) are the primary drugs for lowering serum cholesterol levels.
5. Which class of drugs used to treat hyperlipidemia is the most expensive?	4. Fibric acid agents do not result in substantial reduction of LDL-C, but are effective in lowering triglycerides.
6. Summarize nursing assessments needed for a patient with hyperlipidemia.	5. HMG-CoA drugs, known as *statins*, are the most expensive.
7. Why are supplemental vitamins required with bile acid-binding resins?	6. Nursing assessments needed for patients with hyperlipidemia include risk factors (e.g., family history of increased cholesterol and lipids), smoking, dietary habits, glucose intolerance, elevated serum lipids, obesity, and sedentary lifestyle.
8. What are the signs and symptoms of a vitamin K deficiency?	7. Bile acid-binding resins may deplete the body of its needed supply of fat-soluble vitamins (DEAK).
9. Describe the proper preparation of cholestyramine for administration.	8. Bruising; bleeding gums; dark, tarry stools; and "coffee ground" emesis are signs and symptoms of a vitamin K deficiency.
10. What drug interactions can occur with the use of bile acid-binding resins?	9. To prepare cholestyramine for administration, mix powdered resin with 2–6 oz water, soup, juice, or crushed pineapple; allow to stand until drug is absorbed and dispersed. Follow with an additional glass of water.

11. Discuss patient teaching needed to minimize the common adverse effects with bile acid-binding resins therapy such as constipation, bloating, fullness, nausea, and flatulence.

10. Bile acid-binding resins bind to drugs such as digoxin (Lanoxin), warfarin (Coumadin), thyroid hormones, thiazide diuretics, phenobarbital, nonsteroidal anti-inflammatory drugs, tetracycline (Sumycin), beta blocking agents, gemfibrozil (Lopid), glipizide (Glucotrol), glyburide (DiaBeta), oral contraceptives, and phenytoin (Dilantin). The resins may bind these medicines, which reduces absorption. Minimize this effect by administering these medications 1 hour before or 4 hours after giving a resin. (See also textbook p. 345.)

12. What is the primary desired therapeutic outcome from niacin?

11. See drug monograph, textbook pp. 344-345.

13. What premedication assessments should be performed before administration of niacin?

12. The primary desired therapeutic outcome of niacin is decreased LDL and total cholesterol, decreased triglycerides, and increased HDL levels.

14. Why is niacin not used with diabetic patients?

13. Before administering niacin, assess serum triglyceride and cholesterol levels, liver function, baseline uric acid and blood glucose levels, and vital signs. Document existing gastrointestinal symptoms.

14. Niacin is not recommended for diabetics because of glucose intolerance.

15. What suggestions can be given to patients taking niacin to minimize the adverse effects of flushing, itching, rash, tingling, and headache?

16. Cite the premedication assessments that should be done before niacin therapy.

15. Take niacin with food, take aspirin (325 mg) or ibuprofen (200 mg) 30 minutes before each dose of niacin (unless contraindicated). Tell the patient that tolerance develops quickly.

16. See textbook, p. 346.

17. Name three statin drugs. Name three statin combination products.

18. What are common adverse effects from antilipemic therapy?

17. The statin drugs include atorvastatin (Lipitor), fluvastatin (Lescol), lovastatin (Mevacor, Altoprev), pravastatin (Pravachol), rosuvastatin (Crestor) and simvastatin (Zocor). Statin combination products include atorvastatin-amlodipine (Caduet), lovastatin-niacin (Advicor), and simvastatin-ezetimibe (Vytorin).

18. Nausea, diarrhea, flatulence, bloating, and abdominal distress are common adverse effects with antilipemic therapy.

19. What is the effect of fibric acid agents on triglycerides?

20. What anticipated alterations may occur in the blood glucose level when administering sulfonylureas and insulin with gemfibrozil (Lopid)?

19. The mechanism of action of the fibric acids is unknown; however, they do lower triglyceride levels by 20% to 40%. In patients with hypertriglyceridemia they raise HDL levels by 10% to 15%. They also reduce LDL-C levels by 10% to 15% in patients with elevated cholesterol.

21. What is the mechanism of action of ezetimibe (Zetia)?

20. Gemfibrozil may increase the pharmacologic effect of these agents. Monitor for signs of hypoglycemia and reduce the dose of the insulin or sulfonylurea as needed.

21. Ezetimibe is the first of a new class of agents used to reduce atherosclerosis. It does not bind to cholesterol and reduce absorption as the bile acid resins do, but instead acts on the small intestine to inhibit the absorption of cholesterol present in the small intestine that derives from cholesterol secreted in the bile and from the diet.

Drugs Used to Treat Dyslipidemias

Learning Activities

FILL-IN-THE-BLANK

Finish each of the following statements using the correct term.

1. _____ is characterized by the accumulation of fatty deposits on the inner walls of arteries and arterioles throughout the body that reduces the blood supply to vital organs resulting in strokes, angina pectoris, myocardial infarction, and peripheral vascular disease.

2. _____ is sometimes referred to as "good" lipoproteins because high levels indicate that cholesterol is being removed from vascular tissue where it may participate in the development of coronary artery disease.

3. It is becoming recognized that our _____ may be the greatest contributor to causing hyperlipidemia.

4. Pharmacologic antilipemic therapy is often started with the _____ _____ _____ because of their safety record and success in lowering cholesterol levels.

5. The primary medicines used to lower elevated cholesterol levels are the bile acid-binding resins, _____, and _____.

6. _____ is the first of a new class of agents used to reduce atherosclerosis by blocking the absorption of cholesterol by the small intestine.

7. _____ was the first of a new class of drugs used to decrease atherosclerosis by combining two omega-3 fatty acids which act to decrease the synthesis of triglycerides in the liver.

8. _____ is the only form of vitamin B_3 that is approved by the FDA for the treatment of dyslipidemias.

MATCHING

Match the generic drug name with its corresponding brand name. Each option will be used only once.

_____ 9. simvastatin

_____ 10. lovastatin

_____ 11. fluvastatin

_____ 12. atorvastatin

_____ 13. rosuvastatin

_____ 14. pravastatin

_____ 15. simvastatin-ezetimibe

_____ 16. atorvastatin-amlodipine

_____ 17. lovastatin-niacin

a. Lipitor
b. Zocor
c. Lescol
d. Mevacor
e. Vytorin
f. Advicor
g. Caduet
h. Crestor
i. Pravachol

TRUE OR FALSE

Write "T" for true and "F" for false for each statement. Correct all false statements.

_____ 18. Coronary artery disease is a major cause of premature death in the United States.

_____ 19. Drug therapy for the treatment of hyperlipidemias usually lasts for a few weeks and is then discontinued.

_____ 20. The most cost-effective and successful forms of treatment for hyperlipidemias are smoking cessation, weight reduction, exercise, and dietary modifications.

_____ 21. The primary therapeutic outcome expected from bile acid-binding resin therapy is reduction of LDL and total cholesterol levels.

_____ 22. Antilipemic agents may be used to treat hyperlipidemias only if diet, exercise, and weight reduction are not successful in adequately lowering LDL-C levels.

_____ 23. The statins are the most potent antilipemic agents available with the added benefits of decreasing inflammation, decreasing platelet aggregation, decreasing thrombin formation, and decreasing platelet viscosity resulting in decreased heart attacks and stroke.

_____ 24. HDLs (high-density lipoproteins) are also referred to as "good cholesterol" because they are beneficial in preventing coronary heart disease.

_____ 25. Niacin is effective in lowering triglycerides and cholesterol and raises LDL cholesterol levels.

_____ 26. Smoking contributes to the development and progression of coronary artery disease.

_____ 27. The use of bile acid-binding resins could potentially result in the development of a bleeding disorder if vitamins or a balanced diet are not taken regularly.

_____ 28. Bile acid-binding resins may bind with warfarin (Coumadin), NSAIDs, tetracycline (Sumycin), and beta blockers, thereby enhancing the drugs' effectiveness.

_____ 29. Common adverse effects of niacin use are headache and flushing.

_____ 30. Gemfibrozil (Lopid) may cause hypoglycemia.

_____ 31. Vitamins A, C, and B are significantly affected by bile acid-binding resin drugs.

Drugs Used to Treat Dyslipidemias

Practice Questions for the NCLEX® Examination

_____ 1. Which statement does the nurse include when teaching a patient who is receiving bile acid-binding resins?
   1. "You should limit your water intake to four glasses a day."
   2. "Eat foods that are low in bulk to avoid diarrhea."
   3. "You may need to take supplemental vitamins."
   4. "Now that you are on a medication to lower your lipids, there is no need to monitor your cholesterol intake."

_____ 2. Patients taking bile acid-binding resins are most at risk for the development of which condition?
   1. Hypertension
   2. Tachycardia
   3. Nephrotoxicity
   4. Vitamin K deficiency

_____ 3. A patient has been prescribed the following medications: digoxin (Lanoxin), furosemide (Lasix), and cholestyramine. Which action does the nurse take?
   1. Administers all of the medications together to avoid unnecessary interruption of the patient's rest
   2. Mixes the cholestyramine with soda pop and has the patient immediately consume it
   3. Administers the furosemide and digoxin 1 hour before or 4 hours after administration of cholestyramine
   4. Limits water intake with the administration of cholestyramine to 2 ounces

_____ 4. What is a patient taking HMG-CoA reductase inhibitors for the treatment of hyperlipidemia instructed to do by the nurse?
   1. Avoid grapefruit juice.
   2. Increase any anticoagulants taken by twice as much.
   3. Expect muscle weakness as a common adverse effect.
   4. Take the medication on an empty stomach to increase absorption.

_____ 5. Patients with a deficiency of which vitamin are most at risk for the development of bleeding disorders?
   1. A
   2. D
   3. E
   4. K

_____ 6. Which drug class used to treat hyperlipidemias has the common adverse effects of flushing, itching, rash, tingling, and headache associated with its use?
   1. Niacin
   2. HMG-CoA reductase inhibitors
   3. Fibric acids
   4. Bile acid-binding resins

_____ 7. What is the most common adverse effect of drugs used to treat hyperlipidemias?
   1. Abdominal discomfort and gas
   2. Myopathy
   3. Jaundice
   4. Sweating

_____ 8. When assessing a patient with vitamin K deficiency, which signs does the nurse expect to find? *(Select all that apply.)*
1. Bleeding gums
2. Bruising
3. Dark tarry stools
4. "Coffee-ground" emesis
5. Pink-tinged urine

_____ 9. A patient taking a bile acid-binding resin for the treatment of dyslipidemia tells the nurse that ever since he began taking the medication, he experiences bloating and fullness. What does the nurse instruct the patient to do? *(Select all that apply.)*
1. Swallow the medication without gulping air.
2. Maintain adequate fiber in the diet.
3. Limit fluid intake.
4. Take the medication with a carbonated beverage.
5. Use a daily laxative.

_____ 10. When teaching a patient about niacin therapy, the nurse tells the patient to report which adverse effects to the primary care provider? *(Select all that apply.)*
1. Flushing
2. Tingling
3. Fatigue
4. Muscle aches
5. Jaundice

_____ 11. Which statements about HMG-CoA reductase inhibitors are true? *(Select all that apply.)*
1. They are the most potent antilipemic agents available.
2. They reduce inflammation, platelet aggregation, thrombin formation, and plasma viscosity.
3. Rhabdomyolysis and myoglobinuria have been reported as adverse effects of these drugs.
4. Patients who are pregnant should not take these medications.
5. Renal toxicity is a common complication of this therapy.

12. A patient is prescribed gemfibrozil (Lopid) 1200 mg PO bid to be administered at 0800 and 1900. The medication is available as 600 mg in a container of 500 tablets. How many tablets does the nurse administer at 1900? _____ tablet(s)

13. A patient who is taking omega-3 fatty acids (Lovaza) 4 g/day PO tells the nurse that he forgot to take the prescribed dose yesterday. The drug is available as 1 g per capsule. How many capsules does the nurse instruct the patient to take that day? _____ capsule(s)

_____ 14. A student nurse is planning the care of a patient who is prescribed rosuvastatin (Crestor) and antacids. Which care plan by the new nurse requires the supervising nurse to intervene?
1. Administer the drug at 0800.
2. Establish baseline serum lipid levels and liver function tests before starting therapy.
3. Consult with the nutritionist about a low-cholesterol diet.
4. Schedule antacids at least 2 hours after administering rosuvastatin.

Drugs Used to Treat Hypertension

Review Sheet

The QUESTION column and the ANSWER column have been offset so that you can cover the answer while reading the questions, allowing you to assess your knowledge.

Question	Answer
1. What are systolic and diastolic blood pressure?	
2. How is the mean arterial pressure or average pressure calculated?	1. Systolic blood pressure is pressure exerted as blood is pumped from the heart; diastolic blood pressure is the pressure present during the resting phase of the heartbeat.
3. What are the primary determinants of systolic and diastolic blood pressure?	2. See textbook, p. 353.
4. What is the definition of *hypertension*?	3. The primary determinant of systolic blood pressure is cardiac output, and the determinant for diastolic blood pressure is peripheral vascular resistance.
	4. Hypertension is an elevation in either the systolic or diastolic blood pressure or both. See textbook, pp. 354-355, for discussion of recommended screening in adults.
5. Differentiate among prehypertension, primary hypertension, and secondary hypertension.	5. Prehypertension is a range of blood pressure readings that indicates a high probability of developing a heart attack, heart failure, stroke, or renal disease. Primary hypertension is a controllable but not curable form of hypertension of unknown etiology. There are known risk factors that contribute to the development of primary hypertension. Secondary hypertension occurs following the development of another disorder in the body (e.g., renal disease, head trauma).
6. State the procedure for measuring blood pressure as recommended by JNC 7 guidelines.	
7. Identify the goals of blood pressure therapy.	6. Sit the patient in a chair with feet on the floor and the arm supported at heart level for at least 5 minutes. Use an appropriate size cuff (cuff bladder encircles at least 80% of the arm).
	Verify readings in the opposite arm. The person needs two or more readings on separate occasions to be classified as having hypertension.
	When readings of the systolic and diastolic fall into two different stages, the higher of the two stages is used to classify the degree of hypertension present.

8. List the drug classifications used in the treatment of hypertension.

9. What is therapeutic outcome for antihypertensive therapy?

10. Describe significant nursing processes for people with hypertension.

11. Summarize the classification and management of blood pressure for adults according to the Seventh Report of the Joint National Committee on Prevention, Detection, Evaluation, and Treatment of High Blood Pressure.

12. What class of drugs is used initially in the treatment of uncomplicated hypertension when lifestyle changes are not effective?

13. Summarize the treatment algorithm used for hypertension.

14. What are the nutritional goals for the treatment of hypertension?

15. Summarize the premedication assessments used prior to administration of antihypertensive drugs. (Examine differences among the various types of agents usually prescribed.)

16. What are the four classes of diuretic agents used to treat hypertension?

17. What laboratory test is used as a guide to indicate when a patient needs to switch from a thiazide-type to a loop diuretic?

18. What are the common and serious adverse effects of beta-adrenergic blocking agents?

19. What types of patients should avoid the use of beta blocking agents?

7. Reduction and maintenance of BP below 140/90 mm Hg. Patients with concurrent conditions—e.g., diabetes mellitus, heart failure, and renal disease—less than 130/80. Weight reduction, DASH diet, dietary sodium reduction, physical activity, and moderation of alcohol consumption are recommended. Smoking cessation and stress reduction are also recommended.

8. Hypertension is treated primarily with preferred agents: diuretics and beta-adrenergic blockers; alternative agents: angiotensin-converting enzyme (ACE) inhibitors, angiotensin II receptor antagonists, calcium channel blockers, $alpha_1$-adrenergic blockers; and adjunctive agents: centrally acting $alpha_2$ agonists, peripheral-acting adrenergic antagonists, and direct vasodilators.

9. The therapeutic outcome for antihypertensive therapy is to lower blood pressure by reducing peripheral resistance.

10. See textbook, pp. 358-362.

11. See Table 23-1.

12. If lifestyle changes do not sufficiently reduce blood pressure, a diuretic or a beta blocker is generally the initial treatment of choice.

13. See Figure 23-2.

14. See textbook, pp. 355-356.

15. See sections labeled "premedication assessments" in the drug monographs throughout Chapter 23.

16. The four classes of diuretic agents used to treat hypertension are carbonic anhydrase inhibitors, thiazide and thiazide-like agents, loop diuretics, and potassium-sparing diuretics. Thiazide diuretics are most often used. Carbonic anhydrase inhibitors are rarely used to treat hypertension.

17. The creatinine clearance test is used when a patient needs to switch from a thiazide-like to a loop diuretic.

18. The common and serious adverse effects of beta-adrenergic agents include bradycardia, peripheral vasoconstriction, bronchospasm, wheezing, hypoglycemia in diabetic patients, and heart failure.

20. What precautions should be instituted when beta blocker therapy is to be discontinued?

21. What effect does angiotensin II have on blood vessels?

22. What effect does an increase in aldosterone secretion have on blood pressure?

23. Summarize the common and serious adverse effects of the use of ACE inhibitors.

24. What is the action of angiotensin II receptor antagonists?

25. What is the action of eplerenone (Inspra), the aldosterone receptor blocking agent?

26. What are contraindications to the administration of the aldosterone receptor blocking agent eplerenone (Inspra)?

27. Review the serious adverse effects of the use of eplerenone (Inspra), the aldosterone receptor blocking agent.

28. Which herbal product and fruit juice slows the absorption of eplerenone (Inspra)?

29. What is the action of calcium channel blockers on blood pressure?

30. What are common adverse effects of alpha$_1$ adrenergic blockers?

31. Why should centrally acting alpha$_2$ agonists (e.g., clonidine [Catapres], guanabenz [Wytensin], guanfacine [Tenex], and methyldopa) be discontinued gradually?

32. What is an anticipated adverse effect seen with minoxidil (Loniten)?

19. Beta blocking agents are not as effective in African-American patients and should be avoided in patients with asthma, type 1 diabetes mellitus, heart failure with an etiology of systolic dysfunction, and in patients with peripheral vascular disease.

20. After long-term treatment with beta blockers, discontinue gradually over 1–2 weeks and monitor for anginal symptoms.

21. Angiotensin II produces vasoconstriction, which results in an increase in blood pressure.

22. Aldosterone results in sodium retention, which causes water retention and increased cardiac output, thereby increasing blood pressure.

23. Common adverse effects of ACE inhibitors include nausea, fatigue, headache, diarrhea, and orthostatic hypotension. Serious adverse effects include swelling face, eyes, lips; dyspnea; neutropenia; nephrotoxicity; hyperkalemia; chronic cough; and can cause fetal and neonatal harm during pregnancy.

24. Angiotensin II receptor inhibitors block the angiotensin II from binding to receptor sites in vascular smooth muscle and the adrenal glands. This prevents elevation of pressure and sodium-retaining properties of angiotensin II.

25. Eplerenone, an aldosterone receptor blocking agent, blocks the stimulation of the mineralocorticoid receptors by aldosterone, thereby preventing sodium reabsorption.

26. Eplerenone is contraindicated in patients with serum potassium greater than 5.5 mEq/L, type 2 diabetes with microalbuminuria, serum creatinine greater than 2.0 mg/dL in males or 1.8 mg/dL in females; creatinine clearance less than 50 mL/min, patients taking potassium-sparing diuretics (e.g., amiloride, triamterene), and patients taking strong metabolic enzyme inhibitors (e.g., ketoconazole, cimetidine, others).

27. See textbook, p. 372.

28. Grapefruit juice and St. John's wort.

29. Calcium channel blockers inhibit the movement of calcium ions across cell membranes. This causes slower rate of heart contraction and relaxation of smooth muscles of blood vessels, resulting in vasodilation and reduction of the blood pressure.

30. Common adverse effects of alpha$_1$ adrenergic blockers include drowsiness, headache, dizziness, weakness, tachycardia, and fainting.

31. Sudden discontinuation of centrally acting alpha$_2$ agonists can produce a rebound effect with sudden increase in blood pressure.

33. What is the ending of generic drug names belonging to the class of ACE inhibitors?

34. What is the ending of generic drug names belonging to the class of angiotensin II receptor antagonists?

35. What is the ending of generic drug names belonging to the class of calcium ion antagonists?

36. What is the ending of generic drug names belonging to the class of alpha$_1$ adrenergic blocking agents?

32. The anticipated adverse effect seen with minoxidil is hair growth on the body.

33. Generic drug names of ACE inhibitors end in "-pril" (enalapril, captopril, etc.).

34. Generic drug names of angiotensin II receptor antagonists end in "-sartan" (e.g., candesartan, losartan).

35. Generic drug names of calcium ion antagonists end in "-pine," with the exceptions of diltiazem and verapamil.

36. Generic drug names of alpha$_1$ adrenergic blocking agents end in "-azosin."

Student Name _____

Drugs Used to Treat Hypertension

Learning Activities

FILL-IN-THE-BLANK

Finish each of the following statements using the correct term.

1. The difference between the systolic and diastolic pressure is called the _____ pressure.

2. To reduce the frequency of cardiovascular disease in patients with conditions such as diabetes mellitus, heart failure, or renal disease, a goal blood pressure of _____ mm Hg is suggested.

3. The Dietary Approaches to Stop Hypertension (DASH) diet includes dietary _____ reduction, physical activity, and moderation of _____ consumption.

4. The _____ act as antihypertensive agents by causing volume depletion, sodium excretion, and vasodilatation of peripheral arterioles.

5. After a first dose of an ACE inhibitor, a patient develops swelling of the face, eyes, lips, tongue, and difficulty breathing. This is referred to as _____.

6. Patients should be cautioned against the sudden discontinuation of beta-adrenergic blocking agents for the treatment of hypertension because exacerbation of _____ symptoms may occur, followed in some cases by myocardial infarction.

7. The physiologic goal of antihypertensive therapy is a decrease in blood pressure through reduction in _____ _____.

8. Smoking causes _____ of blood vessels and results in increased peripheral resistance.

MATCHING

Match the generic drug name with its corresponding brand name. Each option will be used only once.

_____ 9. enalapril

_____ 10. valsartan

_____ 11. diltiazem

_____ 12. prazosin

a. Minipress
b. Cardizem
c. Diovan
d. Vasotec

Select the correct statement associated with the terms.

_____ 13. diuretics

_____ 14. beta-adrenergic blockers

_____ 15. angiotensin-converting enzyme (ACE) inhibitors

_____ 16. calcium antagonists

a. Block beta receptors to inhibit cardiac response to sympathetic nerve stimulation
b. Block flow of calcium ions across cell membranes
c. May produce swelling lips and tongue, dyspnea, neutropenia, nephrotoxicity, and/or chronic cough
d. Depletes norepinephrine from adrenergic nerve endings
e. Enhances fluid volume excretion, sodium excretion, and vasodilation of peripheral arterioles

Select the correct drug class associated with the drug names.

_____ 17. thiazide diuretic

_____ 18. beta-adrenergic blocker

_____ 19. angiotensin-converting enzyme (ACE) inhibitor

_____ 20. angiotensin II receptor antagonist

_____ 21. calcium ion antagonist

a. atenolol (Tenormin)
b. hydrochlorothiazide (HydroDIURIL)
c. nifedipine (Procardia)
d. doxazosin (Cardura)
e. clonidine (Catapres)
f. captopril (Capoten)
g. losartan (Cozaar)

TRUE OR FALSE

Write "T" for true and "F" for false for each statement. Correct all false statements.

_____ 22. Peripheral vascular resistance is regulated primarily by contraction and dilation of arterioles.

_____ 23. The cause of most cases of hypertension is unknown.

_____ 24. The most accurate method of obtaining a blood pressure is to have the patient sit on an examination table with the legs dangling over the side.

_____ 25. Recent evidence indicates that systolic hypertension is the least common form of hypertension, and is present in about 2% of individuals older than 60 years of age.

_____ 26. Patients taking beta-adrenergic blocking agents are most at risk for the development of tachycardia.

_____ 27. The ACE inhibitors reduce blood pressure, preserve cardiac output, and increase renal blood flow.

_____ 28. The chronic, dry, nonproductive, persistent cough associated with ACE inhibitor therapy is thought to be due to an accumulation of bradykinin.

_____ 29. The ACE inhibitors are safe to use for the treatment of hypertension in pregnancy.

_____ 30. Orthostatic hypotension is a possible adverse effect seen with most antihypertensive drugs.

_____ 31. Primary hypertension is caused by such disorders as renal disease or head trauma.

_____ 32. The primary goal of antihypertensive therapy is to reduce morbidity and mortality.

_____ 33. ACE inhibitors and diuretics are the preferred agents for initiating treatment of hypertension.

_____ 34. The lifestyle changes required to reduce blood pressure are increased exercise, diet, and weight reduction.

_____ 35. The action of smoking on the blood vessels is vasodilation.

_____ 36. An order stating "take orthostatic blood pressure readings" means to take blood pressure every shift without fail.

_____ 37. An important nursing diagnosis when initiating antihypertensive therapy would be *Injury, risk for, r/t antihypertensive therapy.*

_____ 38. Drowsiness and fatigue are common during the first 2 weeks of antihypertensive therapy.

_____ 39. Potassium-sparing and loop diuretics are commonly used for initiating the step approach to antihypertensive therapy.

_____ 40. Blood pressure readings in supine and standing positions are all the data needed to initiate antihypertensive therapy with a diuretic.

Drugs Used to Treat Hypertension

Practice Questions for the NCLEX® Examination

_____ 1. A patient has a blood pressure reading of 170/102 mm Hg. The nurse identifies this patient as having which classification of hypertension?
1. Normal
2. Prehypertension
3. Stage 1
4. Stage 2

_____ 2. The nurse obtains a blood pressure of 182/112 mm Hg on an individual at a community health fair. What does the nurse inform the patient to do?
1. Have their blood pressure rechecked in 2 years.
2. Have their blood pressure rechecked in 1 year.
3. Evaluate or refer to their source of care within 1 month.
4. Evaluate or refer to their source of care immediately or within 1 week, depending on the clinical situation.

_____ 3. Which statement does the nurse include when providing patient teaching on the use of beta-adrenergic blockers for the treatment of hypertension?
1. "Do not suddenly discontinue beta-adrenergic therapy, because increased angina and myocardial infarction can develop."
2. "Beta-adrenergic blockers are the antihypertensive drug of choice for patients with diabetes mellitus because they help to lower blood sugar."
3. "Wheezing is a normal response to this drug. If wheezing occurs, continue taking the medication and see your primary health care provider at the next scheduled visit."
4. "If you are taking NSAIDs and beta-adrenergic blockers for the treatment of hypertension, the dose of NSAID will need to be increased because beta-adrenergic blockers decrease the effectiveness of NSAIDs."

_____ 4. Patients on angiotensin-converting enzyme (ACE) inhibitor therapy for the treatment of hypertension are monitored for the development of which common electrolyte imbalance?
1. Hyperkalemia
2. Hypocalcemia
3. Hypernatremia
4. Hypomagnesemia

_____ 5. A patient has been ordered an angiotensin II receptor blocker for the treatment of hypertension. The nurse contacts the prescriber for specific approval after discovering that the patient has also been ordered which medication?
1. Digoxin (Lanoxin)
2. Spironolactone (Aldactone)
3. Furosemide (Lasix)
4. Vitamin D

_____ 6. What is the action of hydralazine (Apresoline) in lowering blood pressure?
1. Inhibiting the release of norepinephrine
2. Blocking aldosterone receptors
3. Directing arteriolar smooth muscle relaxation
4. Volume depletion

_____ 7. Patients taking which medication should be informed that the medication or its metabolites may discolor the urine, causing it to darken on exposure to air?
1. Nitroprusside sodium (Nipride)
2. Clonidine (Catapres)
3. Methyldopa
4. Diltiazem (Cardizem)

_____ 8. The nurse is teaching a patient about the use of minoxidil (Loniten) for the treatment of hypertension. Which statement made by the patient indicates a need for further instruction?
1. "I can expect to have an increase in fine body hair due to this drug."
2. "My salt intake will not need to be monitored."
3. "I should take my pulse every day."
4. "I should report weight gain to my primary care provider."

_____ 9. Which statements does the nurse incorporate into the teaching plan for a patient with type 2 diabetes mellitus and asthma who is starting on a beta-adrenergic blocking agent for the treatment of hypertension? (Select all that apply.)
1. "Monitor for hyperglycemia, because beta-adrenergic blocking agents often cause this."
2. "You should notice an improvement in your asthma symptoms because these drugs will help your airways to dilate."
3. "Call your primary care provider if you experience any swelling in your feet."
4. "Do not suddenly discontinue use of this medication."
5. "Increase your diabetes and asthma medications while taking the beta-blocker."

_____ 10. The nurse informs patients taking ACE inhibitors to report which adverse effects to their health care provider? (Select all that apply.)
1. Swelling of the face
2. Rash
3. Difficulty breathing
4. Depression
5. Swelling of the hands

_____ 11. Which conditions are identifiable causes of hypertension? (Select all that apply.)
1. Sleep apnea
2. Chronic kidney disease
3. Primary aldosteronism
4. Marfan's syndrome
5. Thyroid disease

_____ 12. Which drugs are direct vasodilators? (Select all that apply.)
1. Methyldopa
2. Minoxidil (Loniten)
3. Guanadrel (Hylorel)
4. Hydralazine (Apresoline)
5. Aliskiren (Tekturna)

_____ 13. Which statements does the nurse include when teaching a patient about eplerenone (Inspra)? (Select all that apply.)
1. "Do not take this drug with grapefruit juice."
2. "Do not take this medication with St. John's wort."
3. "Avoid the use of salt substitutes in seasoning your food."
4. "Avoid foods that are marketed as low sodium."
5. "If you have a headache, immediately stop taking the drug."

14. A 125-pound patient is prescribed 50 mg of nitroprusside sodium (Nitropress) in 500 mL of D_5W for infusion at 3 mcg/kg/min. How many mL per hour does the nurse infuse?
_____ mL/hr

_____ 15. A patient has been on minoxidil (Loniten) therapy. Which lab result requires follow-up by the nurse?
1. White blood cell (WBC) count of 4000 uL
2. Potassium level of 4.0 mEq/L
3. Serum digoxin level of 1 ng/mL
4. Sodium level of 130 mEq/L

Drugs Used to Treat Dysrhythmias

Review Sheet

The QUESTION column and the ANSWER column have been offset so that you can cover the answer while reading the question, allowing you to assess your knowledge.

Question	Answer
1. Describe *dysrhythmia*.	
2. What function does the electrical system of the heart have on heart action?	1. A dysrhythmia is sometimes called an *arrhythmia*. It occurs when there is a disturbance of the normal electrical conduction of the heart, resulting in an abnormal heart muscle contraction or heart rate.
3. Review the sequence of the heart's conduction system.	2. The electrical system of the heart sequences the muscle contractions of the heart to provide an optimal volume of blood per beat of the heart.
4. What causes dysrhythmias?	3. The heart's conduction system goes from SA node to AV node to bundle of His to Purkinje fibers to ventricular muscle tissue.
5. Describe supraventricular and ventricular dysrhythmias.	4. Dysrhythmias are caused by the firing of abnormal pacemaker cells, the blockage of normal electrical pathways, or a combination of both.
6. What is a *pulse deficit*?	5. Dysrhythmias that develop above the bundle of His are called *supraventricular dysrhythmias*. Examples include atrial flutter, atrial fibrillation, premature atrial contractions (PAC), sinus tachycardia, sinus bradycardia, and paroxysmal supraventricular tachycardia. Dysrhythmias developing below the bundle of His are referred to as *ventricular dysrhythmias*. These include premature ventricular contractions (PVCs), ventricular tachycardia (VT), and ventricular fibrillation (VF).
7. What electrolyte is responsible for electrical system conduction for the SA and AV nodes?	6. *Pulse deficit* is the difference between the apical and radial pulse rates; radial is generally lower than apical. For example: apical pulse = 74, radial pulse = 64, pulse deficit = 10.
8. What electrolyte is responsible for electrical system conduction for the atrial muscle, the His-Purkinje system, and the ventricular muscle?	7. Calcium ions are responsible for electrical system conduction for the SA and AV nodes.
9. What is the goal of treatment for dysrhythmias?	8. Sodium is responsible for electrical system conduction for the atrial muscle, the His-Purkinje system, and the ventricular muscle.

10. What effect do Class I, Ia, Ib, and Ic agents have on the electrical conduction system of the heart?

11. What methods are used to assess dysrhythmias?

12. Review the six cardinal signs of cardiovascular disease.

13. Why can mental status/level of consciousness (LOC) be important when assessing a cardiac patient?

14. What vital signs should be taken as often as necessary to monitor the status of a patient who has a dysrhythmia?

15. Why is it important to monitor hourly urine output in a patient with dysrhythmias?

16. When is the use of disopyramide (Norpace) indicated?

17. What is the interaction between quinidine and neuromuscular blockade?

18. When lidocaine (Xylocaine) is ordered for a dysrhythmia, what should the nurse check on the bottle BEFORE using the medication for IV administration?

19. What serious adverse effects may be seen with the administration of lidocaine (Xylocaine)?

20. What effect does flecainide acetate (Tambocor) have on patients with heart failure and dysrhythmias?

21. Patients should be assessed for what condition before administration of propafenone (Rhythmol)?

9. The goal of treatment for dysrhythmias is to restore normal sinus rhythm and maintain adequate cardiac output to maintain tissue perfusion.

10. The effects of Class I, Ia, Ib, and Ic agents are as follows: I is a myocardial depressant (inhibits sodium ion movement); Ia causes prolonged duration of electrical stimulation on cells and refractory time between electrical impulses; Ib shortens duration of electrical stimulation and time interval between electrical impulses; Ic is the most potent antidysrhythmic, causing myocardial depression and slowing conduction rate through the atria and the ventricles.

11. ECG monitoring, EPS (electrophysiologic studies), exercise electrocardiography, and laboratory values are used to assess for cardiac dysrhythmias.

12. The six cardinal signs of cardiac disease are dyspnea, chest pain, fatigue, edema, syncope, and palpitations.

13. Mental status/LOC indicates whether there is adequate cerebral tissue perfusion.

14. Vital signs include blood pressure in arms, pulse, respirations, temperature, and oxygen saturation.

15. Hourly outputs reflect whether the kidney tissues are being adequately perfused.

16. Disopyramide (Norpace) is used to treat atrial fibrillation, Wolff-Parkinson-White syndrome, paroxysmal supraventricular tachycardia, premature ventricular tachycardia, and ventricular tachycardia.

17. Quinidine may prolong the effects of surgical muscle relaxants (tubocuraine, succinylcholine) and aminoglycoside antibiotics (gentamicin, tobramycin, kanamycin). The patient's respiratory rate and depth should be monitored. The patient should be observed for signs of cyanosis and additional dysrhythmias. Patients on ventilators may require additional time to be weaned from ventilatory assistance.

18. The bottle must be labeled "Xylocaine for dysrhythmia" or "Lidocaine without preservatives."

19. Light-headedness, muscle twitching, hallucinations, agitation, euphoria, respiratory depression.

20. Flecainide acetate has a negative inotropic effect and may cause or worsen heart failure, particularly in patients with pre-existing severe heart failure. Flecainide may also aggravate an existing dysrhythmia and precipitate new ones, especially in patients with underlying heart disease.

22. What are the drawbacks of using amiodarone hydrochloride (Cordarone)?

23. What are the actions and uses of calcium channel blocking agents in the treatments of dysrhythmias?

24. For what condition is adenosine (Adenocard) recommended as a treatment?

25. Digoxin (Lanoxin) is used to treat which kind of dysrhythmias?

21. Because propafenone has mild beta-adrenergic blocking properties, it should not be used in patients with asthma.

22. Amiodarone hydrochloride requires hospitalization during loading dose and the maintenance dose is difficult to establish. Life-threatening dysrhythmias may recur at unpredictable intervals. Once the drug is used, switching to a different antidysrhythmic is difficult because the body may store the drug; therefore, a drug interaction with the newly prescribed antidysrhythmic may occur.

23. Calcium channel blockers (verapamil, diltiazem) are widely used as antidysrhythmic agents. They inhibit cardiac response by blocking the L-type calcium channels in the SA and AV nodal tissue. This slows AV conduction, prolongs refractoriness, and decreases automaticity. These agents are effective in the treatment of automatic and re-entrant tachycardias. They are contraindicated in systolic heart failure.

24. Because of its strong depressant effects on the SA and AV nodes, adenosine is recommended for the treatment of paroxysmal supraventricular tachycardia that involves conduction through the SA node, atrium, or AV node.

25. Digoxin may be used to treat atrial fibrillation, atrial flutter, and paroxysmal tachycardia.

Drugs Used to Treat Dysrhythmias

Learning Activities

FILL-IN-THE-BLANK

Finish each of the following statements using the correct term.

1. Adenosine (Adenocard) is recommended for the treatment of paroxysmal supraventricular tachycardia because of its strong depressant effects on the _____ and _____ nodes of the heart.

2. The therapeutic blood level of procainamide hydrochloride (Procanbid) is _____ to _____ mg/L.

3. The mechanism of action of digoxin (Lanoxin) is _____ stimulation.

4. Rash, chills, fever, increasing mental confusion and tinnitus caused by the use of quinidine are known as _____.

5. The six cardinal signs of cardiovascular disease include _____, _____, _____, _____, _____, and _____.

6. Lidocaine is used in the treatment of _____, _____, and _____.

MATCHING

Match the generic drug name with its corresponding brand name. Each option will be used only once.

_____ 7. flecainide acetate

_____ 8. disopyramide

_____ 9. propafenone

_____ 10. amiodarone hydrochloride

_____ 11. adenosine

a. Adenocard
b. Rhythmol
c. Cordarone
d. Tambocor
e. Norpace

TRUE OR FALSE

Write "T" for true and "F" for false for each statement. Correct all false statements.

_____ 12. Antidysrhythmic agents are classified according to their effects on the electrical conduction system of the heart.

_____ 13. Currently there are two classifications of antidysrhythmic agents used in clinical practice.

_____ 14. Adenosine is a naturally occurring chemical found only in cardiac cells.

_____ 15. Patients must be hospitalized while the loading dose of amiodarone (Cordarone) is administered.

_____ 16. Digoxin (Lanoxin) slows conduction through the AV node, reducing conduction velocity and automaticity.

_____ 17. Patients taking amiodarone hydrochloride (Cordarone) should be cautioned about photosensitivity.

_____ 18. With amiodarone hydrochloride (Cordarone) therapy, it is difficult to predict the degree and duration of antidysrhythmic response.

_____ 19. Because propafenone (Rhythmol) has mild beta-adrenergic blocking properties, it should not be used in patients with asthma.

_____ 20. Flecainide acetate (Tambocor) must be administered intravenously.

Drugs Used to Treat Dysrhythmias

Practice Questions for the NCLEX® Examination

_____ 1. A patient starting amiodarone hydro-chloride (Cordarone) therapy for treatment of a dysrhythmia asks the nurse how long it will take to find out if this drug will work. What is the nurse's best response?
1. "In 24 hours, we will know if the drug is working for you."
2. "It takes at least 3 days for the full therapeutic effect of the drug to be known."
3. "The response to this drug requires 2 weeks or more."
4. "A blood test has already been completed for you and we are certain this drug will be effective for you."

_____ 2. When caring for a patient taking warfarin (Coumadin) as well as amiodarone hydrochloride (Cordarone), the nurse monitors the status and results of which laboratory test?
1. PT
2. aPTT
3. AST
4. BUN

_____ 3. What is a common adverse effect of quinidine that usually subsides?
1. Diarrhea
2. Rash
3. Tinnitus
4. Fever

_____ 4. Patients on procainamide hydrochloride (Procanbid) therapy are at risk for the development of neuromuscular blockade and respiratory depression when taking which types of antibiotics?
1. Penicillins
2. Tetracyclines
3. Macrolides
4. Aminoglycosides

_____ 5. Before administering disopyramide (Norpace) therapy, it is most important for the nurse to ask the patient about a history of which condition?
1. Atrial fibrillation
2. Digitalis use
3. Diabetes mellitus
4. Urinary obstruction

_____ 6. Patients taking flecainide acetate (Tambocor) should report which adverse effect to the health care provider immediately?
1. Nausea
2. Dizziness
3. Increasing dyspnea
4. Headache

_____ 7. Which statements about amiodarone hydrochloride (Cordarone) therapy for the treatment of dysrhythmias are true? *(Select all that apply.)*
1. Patients must be hospitalized while the loading dose is given.
2. Amiodarone therapy is contraindicated in the treatment of patients who have pacemakers.
3. Response from amiodarone therapy often requires 2 weeks or more of treatment.
4. Amiodarone should be administered with food or milk if gastric irritation develops.
5. Yellow-brown pigmentations of the cornea have developed in patients taking amiodarone.

_____ 8. A patient has been ordered digoxin (Lanoxin) 0.125 mg PO daily. The medication is available as 250 mcg per tablet. How many tablets does the nurse administer?
1. 1/4
2. 1/2
3. 1
4. 1 1/2

9. A patient is ordered to receive lidocaine 2 mg/min via an infusion pump. The medication is available as 2 grams in 500 mL of D₅W. The nurse regulates the flow rate to how many mL/h to deliver 2 mg/min of lidocaine?
_____ mL/h

10. A patient is ordered an IV initial bolus dose of 100 mg of lidocaine. The medication is available as 2% (20 mg/mL) in a 5-mL syringe. How many mL of the medication does the nurse administer? _____ mL

Drugs Used to Treat Angina Pectoris

Review Sheet

The QUESTION column and the ANSWER column have been offset so that you can cover the answer while reading the questions, allowing you to assess your knowledge.

Question	Answer
1. Explain the underlying cause of anginal pain.	
2. Review the various presenting symptoms of angina.	1. The pain and discomfort of angina is caused by the lack of an adequate oxygen supply to the cells in the heart (ischemic heart disease). The underlying etiology is vasospasm of a coronary artery that reduces blood flow through the coronary arteries to the heart tissue.
3. What are the American Heart Association (2005) recommendations for seeking medical attention for chest pain and nitroglycerin administration?	2. See textbook, p. 397.
4. Compare the precipitating factors associated with chronic stable angina, unstable angina, and variant angina.	3. In 2005, the American Heart Association recommended that if chest pain is not relieved by one sublingual nitroglycerin tablet within 5 minutes, the patient should seek medical attention (call 911).
5. What are the desired therapeutic outcomes during treatment of angina?	4. Chronic stable angina is precipitated by physical exertion or stress. Unstable angina is precipitated by unpredictable factors such as atherosclerotic narrowing, vasospasm, or thrombus formation. Variant angina occurs at rest. The underlying etiology is vasospasm of a coronary artery that reduces blood flow through the coronary arteries to the heart tissue.
6. What questions should be asked during a nursing assessment related to an angina attack?	5. The goals in treatment of angina pectoris are to prevent myocardial infarction and death, thereby prolonging life, and to relieve anginal pain symptoms, thereby improving the quality of life.
7. What are the seven groups of drugs that may be used to treat angina?	6. See textbook, pp. 398-399.
8. Compare the premedication assessments required for nitrates, beta-adrenergic blockers, calcium channel blockers, and angiotensin-converting enzyme (ACE) inhibitors.	7. Nitrates, beta-adrenergic blocking agents, ACE inhibitors, calcium channel blockers, statins, platelet-active agents, and fatty oxidase enzyme inhibitors.
9. What is the drug of choice for acute attacks of angina pectoris?	8. See textbook, pp. 401-406.

10. Why is it important to teach patients taking nitroglycerin not to consume alcohol?

11. What dose forms are available for nitroglycerin?

12. What side effects can be expected when rapid-acting nitrates (e.g., nitroglycerin, amyl nitrite) are used?

13. What premedication assessments should be performed prior to therapy with nitrates?

14. Describe the procedure for administering nitroglycerin sublingually, via translingual spray, topical ointment, transmucosal tablets, and topical disk.

15. How does one evaluate anginal attacks and what health teaching is needed for an individual who has anginal attacks?

16. What are some guidelines used during the preparation and administration of IV nitroglycerin?

17. What are the desired therapeutic outcomes for the use of beta-adrenergic blocking agents in the treatment of anginal pain?

18. What is the desired result of the use of calcium channel blockers to treat angina?

19. What are common adverse effects associated with angiotensin-converting enzyme inhibitors?

20. Describe uses of ranolazine (Ranexa). Which types of patients benefit most from this therapy?

9. Nitroglycerin, administered sublingually, is the drug of choice for acute attacks of angina pectoris.

10. Alcohol use results in vasodilation and may lead to postural hypotension.

11. Sublingual tablets, transmucosal tablets, translingual spray, topical disks, sustained-release capsules, topical ointment, and intravenous forms of nitroglycerin are available.

12. Headache and hypotension caused by vasodilation are side effects of nitroglycerin and amyl nitrite treatment.

13. Assess for pain level, location, duration, intensity, and pattern, and obtain a history of most recent nitrate use before beginning amyl nitrate therapy.

14. Procedure for administration of the various forms of nitroglycerin can be found in the textbook in Chapter 8 and pp. 401-403.

15. See textbook, pp. 398-400.

16. See textbook, p. 403.

17. The desired therapeutic outcomes of beta blocker therapy are decreased frequency and severity of anginal attacks, increased tolerance of activities, and decreased use of nitroglycerin for acute anginal attacks. Before administering beta blockers, take BP in supine and standing position, check for history of respiratory disorders such as COPD, and check for history of diabetes. If patient is a diabetic, determine whether the physician wants baseline blood glucose studies before initiating the medication.

18. The desired action of calcium channel blockers in the treatment of angina is to decrease myocardial oxygen demands by increasing myocardial blood supply via coronary arteries and decrease resistance to blood flow and dilate peripheral vessels, resulting in decreased workload of the heart.

19. ACE inhibitors cause hypotension with dizziness, tachycardia, fainting, and nonproductive cough.

20. Ranolazine is used to treat chronic stable angina. It does not affect blood pressure or heart rate. It will prolong QT interval; therefore, it should only be used to treat angina in patients who have not achieved an antianginal response from other agents or cannot tolerate the adverse effects of those medicines. Ranolazine will not reduce the symptoms of an acute anginal attack.

Drugs Used to Treat Angina Pectoris

Learning Activities

FILL-IN-THE-BLANK

Finish each of the following statements using the correct term.

1. Patients taking nitroglycerin should be instructed to not ingest alcohol, because alcohol consumed in combination with nitroglycerin causes _____, potentially resulting in postural _____.

2. _____ is currently the drug of choice for treatment of angina pectoris.

3. The initial dose of angiotensin-converting enzyme inhibitors may cause hypotension with dizziness, _____, and fainting.

MATCHING

Match the generic drug name with its corresponding brand name. Each option will be used only once.

_____ 4. verapamil

_____ 5. nifedipine

_____ 6. diltiazem

_____ 7. amlodipine

_____ 8. isosorbide mononitrate

_____ 9. ranolazine

a. Procardia, Adalat
b. Calan, Isoptin
c. Norvasc
d. Cardizem
e. Monoket
f. Ranexa

TRUE OR FALSE

Write "T" for true and "F" for false for each statement. Correct all false statements.

_____ 10. Cancer is the leading cause of disability, socioeconomic loss, and death in the United States.

_____ 11. Calcium ion antagonists decrease myocardial oxygen demand, and increase myocardial blood supply by coronary artery dilation.

_____ 12. Isosorbide dinitrate (Isordil) is available for inhalation administration.

_____ 13. Transdermal disk administration of nitrates provides controlled release of nitroglycerin for a 48-hour period when applied to intact skin.

_____ 14. Sildenafil (Viagra) is commonly administered with nitrates to provide optimal therapeutic effects.

_____ 15. Statins are used to lower LDL cholesterol levels.

_____ 16. If more than three nitroglycerin tablets within 15 minutes are required to control pain, the patient should seek medical attention.

_____ 17. Patients must be taught that nitroglycerin tablets must be replaced every month.

Drugs Used to Treat Angina Pectoris

chapter

25

Practice Questions for the NCLEX® Examination

____ 1. What does the nurse teach a patient to do at the first sign of an anginal attack?
1. Call 911.
2. Sit or lie down
3. Take two nitroglycerin tablets.
4. Take an extra dose of transdermal nitroglycerin.

____ 2. Which statement does the nurse include when teaching a patient about the use of isosorbide dinitrate (Isordil)?
1. "Store the medication in the original, dark-colored glass container with a tight lid."
2. "Four tablets may be taken a few minutes before engaging in activities that may trigger an anginal attack."
3. "If a slight stinging or burning sensation occurs when you take the medication, report this to the health care provider at once."
4. "If you develop a headache from taking this medication, take aspirin as indicated."

____ 3. Which statements does the nurse include when teaching a patient about the use of nitroglycerin spray (Nitrolingual)? (Select all that apply.)
1. "Do not shake the container before administration."
2. "Hold the canister vertically when administering the medication."
3. "Spray the dose onto the roof of your mouth."
4. "Do not inhale or swallow the spray."
5. "Call 911 if chest pain is not relieved by one dose within 5 minutes."

____ 4. Which action does the nurse take when administering IV nitroglycerin (Nitro-Bid IV) to a patient?
1. Administer the nitroglycerin with another IV medication to avoid fluid overload.
2. Use standard plastic containers and administration sets when infusing the medication.
3. Follow the practice of gradual weaning under controlled conditions.
4. Administer the medication via gravity drip.

____ 5. When applying transdermal nitroglycerin using a disk, which sites does the nurse consider using? (Select all that apply.)
1. Newly shaved area of the chest
2. Pelvis
3. Inner arm
4. Side of the chest
5. Upper chest

____ 6. What is the most common adverse effect of nitrate therapy?
1. Excessive hypotension
2. Tolerance
3. Nausea
4. Prolonged headache

____ 7. The nurse can administer nitroglycerin to a patient using which routes? (Select all that apply.)
1. Transmucosal tablets
2. Transdermal patches
3. Translingual spray
4. Sustained-release tablet
5. Intramuscular injection

____ 8. The nurse is teaching a patient about the use of nitroglycerin (Nitrostat). Which statement made by the patient indicates a need for further teaching?
1. "Every 3 months the nitroglycerin prescription should be refilled and the old tablets safely discarded."
2. "Nitroglycerin should be stored in the original container it came in."
3. "When taking the drug, I'll feel a slight stinging or burning sensation, which usually indicates that it is still potent."
4. "I'll swallow my saliva immediately after the tablet dissolves."

____ 9. What are the actions of angiotensin-converting enzyme (ACE) inhibitors? *(Select all that apply.)*
1. To prevent thrombus formation
2. To minimize platelet cell aggregation
3. To dissolve clots
4. To promote coronary artery dilation
5. To lower the heart rate

____ 10. A patient with a history of which disorder is at highest risk for complications associated with use of beta-adrenergic blockers for the treatment of angina?
1. High blood pressure
2. Gastric ulcer
3. Anemia
4. Respiratory disorders

____ 11. Which statements does the nurse include when teaching a patient about ranolazine (Ranexa) therapy? *(Select all that apply.)*
1. "Use ranolazine at the first sign of an anginal attack."
2. "Monitor your pulse before taking ranolazine because low heart rate is a common adverse effect of this medication."
3. "This medication should reduce the frequency and severity of anginal attacks you experience."
4. "You will have routine electrocardiograms to assess for possible adverse effects of this medication."
5. "Crush the ranolazine tablet if you have difficulty swallowing it."

____ 12. A patient is ordered nifedipine (Procardia) sustained-release tablets 120 mg PO daily. The drug is available in 30-mg, 60-mg, and 90-mg tablets. How many tablets does the nurse administer?
1. Four 30-mg tablets
2. Two 30-mg tablets and one 60-mg tablet
3. One 30-mg tablet and one 90-mg tablet
4. One 90-mg tablet and one-half 60-mg tablet

13. A patient is ordered nicardipine (Cadene) 40 mg three times a day. The medication is available as 20 mg per capsule. How many capsules will the patient take in a one-week period?
_____ capsules

____ 14. A patient is ordered isosorbide dinitrate (Isordil) oral tablets 2.5 mg three times a day. The medication is available as 5 mg per tablet. How many tablets will the patient take in a 24-hour period?
1. 1
2. 1 1/2
3. 2
4. 2 1/2

Drugs Used to Treat Peripheral Vascular Disease

Review Sheet

The QUESTION column and the ANSWER column have been offset so that you can cover the answer before reading the questions, thus allowing you to assess your knowledge.

Question	Answer
1. Explain the pathophysiology of intermittent claudication, vasospasm, paresthesia, arteriosclerosis obliterans, and Raynaud's disease.	
2. What are the goals of treatment of arteriosclerosis obliterans?	1. See textbook, pp. 409-410.
3. List the agents specifically approved by the FDA to treat chronic occlusive arterial disease.	2. Improve blood flow, relieve pain, and prevent skin ulcerations and/or gangrene.
4. Name the three calcium ion antagonists used in the treatment of Raynaud's disease.	3. Pentoxifylline and cilostazol
5. What is the action of an ACE inhibitor in the treatment of peripheral vascular disease?	4. Diltiazem, verapamil, and nifedipine
6. What preventive actions can be taken by a patient with Raynaud's disease to reduce or stop vasospastic attacks?	5. The ACE inhibitors cause an increase in bradykinin, which is a potent vasodilator.
7. What nursing assessments should be made on a regular basis when peripheral vasodilators are prescribed?	6. Avoid cold temperature, emotional stress, tobacco, and drugs known to induce attacks.
8. Describe the health teaching needed when peripheral vascular disease is diagnosed that would promote improved tissue perfusion.	7. Assess for color and temperature of the hands, fingers, legs, and feet. Check for signs and symptoms of skin breakdown, presence of limb pain, or a reduction in sensation in the extremities. Pedal pulses and radial pulse rates should be taken and recorded every 4 hours during hospitalization and twice a day upon discharge.
9. What is the action of pentoxifylline (Trental) and cilostazol (Pletal)?	8. See textbook, pp. 412-413.
10. What type of vascular conditions may be treated using peripheral vasodilating agents?	9. Trental increases RBC (red blood cell) flexibility, decreases concentration of fibrinogen in the blood, and prevents aggregation of RBCs and platelets, thus preventing blood clotting. Cilostazol inhibits platelet aggregation and promotes vasodilation.
11. What is the mechanism of action of vasodilators used to treat peripheral vascular disease?	10. Intermittent claudication, arteriosclerosis obliterans, vasospasms associated with thrombophlebitis, nocturnal leg cramps, and Raynaud's disease.

12. What are the adverse effects to expect with the administration of vasodilating agents?

13. List the premedication assessments required for all prescribed medications for peripheral vascular disease.

11. Relaxation of peripheral arterial blood vessels, thereby increasing blood flow to the extremities.

12. Flushing, tingling, sweating. May also produce orthostatic hypotension and tachycardia. Also may cause possible nervousness and weakness as therapy progresses.

13. Baseline assessment of symptoms of peripheral vascular disease and degree of pain present; take baseline vital signs and assess for tissue perfusion.

Drugs Used to Treat Peripheral Vascular Disease

Learning Activities

FILL-IN-THE-BLANK

Finish each of the following statements using the correct term.

1. Major treatable causes of peripheral vascular disease include _____, cigarette smoking, and _____.

2. The most common form of obstructive arterial disease is _____ _____.

3. Peripheral vascular disease caused by arterial vasospasm is known as _____ disease.

4. _____ and _____ are the only agents approved by the FDA that are specifically indicated for the treatment of intermittent claudication caused by chronic occlusive arterial disease of the limbs.

5. Patients with peripheral vascular disease should be taught to not elevate their extremities above the level of the _____ without specific orders to do so from the health care provider.

MATCHING

Match the generic drug name with its corresponding brand name. Each option will be used only once.

_____ 6. pentoxifylline

_____ 7. cilostazol

a. Trental
b. Pletal

TRUE OR FALSE

Write "T" for true and "F" for false for each statement. Correct all false statements.

_____ 8. The most cost-effective and successful forms of treatment for peripheral vascular disease are smoking cessation, weight reduction, exercise, and dietary modification.

_____ 9. The typical pain pattern described by a person with peripheral vascular disease is sharp, stabbing pain at rest.

_____ 10. Peripheral vascular disease is often accompanied by increased blood viscosity.

_____ 11. The ACE inhibitors are used in the treatment of peripheral vascular disease because they cause an increase in bradykinin which is a potent vasodilator.

_____ 12. When positioning a patient who has peripheral vascular disease in bed, the nurse should flex the knees and place pillows in the popliteal space.

_____ 13. Part of the assessment process for peripheral vascular disease includes reviewing laboratory data relating to serum glucose levels and serum lipids.

_____ 14. Foot care for an individual with peripheral vascular disease should include regular trimming of toenails and corns.

_____ 15. Improvement in the symptoms of peripheral vascular disease includes reduction in frequency and degree of pain, intolerance to exercise, and an overall improvement in quality of the peripheral pulses.

_____ 16. Vasodilating agents have the potential for initiating orthostatic hypotension.

_____ 17. Flushing of the face, neck, and chest is a common adverse effect of vasodilators.

Drugs Used to Treat Peripheral Vascular Disease

Practice Questions for the NCLEX® Examination

_____ 1. What are the mechanisms of action for pentoxifylline (Trental) in the treatment of peripheral vascular disease? *(Select all that apply.)*
1. It increases erythrocyte flexibility.
2. It decreases the concentration of fibrinogen in the blood.
3. It prevents aggregation of red blood cells and platelets.
4. It increases the viscosity of blood.
5. It causes vasodilation.

_____ 2. Which statement does the nurse include when teaching a patient about pentoxifylline (Trental) for treatment of peripheral vascular disease?
1. "You will need to have a blood test called an INR to monitor the effects of this drug."
2. "This drug must be taken on an empty stomach."
3. "This drug may cause your blood pressure to be lower."
4. "If this drug makes you feel dizzy, stop taking it immediately."

_____ 3. Which statement does the nurse include in teaching a patient about papaverine hydrochloride (Pavagen TD) therapy?
1. "Avoid milk products when taking this medication."
2. "Increase consumption of foods high in vitamin C."
3. "Do not take over-the-counter cough and cold preparations without first consulting your health care provider."
4. "Take this medication before bed on an empty stomach."

_____ 4. A patient asks the nurse what can be done to decrease the occurrence and severity of vasospastic attacks of Raynaud's disease. How does the nurse respond? *(Select all that apply.)*
1. "Most attacks of Raynaud's disease can be stopped by the avoidance of hot temperatures."
2. "Tobacco use is highly associated with vasospastic attacks of Raynaud's disease."
3. "It is not known what really triggers the vasospastic attacks seen with Raynaud's disease."
4. "The signs and symptoms associated with Raynaud's disease are due to vasospasm of the arteries of the skin of the hands, fingers, and sometimes toes."
5. "Most people have Raynaud's disease for a few years and then it goes away."

_____ 5. A patient receiving pentoxifylline (Trental) for the treatment of intermittent claudication is taught to contact the health care provider if which adverse effect occurs?
1. Shortness of breath
2. Dizziness
3. Headache
4. Nausea

6. A patient is prescribed pentoxifylline (Trental) 400 mg PO tid with meals. How many mg of the drug does the patient receive in a 24-hour period? _____ mg

7. Cilostazol (Pletal) 100 mg is ordered for a patient at 0800 and 2000. The medication is available in 50-mg tablets. How many tablets does the nurse administer at 0800? _____ tablet(s)

8. A patient is ordered papaverine hydrochloride 300 mg three times a day. The medication is available in 150-mg capsules. How many capsules will the patient take in a 7-day period? _____ capsules

Drugs Used to Treat Thromboembolic Disorders

chapter

27

Review Sheet

The QUESTION column and the ANSWER column have been offset so you can cover the answer while reading the question, allowing you to assess your knowledge.

Question	Answer
1. Differentiate among thromboembolic disease, thrombosis, thrombus, and embolus.	
2. Explain factors that trigger blood clot formation.	1. See textbook, p. 417.
3. List factor(s) that trigger(s) the intrinsic blood clotting pathway.	2. See textbook, p. 417.
4. Identify factor(s) that trigger(s) the extrinsic pathway triggers.	3. Factor XII
5. What is the difference between red and white blood clots?	4. Factor VII to VIIa (factor VIIa can also activate factor X)
6. Describe appropriate nonpharmacologic patient education for prevention and treatment of thromboembolic disease.	5. Red embolus is a venous thrombus. White thrombi develop in arteries. See also textbook, p. 418.
7. Differentiate among the drug actions of platelet inhibitors, anticoagulants, thrombolytic agents, glycoprotein IIb/IIIa inhibitors, and thromboembolic agents.	6. See textbook, pp. 418-419.
8. Summarize the nursing actions that can help in the prevention of clot formation.	7. Platelet inhibitors reduce arterial clot formation by inhibiting platelet aggregation. Anticoagulants prevent new clot formation. Thrombolytic agents dissolve thromboemboli already formed. Glycoprotein IIb/IIIa inhibitors prevent platelet aggregation and are specifically used for patients undergoing percutaneous coronary interventions. Thromboembolic agents either prevent platelet aggregation or inhibit a variety of steps in fibrin clot formation.
9. State hydration information that should be provided to an individual for whom an anticoagulant is prescribed.	8. See textbook, pp. 419-420.
10. Identify laboratory tests used to evaluate anticoagulant therapy.	9. Adequate hydration to maintain fluidity of blood should be encouraged. Check to be certain the patient does not have coexisting disease that precludes forcing fluids.

11. Explain the desired therapeutic outcomes for platelet inhibitors.

12. List premedication assessments that should be performed before administering aspirin as a platelet inhibitor.

13. Differentiate the between the actions of low molecular weight heparins (LMWHs) and heparin.

14. Name three commonly used LMWH drugs.

15. What laboratory studies are used to monitor for adverse effects of LMWHs?

16. What drug is used as an antidote in case of heparin overdose?

17. What is the normal therapeutic range for warfarin (Coumadin) therapy?

18. What is the antidote for hemorrhage that occurs with warfarin (Coumadin) therapy?

19. List six fibrinolytic agents.

20. When are fibrinolytic agents administered?

21. How long a time is required before clopidogrel (Plavix) achieves full antiplatelet activity level?

22. What is the primary use of ticlopidine (Ticlid)?

10. Refer to the anticoagulant monographs in the textbook. Prothrombin time (PT) is reported as international normalized ratio (INR) and is routinely used for warfarin therapy; activated partial thromboplastin time (aPTT) is most commonly used for heparin therapy.

11. Reduce the frequency of transient ischemic attacks (TIAs), strokes, and myocardial infarction.

12. Neurologic assessment, gastrointestinal symptoms present, check for any concurrent anticoagulant therapy being taken; if on oral hypoglycemics, baseline serum glucose levels.

13. Heparin acts at several specific points in the coagulation pathway. LMWHs act at fewer specific steps in the coagulation pathway (factors Xa and thrombin), reducing the potential for hemorrhage. LMWHs also have a longer duration of action. Dalteparin, enoxaparin, and tinzaparin have no antiplatelet activity and only minimal effect on PT and aPTT.

14. Dalteparin (Fragmin), enoxaparin (Lovenox), and tinzaparin (Innohep).

15. Periodic CBC, daily platelet counts, and periodic checking of stools for occult blood are tests used to monitor for adverse effects of LMWHs.

16. Protamine sulfate; see textbook, p. 429, for details.

17. The dosage of warfarin is adjusted based on prolonging the INR. In general, the target range for the INR with warfarin therapy is 2.0 to 3.0 when treating atrial fibrillation, emboli stroke, MI, and DVT. When anticoagulating the patient with a mechanical prosthetic heart valve, the target INR range is 2.5 to 3.5.

18. In most cases of hemorrhage, the dosage of warfarin is withheld until the INR returns to therapeutic levels. In rare cases, vitamin K is administered. In cases of severe hemorrhage, a transfusion with plasma or whole blood may be required.

19. Streptokinase, urokinase, anistreplase, alteplase, reteplase, and tenecteplase.

20. Fibrinolytic agents are used to dissolve clots secondary to an MI, pulmonary or cerebral embolism, or deep vein thrombosis (DVT).

21. Three to seven days of continuous therapy are required.

22. To reduce risk of additional strokes in people who have had a stroke or TIA.

Drugs Used to Treat Thromboembolic Disorders

Learning Activities

FILL-IN-THE-BLANK

Finish each of the following statements using the correct term.

1. _____ is the process of formation of a fibrin blood clot, and _____ is a small fragment of a thrombus that breaks off and circulates until it becomes trapped in a capillary, causing either ischemia or infarction to the area distal to the obstruction.

2. The _____ agents are used to dissolve thromboemboli, once formed.

3. While receiving anticoagulant therapy, patients must limit intake of green leafy vegetables that contain vitamin _____.

4. A unique property of aspirin, when compared with other salicylates, is inhibition of _____ aggregation with prolongation of bleeding time.

5. Enoxaprin (Lovenox) is manufactured from heparin derived from _____ and should not be used in patients allergic to _____ byproducts.

6. Subcutaneous injection of heparin is usually made into the tissue over the _____.

7. _____ _____ is the antidote for heparin.

8. The class of drugs used to dissolve recently formed thrombi is known as _____ agents.

9. The therapeutic effect of heparin is monitored by the use of the laboratory test known as _____ time.

10. The antidote for excessive bleeding during warfarin therapy is _____.

MATCHING

Match the generic drug name with its corresponding brand name. Each option will be used only once.

_____ 11. warfarin

_____ 12. enoxaparin

_____ 13. ticlopidine

_____ 14. clopidogrel

_____ 15. dipyridamole

a. Plavix
b. Persantine
c. Lovenox
d. Coumadin
e. Ticlid

Select the laboratory test(s) used to monitor the drug therapy listed. Some options will not be used.

_____ 16. warfarin

_____ 17. heparin

a. whole blood clotting time
b. PT or INR
c. aPTT
d. bleeding time

TRUE OR FALSE

Write "T" for true and "F" for false for each statement. Correct all false statements.

_____ 18. The pharmacologic agents used to treat thromboembolic disease act either to prevent platelet aggregation or to inhibit a variety of steps in the fibrin clot formation cascade.

_____ 19. The primary purpose of anticoagulants is to dissolve an existing clot.

_____ 20. Patients with thromboembolic disorders of the lower extremities should be positioned in bed with the knees flexed and a pillow under the popliteal space.

_____ 21. The primary therapeutic outcome from dipyridamole (Persantine) therapy is prevention of blood clots secondary to artificial valve placement.

_____ 22. The use of clopidogrel (Plavix) and aspirin concurrently is contraindicated.

_____ 23. Early studies indicate that ticlopidine (Ticlid) is more effective in reducing the risk of strokes than aspirin, but the potential for adverse effects limits its use to patients who cannot tolerate aspirin therapy or who should not take aspirin.

_____ 24. Dalteparin (Fragmin) should not be administered intramuscularly.

_____ 25. To minimize bruising after subcutaneous administration of dalteparin (Fragmin), rub the injection site after completing the injection.

Drugs Used to Treat Thromboembolic Disorders

chapter

27

Practice Questions for the NCLEX® Examination

_____ 1. The anti-aggregatory effect of clopido-grel (Plavix) persists for approximately how many days after discontinuation of therapy?
1. 1
2. 2
3. 3
4. 5

_____ 2. Which herbal medicine will increase the risk for bleeding when administered with ticlopidine (Ticlid)?
1. St. John's wort
2. Ginkgo
3. Green tea
4. Echinacea

_____ 3. Before administering dalteparin (Fragmin), the nurse assesses the patient for an allergy to which substance?
1. Pork
2. Dairy
3. Penicillin
4. Shellfish

_____ 4. Which procedure does the nurse follow when administering heparin subcutane-ously?
1. Checks the current order and PT value before administering heparin
2. Injects within 1 inch of the umbilicus
3. Uses an 18-gauge 1-inch needle for the injection
4. After the needle is injected into the subcutaneous skin, does not aspirate

_____ 5. Which statement is true about type II heparin induced thrombocytopenia (HIT)?
1. Type II HIT should be suspected when the platelet count falls below 10,000/mm^3.
2. Type II HIT is an allergic reaction to heparin that causes aggregation of platelets.
3. Warfarin (Coumadin) therapy is con-traindicated in patients with type II HIT.
4. Aspirin therapy is contraindicated in patients with type II HIT.

_____ 6. Which statement does the nurse include when teaching a patient about warfarin (Coumadin) therapy?
1. "Warfarin is a potent anticoagulant that acts by inhibiting the activity of vitamin K, which is required for the activation of clotting factors in the blood."
2. "Warfarin is used to dissolve clots."
3. "Patients taking warfarin will need to have their PTT blood values moni-tored."
4. "Protamine sulfate is the antidote for warfarin overdose."

_____ 7. Which laboratory value does the nurse identify as ideal in a patient receiving warfarin (Coumadin) therapy?
1. Platelets at 10,000/mm^3
2. aPTT at 4.5 to 5.5 control
3. INR at 2 to 3
4. Serum cholesterol of 220 mg/dL

_____ 8. Which fibrinolytic agent requires concurrent use of heparin therapy?
1. Streptokinase
2. Urokinase
3. Atistreplase
4. Alteplase

_____ 9. When teaching a patient about nutrition related to warfarin (Coumadin) therapy, which statements does the nurse include? *(Select all that apply.)*
1. "Limit your intake of green leafy vegetables."
2. "Drink six to eight 8-ounce glasses of water daily."
3. "Carrots are to be excluded from your diet."
4. "You must not eat more than one serving of protein a day."
5. "Avoid foods that contain potassium."

_____ 10. Which adverse effects of ticlopidine (Ticlid) should be immediately reported to the health care provider? *(Select all that apply.)*
1. Nosebleed
2. Easy bruising
3. Dark, tarry stools
4. Blood in the urine
5. Anorexia

_____ 11. Which statements about enoxaparin (Lovenox) are true? *(Select all that apply.)*
1. Patients who are allergic to pork by-products should not receive enoxaparin.
2. Patients taking enoxaparin are at a higher risk of hemorrhage than patients taking heparin.
3. Enoxaparin is administered intramuscularly.
4. No special monitoring of clotting times such as aPTT are necessary for patients taking enoxaparin.
5. Enoxaparin has high antiplatelet activity.

_____ 12. An order is for heparin 8,000 units subcutaneously stat. The medication is available as 10,000 units/mL. What type of syringe does the nurse use?
1. U-100 insulin
2. U-50 insulin
3. 1 mL
4. 5 mL

13. A patient is ordered heparin 3,500 units subcutaneously every 12 hours. The medication is available as 5,000 units/mL. How many mL of heparin will the nurse administer? _____ mL

14. A patient is ordered warfarin (Coumadin) 5 mg per day by mouth. The medication is available as 2.5 mg per tablet. How many tablets will the patient use in a 7-day period? _____ tablets

Drugs Used to Treat Heart Failure

chapter
28

Review Sheet

The QUESTION column and the ANSWER column have been offset so that you can cover the answers while reading the questions, allowing you to assess your knowledge.

Question	Answer
1. What are the results of systolic dysfunction of the heart?	
2. What is the ultimate problem associated with diastolic dysfunction of the heart?	1. The result of systolic dysfunction of the heart is inability of the heart to contract with sufficient force to pump all the blood (decreased cardiac output) from the heart to maintain sufficient cardiac output to meet the body's oxygenation needs (decreased tissue perfusion).
3. What effect does the sympathetic nervous system's release of epinephrine and norepinephrine have on heart function?	2. Due to diastolic dysfunction of the heart, residual volume remains from the previous contraction and the left ventricle does not fill adequately prior to next contraction. The left ventricle develops a "stiffness," and back-pressure builds up in the lungs and peripheral vasculature that results in symptoms of pulmonary congestion and peripheral edema.
4. What is the effect of the renin-angiotensin-aldosterone system and vasopressin (antidiuretic hormone) in heart failure?	3. Epinephrine and norepinephrine are released producing tachycardia and an increase in cardiac contractility. The increased sympathetic stimulation also increases peripheral vasoconstriction, resulting in an increased afterload against which the heart must pump, causing a further decrease in cardiac output.
5. What is the result of decreased perfusion to the kidneys secondary to low cardiac output from heart failure?	4. The renin-angiotensin-aldosterone system stimulates renal distal tubule sodium and water retention in an effort to increase circulating blood volume, which increases preload to the heart. The increased production of vasopressin (antidiuretic hormone) from the pituitary gland increases water recovery from the kidneys and increases intravascular volume and preload.
6. What are the three main classes of drugs used to treat heart failure?	5. With reduced perfusion, the kidneys increase sodium resorption in the proximal tubules to help expand circulating blood volume. The increased intravascular volume initially improves tissue perfusion, but over time, excessive amounts of sodium and water are retained, causing increased pressure within the capillaries, resulting in edema.

7. What is the role of inotropic agents in the treatment of heart failure?

8. What is the role of diuretic therapy in the treatment of heart failure?

9. Summarize the role of vasodilator therapy in the treatment of heart failure.

10. What is the action of intravenous nitroglycerin, nitroprusside, and nesiritide?

11. List the six cardinal signs of heart disease and give a rationale for their occurrence.

12. What nursing assessments should be performed at regular intervals for the patient undergoing heart failure therapy?

13. Describe essential patient education and health promotion for patients being treated for heart failure.

14. What are the desired therapeutic outcomes of the digitalis glycosides (digoxin) for the treatment of heart failure?

15. What are the signs and symptoms of digitalis toxicity that the nurse would teach a patient to monitor for?

16. What data should be gathered *before* administering digoxin (Lanoxin)?

6. Heart failure is treated with a combination of vasodilator, inotropic, and diuretic therapy.

7. Inotropic agents stimulate the heart to increase the force of contraction, thus boosting cardiac output. This also helps reduce pulmonary congestion and improve tissue perfusion.

8. As renal perfusion is improved, potent diuretics are administered to enhance sodium and water excretion. This provides substantial symptomatic relief to the patient in addition to reducing the workload on the heart.

9. The vasodilators are used to reduce preload and afterload in patients with heart failure.

10. These drugs are vasodilators that reduce cardiac preload and afterload.

11. The six cardinal signs of heart disease are dyspnea, associated with inadequate tissue perfusion and diastolic dysfunction; chest pain, resulting from inadequate oxygen to support myocardium function; fatigue, due to depleted oxygen to body tissue; edema, because the left ventricle is not pumping adequate volumes of blood and a back-pressure builds up in the lungs (causing dyspnea) and the peripheral blood vessels, causing interstitial edema; syncope, due to insufficient oxygen to meet the brain's needs; and palpitations, caused by sympathetic nervous system's release of epinephrine and norepinephrine that produces tachycardia and dysrhythmias.

12. Mental status, vital signs (T, P, R), blood pressure, heart and lung sounds, skin color, neck vein status, presence of clubbing, central venous pressure, abdomen size, fluid volume status, nutrition, activity and exercise tolerance, anxiety level, and laboratory tests should be checked regularly to assess cardiac function.

13. See textbook, pp. 441-442.

14. The primary therapeutic outcomes expected from digoxin therapy are improved cardiac output resulting in improved tissue perfusion, and improved tolerance to activity as demonstrated by the ability to perform ADLs without supplemental oxygen therapy or fatigue.

15. The nurse would teach the patient that common symptoms of digoxin toxicity include anorexia, nausea, vomiting, bradycardia, visual disturbances, and psychiatric disturbances.

17. Under what conditions should two qualified nurses check a dose of digoxin?

18. When should serum levels of digoxin be obtained?

19. Why should a patient taking digoxin be cautioned not to take an antacid within 2 hours of taking the digitalis without first consulting the physician?

20. What effect can the concurrent use of a digoxin and a diuretic have?

21. What is the treatment for digoxin toxicity?

22. What is the action of phosphodiesterase inhibitors (inamrinone) in the treatment of heart failure?

23. Name two phosphodiesterase inhibitors used to treat heart failure.

24. What is the action of ACE inhibitors in the treatment of heart failure?

25. What is the action of nesiritide (Natrecor)?

16. Before administering digoxin, the apical pulse should be taken for one full minute. Institution guidelines for withholding the drug should be followed; for example, if pulse is fewer than 60 or greater than 100 beats per minute. Consult the physician before administering the prescribed dose if the apical rate is below 60 beats per minute in an adult, or below 90 beats per minute in a child. In the long-term care setting, radial pulse may be acceptable. Before initiating therapy, baseline data such as vital signs, lung sounds, weight, and laboratory studies should be obtained. The patient should be monitored for development of digitalis toxicity, hypokalemia, hypomagnesemia, or sudden increase in pulse rate that previously had been normal.

17. Any time the dose requires calculation, two qualified nurses should check the dose.

18. Draw blood to measure the level of digoxin before the daily dose or at least 6 hours after administration of the last dose of digoxin.

19. An antacid taken with digoxin reduces the absorption of digoxin.

20. Diuretics may induce hypokalemia, which may result in signs of digoxin toxicity.

21. To treat for digoxin toxicity, stop digoxin, stop potassium-depleting diuretic, check potassium level, and administer prescribed potassium if deficient. If signs of toxicity are severe and life-threatening, the antidote for digoxin, digoxin immune Fab (Digibind), may be administered.

22. Phosphodiesterase inhibitors (inamrinone) are inotropic agents that increase the force and velocity of myocardial contractions by inhibiting cyclic adenosine monophosphate (cAMP) phosphodiesterase activity, and increase cellular levels of cAMP in the heart muscle. It is also a vascular smooth muscle relaxant that causes vasodilatation, reducing preload and afterload.

23. Two phosphodiesterase inhibitors used to treat heart failure are inamrinone and milrinone (Primacor).

24. ACE inhibitors reduce afterload by blocking angiotensin II-mediated peripheral vasoconstriction promoting vasodilation; they also reduce circulating blood volume by inhibiting aldosterone, allowing excretion of excess water.

25. It is a human B-type natriuretic peptide (hBNP) that is a hormone normally secreted by the cardiac ventricles in response to fluid and pressure overload. It helps the heart recover from deteriorating cardiac function by reducing preload and afterload pressures, increasing diuresis and sodium excretion, suppressing the renin-angiotensin-aldosterone system, and reducing secretion of norepinephrine.

Drugs Used to Treat Heart Failure

Learning Activities

FILL-IN-THE-BLANK

Finish each of the following statements using the correct term.

1. _____ agents are used in the treatment of heart failure to increase the force of contractions, thus boosting cardiac output.

2. The two primary actions of digoxin glycosides on the heart are positive _____ and negative _____.

3. _____ is the term used to describe giving a loading dose of digitalis to a patient over the period of hours or days necessary to produce the desired cardiac effect.

4. The antidote for severe digoxin intoxication is _____.

5. _____ is the first of a new class of drugs, the human B-type natriuretic peptides.

6. The most commonly reported adverse effects of inamrinone therapy include _____ and _____.

7. The _____ pulse should be taken for _____ minute before administering digoxin in a hospital setting.

8. The _____ represent a major breakthrough in the treatment of heart failure.

MATCHING

Match the drug class with the corresponding drug. Each definition will be used only once.

_____ 9. inamrinone

_____ 10. captopril (Capoten)

_____ 11. nesiritide (Natrecor)

_____ 12. digoxin (Lanoxin)

a. digitalis glycoside
b. phosphodiesterase inhibitor
c. ACE inhibitor
d. natriuretic peptide

TRUE OR FALSE

Write "T" for true and "F" for false for each statement. Correct all false statements.

_____ 13. Nesiritide (Natrecor) is used as a vasodilator in patients with severe heart failure who have dyspnea at rest or with minimal activity.

_____ 14. Large studies have shown that ACE inhibitors reduce morbidity and mortality associated with heart failure.

_____ 15. Inamrinone has been found to be the most effective treatment for diastolic heart failure.

_____ 16. If heart failure is acute, most therapy will be administered intravenously in an intensive care unit.

_____ 17. Inamrinone should be diluted with dextrose solutions.

_____ 18. The beta blockers used in the treatment of heart failure inhibit renin release, diminishing the cascade of the renin-angiotensin-aldosterone systems that would induce vasoconstriction and sodium reabsorption.

Drugs Used to Treat Heart Failure

Practice Questions for the NCLEX® Examination

_____ 1. A patient receives a daily dose of digitalis at 0800 hours. At what time does the nurse perform a blood draw to assess the serum digitalis level?
   1. 0800
   2. 1000
   3. 1200
   4. 1400

_____ 2. What is a common early symptom of digitalis toxicity in the older adult?
   1. Gastric irritation
   2. Low blood pressure
   3. Anorexia and mild nausea
   4. Urticaria

_____ 3. Which daily oral maintenance doses of digoxin (Lanoxin) does the nurse question before administering the medication to an adult? *(Select all that apply.)*
   1. 0.125 mg
   2. 0.25 mg
   3. 0.50 mg
   4. 1.25 mg
   5. 1.50 mg

_____ 4. The nurse teaches patients with heart failure to make which dietary modification?
   1. Restrict sodium intake.
   2. Limit protein intake.
   3. Avoid carbohydrates.
   4. Drink 10 to 12 glasses of fluid daily.

_____ 5. Which position is most beneficial for a patient experiencing signs and symptoms of heart failure?
   1. Sims'
   2. Trendelenberg
   3. Semi-Fowler's
   4. Lithotomy

_____ 6. Which factor is the best indicator of fluid gain or loss in a patient with heart failure?
   1. Daily weight
   2. Intake and output record
   3. Hematocrit and hemoglobin
   4. Blood pressure

_____ 7. Which statement does the nurse include while teaching proper therapeutic regimen management for a patient with heart failure?
   1. "Take your medications only on the days when you feel you need them."
   2. "Report signs of digitalis toxicity such as anorexia, nausea, slow heart rate below 60 or high heart rate above 100, or changes in your mental status."
   3. "Weigh yourself every 3 days."
   4. "Take diuretics at bedtime for the most beneficial effect."

_____ 8. Prior to administration of digitalis, what is most important for the nurse to assess?
   1. Hypokalemia
   2. Hypocalcemia
   3. Hypomagnesemia
   4. Hyponatremia

_____ 9. Which drug used to treat heart failure is most likely to cause thrombocytopenia?
   1. Inamrinone
   2. Nesiritide (Natrecor)
   3. Digoxin (Lanoxin)
   4. Metoprolol (Toprol)

_____ 10. A patient receiving digoxin (Lanoxin) for heart failure informs the nurse that he also takes St. John's wort. What is most important for the nurse to assess?
1. Altered electrolyte balance
2. Enhanced therapeutic and toxic effect of digoxin
3. Reduced therapeutic effect of digoxin
4. Increased urinary output

_____ 11. Which are signs and symptoms of digitalis toxicity? (*Select all that apply.*)
1. Anorexia
2. Nausea and vomiting
3. Bradycardia
4. Thrombocytopenia
5. Psychiatric disturbances

_____ 12. The nurse is preparing to administer digoxin (Lanoxin) to a child. The nurse informs the health care provider after the child's pulse rate is measured at how many beats per minute?
1. 85
2. 95
3. 100
4. 105

_____ 13. Which statements about milrinone (Primacor) are true? (*Select all that apply.*)
1. It is a negative inotropic agent.
2. It causes vasoconstriction.
3. It should not be infused in the same IV line as furosemide.
4. Its most common adverse effects are dysrhythmias and hypotension.
5. It is a natriuretic peptide.

_____ 14. Which statements does the nurse include when teaching a patient about digoxin (Lanoxin) therapy for the treatment of heart failure? (*Select all that apply.*)
1. "Take your pulse for one full minute before taking the digoxin. If your pulse is fewer than 80 beats per minute, do not take the medicine."
2. "Weigh yourself every other day and report a weight gain of 5 pounds or more in a 2-day period."
3. "Call your health care provider if you develop a cough."
4. "You will need to take these medications as lifelong treatment and adhere to them as prescribed to gain control of the disease."
5. "Inform your health care provider if you have difficulty with red-green color perception."

15. A patient is ordered digoxin elixir (Lanoxin) 0.25 mg PO daily at 0800. The medication is available as 50 mcg/mL. How many mL does the nurse administer? _____ mL

16. A patient is ordered digoxin (Lanoxin) 600 mcg IV stat. The medication label reads digoxin injection 2 mL 500 mcg (0.5 mg) in 2 mL. How many mL of the medication does the nurse administer? _____ mL

Drugs Used for Diuresis

Review Sheet

The QUESTION column and the ANSWER column have been offset so you can cover the answer while reading the question, allowing you to assess your knowledge.

Question	Answer
1. Explain the therapeutic outcomes associated with diuretic therapy.	
2. What laboratory tests should be performed to determine if kidney function is impaired?	1. The therapeutic outcomes of diuretic therapy are diuresis with reduction of edema and improvement in the symptoms of fluid overload and reduced blood pressure.
3. What laboratory studies should be performed whenever a diuretic is prescribed?	2. Check for elevated BUN and serum creatinine; also check for decreased creatinine clearance, decreased urine output, and increasing edema.
4. What patient assessments should be performed on a regular basis when diuretics are being taken?	3. Check Hct, serum electrolytes, blood glucose, uric acid, BUN, and serum creatinine.
5. What is the action of a diuretic?	4. Assess intake and output of fluids, state of hydration, presence of edema, heart rate and rhythm, blood pressure bid or qid, and daily weights. Check for signs and symptoms of electrolyte imbalance, gastric irritation, rash, hyperuricemia, and hyperglycemia. Monitor for drug interactions (e.g., digitalis glycosides, corticosteroids, lithium).
6. What are the five classes of diuretics?	5. Diuretics inhibit the reabsorption of sodium, increasing the loss of water.
7. Which class of diuretic has the most rapid onset of action? (List three loop diuretics.) What three routes of administration can be used for loop diuretics?	6. The five classes of diuretics are; carbonic anhydrase inhibitors, sulfonamide-type (loop diuretics), thiazide, potassium-sparing, and combination diuretics. Thiazides and potassium-sparing diuretics are available as combination products.
8. What is the primary therapeutic outcome associated with sulfonamide loop diuretic therapy?	7. Sulfonamide-type loop diuretics are the most rapid-acting diuretics. Furosemide (Lasix), bumetanide (Bumex), and ethacrynic acid (Edecrin). Oral (PO), intramuscular (IM), or intravenous (IV) routes.
9. When would loop diuretics be prescribed?	8. Diuresis with reduction of edema and improvement in symptoms related to excessive fluid accumulation.
10. Of the four loop diuretics, which is most frequently prescribed?	9. When rapid diuresis is needed (e.g., in pulmonary edema) or when renal function is diminished.

11. Would thiazide or loop diuretics be used when renal function is impaired?

12. What classes of diuretics can cause a loss of serum potassium (hypokalemia)?

13. What class(es) of diuretic(s) can cause an increase in serum potassium (hyperkalemia)?

14. Why would a potassium-sparing and another type of diuretic be prescribed simultaneously?

15. What actions can be taken to prevent and/or treat hypokalemia?

16. What actions can be taken to prevent hyperkalemia when potassium-sparing diuretics are prescribed?

17. Are diuretics useful for edema that occurs during pregnancy?

18. What medicine may need to be ordered for patients who have gouty arthritis who require diuretics?

19. Which type of diuretic has been associated with hearing loss when used concurrently with aminoglycoside antibiotics or cisplatin?

20. What class of antibiotics can cause hearing loss and, if combined with loop diuretics, may increase the possibility of ototoxicity?

21. After reading that diuretics can interact with digoxin (Lanoxin) to produce digoxin toxicity, what signs and symptoms would you monitor when therapy is combined?

22. What are the normal values for sodium, potassium, and chloride?

23. List six foods that are good sources of potassium.

24. Why should salicylates not be taken with furosemide (Lasix) for prolonged periods?

25. Describe the signs and symptoms of salicylate toxicity.

26. Which class of diuretics can affect the male libido?

27. Why are potassium-sparing diuretics not used in patients with renal failure?

28. What are the signs and symptoms of circulatory overload?

10. Furosemide (Lasix).

11. Loop diuretics are more effective than other classes of diuretics when renal function is impaired (decreased creatinine clearance).

12. Thiazide and loop diuretics

13. Potassium-sparing diuretics

14. To prevent hypokalemia, improve diuresis, and lower blood pressure

15. Give potassium supplements and/or increase dietary intake of foods rich in potassium.

16. Do not use salt substitutes that contain potassium. Maintain an adequate fluid intake. Do not administer potassium supplements. Use ACE inhibitors, angiotensin II receptor blockers, eplerenone (Inspra), and NSAIDs with extreme caution to prevent hyperkalemia.

17. Diuretics are rarely used for edema associated with pregnancy. Diuretics cross the placental barrier and may be harmful to the fetus. Consult a physician before taking any medication during pregnancy or while breastfeeding.

18. Allopurinol (Zyloprim)

19. Loop diuretics

20. Aminoglycosides: gentamicin (Vancocin), tobramycin, amikacin (Amikin).

21. Anorexia, nausea, fatigue, blurred or colored vision, bradycardia, dysrhythmias.

22. Sodium: 135–145 mEq/L; potassium: 3.5–4.7 mEq/L; chloride: 95–105 mEq/L.

23. Dried almonds; apricots, raw; avocados, raw; bananas, raw; beans, lima (cooked, boiled); carrots, raw; cocoa, plain; potatoes (cooked, boiled).

24. The potential for salicylate toxicity may be increased if taken concurrently for several days.

25. Nausea, tinnitus, fever, sweating, dizziness, mental confusion, lethargy, and impaired hearing

26. Potassium-sparing diuretics (e.g., amiloride [Midamor], spironolactone [Aldactone])

27. They are usually not effective as diuretics in moderate to severe renal failure and may cause hyperkalemia.

29. What premedication assessments should be made before administering any type of diuretic?

28. Bounding, full pulse; jugular vein distention; dyspnea; frothy sputum; cough.

29. Baseline vital signs, lung sounds, weight, assessment of degree of edema, level of consciousness, muscle strength, tremors, general appearance; blood glucose levels for patients with diabetes. Baseline laboratory studies as prescribed by physician.

Drugs Used for Diuresis

Learning Activities

FILL-IN-THE-BLANK

Finish each of the following statements using the correct term.

1. The thiazide and loop diuretics act directly on the _____ _____ to inhibit the reabsorption of sodium and chloride from the lumen of the tubule.

2. _____ is the term used to describe excess fluid accumulation in the extracellular spaces.

3. Furosemide (Lasix) may inhibit the excretion of uric acid, resulting in _____.

4. _____ is a potassium-sparing diuretic that also has weak antihypertensive activity.

5. Because the chemical structure of _____ is similar to that of estrogenic hormones, an occasional male patient will report gynecomastia, reduced libido, and diminished erection.

6. The most common problem associated with thiazide diuretic therapy is _____.

7. The most frequently used loop diuretic is _____.

8. _____ is known to occur when a loop diuretic is combined with an aminoglycoside or cisplatin.

9. Diabetic patients receiving a diuretic must be checked regularly for _____.

10. _____ _____ is a loop diuretic which can be used in conjunction with 0.9% sodium chloride infusions to enhance excretion of calcium in patients with hypercalcemia.

MATCHING

Match the generic drug name with its corresponding brand name. Each option will be used only once.

_____ 11. acetazolamide

_____ 12. bumetanide

_____ 13. ethacrynic acid

_____ 14. furosemide

_____ 15. amiloride

_____ 16. triamterene

a. Dyrenium
b. Midamor
c. Lasix
d. Edecrin
e. Bumex
f. Diamox

TRUE OR FALSE

Write "T" for true and "F" for false for each statement. Correct all false statements.

_____ 17. Diuretics are mainstays of treatment in two major diseases affecting the cardiovascular system: heart failure and hypertension.

_____ 18. Acetazolamide (Diamox) is used to reduce cerebral edema.

_____ 19. When a patient is overhydrated, hematocrit and hemoglobin values drop as a result of hemodilution.

_____ 20. The most appropriate time to administer diuretics to a patient is at bedtime.

_____ 21. Acetazolamide (Diamox) is a weak diuretic that acts by inhibiting the enzyme carbonic anhydrase within the kidney, brain, and eye.

_____ 22. Diuresis is occasionally noted when aminophylline is used in the treatment of asthma.

_____ 23. Furosemide (Lasix) is one of the most potent and effective diuretics currently available.

_____ 24. Patients who are diabetic and taking furosemide (Lasix) therapy must be monitored for the development of hypoglycemia, particularly during the early weeks of therapy.

Drugs Used for Diuresis

chapter

29

Practice Questions for the NCLEX® Examination

_____ 1. When assessing a patient who is overhy-drated, which assessment finding does the nurse expect to see?
   1. Poor skin turgor
   2. Deteriorating vital signs
   3. Deeply furrowed tongue
   4. Neck vein engorgement

_____ 2. A patient who has received IV fluids in excess of fluids excreted is likely to develop which electrolyte imbalance?
   1. Hypokalemia
   2. Hyperkalemia
   3. Hyponatremia
   4. Hypernatremia

_____ 3. Patients taking potassium-sparing diuretics should be instructed to avoid which food or food substitute?
   1. Salt substitutes
   2. Chicken
   3. Sugar substitutes
   4. Milk products

_____ 4. A patient is currently taking digoxin (Lanoxin), aminoglycosides, nonsteroidal anti-inflammatory drugs (NSAIDs), and corticosteroids for multiple medical problems. Bumetanide (Bumex) has now been prescribed. Which principle does the nurse consider in monitoring this patient?
   1. The amount of digoxin will need to be increased.
   2. The potential for ototoxicity from the aminoglycosides is increased.
   3. The dose of bumetanide will need to be decreased when also taking NSAIDs.
   4. The use of corticosteroids and bumetanide may cause hyperkalemia.

_____ 5. A patient taking ethacrynic acid (Edecrin) is most at risk for the development of dizziness, deafness, and tinnitus when he or she also has which condition?
   1. Liver disease
   2. A hearing deficit
   3. Impaired renal function
   4. A history of myocardial infarction

_____ 6. Which electrolyte imbalance is most likely to develop as a result of spironolactone (Aldactone) therapy?
   1. Hyperkalemia
   2. Hypercalcemia
   3. Hypermagnesemia
   4. Hypernatremia

_____ 7. Which statements does the nurse include when teaching a patient about diuretic therapy? _(Select all that apply.)_
   1. "If you are taking Aldactone, avoid the use of salt substitutes in your diet."
   2. "You should rise slowly from a lying or sitting position and lie down if you feel faint, because some diuretics cause you to develop low blood pressure in certain positions."
   3. "You should take your diuretic pill before you go to sleep."
   4. "Weigh yourself every day and call your primary health care provider if you note a one-pound weight gain in one day."
   5. "The purpose of diuretics is to increase the net loss of water."

_____ 8. Which drugs may potentially interact
with bumetanide (Bumex)? *(Select all that
apply.)*
  1. Ibuprofen (Motrin)
  2. Dexamethasone (Decadron)
  3. Digoxin (Lanoxin)
  4. Morphine sulfate
  5. Probenecid

_____ 9. Which electrolytes are most commonly
altered due to furosemide (Lasix) therapy? *(Select all that apply.)*
  1. Potassium
  2. Sodium
  3. Chloride
  4. Magnesium
  5. Calcium

_____ 10. A patient with type 2 diabetes mellitus
and congestive heart failure is being
treated with metformin (Glucophage),
warfarin (Coumadin), and digitalis. The
patient has a new order for bumetanide
(Bumex). Upon review of the chart, the
nurse learns that the patient is allergic to
furosemide (Lasix). What does the nurse
do next? *(Select all that apply.)*
  1. Discontinues the bumetanide because there is a cross-allergy with
furosemide.
  2. Increases the amount of green leafy
vegetables in the patient's diet because bumetanide decreases the anticoagulant effect of warfarin.
  3. Obtains an order to increase the dose
of digitalis because bumetanide reduces the effectiveness of digitalis.
  4. Increases citrus fruits, tomatoes,
bananas, dates, and apricots in the
patient's diet.
  5. Assesses blood sugar because bumetanide may decrease the hypoglycemic effects of metformin.

_____ 11. A male patient with hypertension is prescribed spironolactone (Aldactone) therapy. Which instruction does the nurse
include when teaching the patient about
this therapy?
  1. "Avoid salt in your diet as well as
salt substitutes."
  2. "Take spironolactone on an empty
stomach."
  3. "Be sure to increase the amounts of
tomatoes and citrus in your diet."
  4. "If you develop breast tenderness,
immediately stop taking the spironolactone."

_____ 12. A patient is prescribed acetazolamide (Diamox) 375 mg PO at 1000.
Acetazolamide is available in 125-mg
and 250-mg tablets. What does the nurse
administer to the patient?
  1. Three 125-mg tablets
  2. One 125-mg tablet and one 250-mg
tablet
  3. One 250-mg tablet and one-half of a
250-mg tablet
  4. One-half of a 250-mg tablet and one
250-mg tablet

Drugs Used to Treat Upper Respiratory Disease

Review Sheet

The QUESTION column and the ANSWER column have been offset so you can cover the answer while reading the question, allowing you to assess your knowledge.

Question	Answer
1. What is allergic rhinitis?	1. Inflamed nasal mucosa associated with an allergic reaction.
2. What are the drugs of choice for treating allergic rhinitis?	2. Antihistamines
3. What is the mechanism of action of decongestants?	3. Decongestants are alpha-adrenergic receptor stimulants that constrict blood vessels in the nasal passages, reducing swollen tissues and obstruction.
4. What is a "rebound" effect associated with nasally administered decongestants?	4. Excessive or prolonged use of nasal decongestants causes a rebound swelling in the nasal passages that requires further use of nasal decongestants to unblock nasal passages. It is difficult to break this cycle, so it is particularly important not to overuse nasal decongestants.
5. Name two commonly used decongestants administered intranasally, and one administered orally.	5. Pseudoephedrine (Sudafed)—oral tablets; phenylephrine (Neo-Synephrine)—nasal spray; oxymetazoline (Afrin)—nasal spray; xylometazoline (Otrivin)—nasal spray. See Table 30-1.
6. Explain how to administer a nasal spray, nose drops, and medications by inhalation.	6. See Chapter 8, pp. 119-121.
7. What response does histamine release have on the mucous membranes?	7. Urticaria (itching), redness, and edema.
8. What is an antigen?	8. A substance that elicits an immunologic response such as the production of a specific antibody against that substance.
9. When is histamine released?	9. In cases of tissue damage (trauma), allergic reactions, and infection.
10. How do antihistamines act?	10. Histamines block the H_1 receptor sites on the target cells; they do not affect the amount or the release of histamine.
11. What adverse effects can be anticipated whenever an antihistamine is administered?	11. Sedation and dryness of mucous membranes (anticholinergic effects)
12. What actions should be initiated to offset the drying effects of antihistamines?	12. Consume an adequate fluid intake of 8–12 8-oz glasses daily.
13. What patient education should accompany the use of antihistamines?	

14. What is the action of cromolyn sodium (Nasalcrom)?

15. What condition is treated with cromolyn sodium (Nasalcrom) that affects the upper respiratory tract?

16. What are the desired therapeutic outcomes from the use of respiratory anti-inflammatory agents?

17. When a drug monograph says that a drug produces anticholinergic effects, what does this mean?

13. Maintain adequate hydration. If the person knows he/she is going to be exposed to an allergen (e.g., pollen outdoors), take the dose 30–45 minutes prior to possible exposure to block receptors before histamine can attach. If exposure is unanticipated, take a dose immediately upon recognition of an allergic response (e.g., runny nose and burning, itchy eyes). Exercise caution when operating any power equipment or while driving because of the medicine's sedative effects.

14. Cromolyn prevents release of histamine from its storage sites, the mast cells.

15. Cromolyn is used with other medications to treat severe allergic rhinitis and prevent release of histamine that causes the symptoms of allergic rhinitis.

16. Reduction in rhinorrhea, rhinitis, itching, and sneezing.

17. Blurred vision; constipation; urinary retention; dryness of mucosa of mouth, throat, and nose.

Drugs Used to Treat Upper Respiratory Disease

chapter

30

Learning Activities

FILL-IN-THE-BLANK

Finish each of the following statements using the correct term.

1. _____ is defined as inflammation of the nasal mucous membranes.

2. The respiratory function of the nose is to _____ , humidify, and _____ the air inhaled to prepare it for the lower respiratory airways.

3. A(n) _____ is a physiologic reflex used by the body to clear the nasal passages of foreign matter.

4. Overuse of topical decongestants may lead to a rebound of nasal secretions known as _____ _____ .

5. _____ are the drugs of choice in treating allergic rhinitis.

6. Decongestants cause the blood vessels in the nasal mucosa to _____ .

MATCHING

Match the generic drug name with its corresponding brand name. Each option will be used only once.

_____ 7. mometasone

_____ 8. fluticasone

_____ 9. budesonide

_____ 10. fexofenadine

_____ 11. ipratropium

_____ 12. oxymetazoline

_____ 13. pseudoephedrine

_____ 14. loratidine

_____ 15. levocetirizine

_____ 16. ciclesonide

a. Afrin
b. Allegra
c. Sudafed
d. Atrovent
e. Claritin
f. Flonase
g. Nasonex
h. Rhinocort Aqua
i. Xyzal
j. Omnaris

TRUE OR FALSE

Write "T" for true and "F" for false for each statement. Correct all false statements.

_____ 17. Cholinergic stimulation causes vasodilatation of the blood vessels lining the nasal mucosa, and sympathetic stimulation causes vasoconstriction.

_____ 18. The common cold is actually a bacterial infection of the upper respiratory tissues.

_____ 19. The medical term used for a runny nose is *rhinorrhea*.

_____ 20. When an antigen-antibody reaction takes place and histamine is released, it reacts with the H_1 receptors in the bronchioles resulting in bronchodilation.

_____ 21. A paradoxical effect from antihistamines often seen in children and older adults is central nervous system stimulation rather than sedation, which may cause insomnia, nervousness, and irritability.

_____ 22. Adult patients with blocked nasal passages should be encouraged to use a decongestant just before intranasal cromolyn sodium (Nasalcrom) administration to ensure adequate penetration.

Drugs Used to Treat Upper Respiratory Disease

Practice Questions for the NCLEX® Examination

_____ 1. What findings does the nurse typically assess in a patient experiencing a severe allergic reaction? *(Select all that apply.)*
   1. Hypertension
   2. Dry skin
   3. Urticaria
   4. Bronchospasms
   5. Tachycardia

_____ 2. Antihistamines used for the treatment of allergic rhinitis reduce which manifestations in a patient? *(Select all that apply.)*
   1. Nasal pruritus
   2. Sneezing
   3. Rhinorrhea
   4. Nasal congestion
   5. Lacrimation

_____ 3. The nurse consults with the prescriber before administering a sympathomimetic decongestant to a patient with which conditions? *(Select all that apply.)*
   1. Diabetes mellitus
   2. Glaucoma
   3. Allergy to shellfish
   4. Hypothyroidism
   5. Prostatic hyperplasia

_____ 4. What are potential anticholinergic adverse effects of antihistamine therapy? *(Select all that apply.)*
   1. Diarrhea
   2. Blurred vision
   3. Dry mouth
   4. Urinary retention
   5. Stuffy nose

_____ 5. Which statement does the nurse include when teaching a patient about the use of cromolyn sodium (Nasalcrom)?
   1. "Cromolyn sodium should be administered after the body receives a stimulus to release histamine."
   2. "Cromolyn sodium causes bronchodilation."
   3. "A 2- to 4-week course of therapy is usually required to determine clinical response."
   4. "Cromolyn sodium should be discontinued when the desired therapeutic response is achieved."

_____ 6. Which statements does the nurse include when teaching a patient about the use of topical decongestants and intranasal corticosteroids for allergic seasonal rhinitis? *(Select all that apply.)*
   1. "Take your intranasal corticosteroid first, followed by the topical decongestant."
   2. "Be sure to blow your nose thoroughly before administering the nasal therapy."
   3. "Immediately discontinue the therapy if you experience nasal burning."
   4. "The therapeutic effect is usually not immediate, so be sure to follow the medical regimen fully, as most patients usually do not experience full benefit of the therapy for a few days."
   5. "Take the medication all year to maintain a steady blood level of the drug."

_____ 7. Which statements about cromolyn sodium (Nasalcrom) are true? *(Select all that
apply.)*
  1. Cromolyn must be taken before exposure to the stimulus that initiates
an attack of allergic rhinitis.
  2. Cromolyn has no direct bronchodila-
tory or antihistaminic activities.
  3. Cromolyn does not relieve nasal congestion.
  4. Patients who experience coughing
when taking cromolyn should notify
their primary health care provider.
  5. The full therapeutic benefit is usually
not evident until after 3 to 6 weeks of
therapy.

8. A patient is prescribed mometasone (Nasonex)
2 sprays (100 mcg) in each nostril once daily.
The medication is available in 120 actuations/
bottle. The nurse expects this bottle of medication to last the patient how many days before a
refill is needed? _____ day(s)

9. A patient is prescribed desloratadine (Clarinex)
5 mg PO daily at 1000. The medication is available as 5 mg/10 mL syrup. How many mL of
the medication does the nurse administer?
_____ mL

Drugs Used to Treat Lower Respiratory Disease

Review Sheet

The QUESTION column and the ANSWER column have been offset so that you can cover the answers while reading the questions, allowing you to assess your knowledge.

Question	Answer
1. Define *ventilation, perfusion,* and *diffusion*.	
2. What are the differences between obstructive and restrictive respiratory diseases?	1. Ventilation is the movement of air in and out of the lungs; perfusion is blood flow through the pulmonary arteries to the capillaries surrounding the alveoli to the pulmonary veins; and diffusion is the process by which oxygen passes across the alveolar membrane to the blood in the capillaries and carbon dioxide passes from the blood to the alveolar sacs.
3. Why are pulmonary function tests performed?	2. Obstructive disease is associated with narrowed air passages and increasing resistance to air flow (e.g., asthma, acute bronchitis). Restrictive airway disease is characterized by restricted alveolar expansion due to loss of elasticity of tissue or physical deformity of the chest itself.
4. Why is the SaO_2 ratio valuable in an assessment of respiratory function?	3. To assess ventilation and diffusion capacity of the lungs and to determine whether medicines are having a therapeutic effect.
5. What is asthma?	4. It reflects the percent of oxygen bound to the hemoglobin compared with the maximum amount of oxygen that could be attached.
6. What is bronchitis?	5. Asthma is a common chronic airway disease characterized by inflammation of the bronchi and bronchioles.
7. What is emphysema?	6. Bronchitis is a condition in which chronic irritation causes inflammation and edema with excessive mucus secretion leading to airflow obstruction.
8. What are the goals of therapy for asthma?	7. Emphysema is a disease of alveolar destruction without fibrosis. Alveolar sacs lose elasticity and collapse during exhalation, trapping air within the lung.
9. What is the action of expectorants?	8. Goals are: maintain normal activity levels, maintain near-normal pulmonary function rates, prevent chronic and troublesome symptoms, prevent recurrent exacerbations, and avoid adverse effects from asthma medications.

10. What is the action of an antitussive agent?

11. What is the action of a mucolytic agent?

12. What is the purpose of administering a bronchodilator?

13. What types of drugs are known as *anti-inflammatory agents*?

14. What data should be collected as part of a respiratory assessment?

15. Explain desirable peak expiratory flow (PEF) used to assess the severity of asthma symptoms.

16. What dietary considerations should be made for a person with a respiratory disease?

17. How should people with known respiratory disease prevent infection?

18. What medication administration considerations should be made for the delivery of aerosol therapy to a child or older adult?

19. Cite important aspects of patient education and health promotion for individuals with a lower respiratory disease.

20. What posture does a dyspneic patient assume?

21. Describe appropriate health teaching for patients requiring respiratory therapy.

22. What is the primary action of guaifenesin (Robitussin)?

23. What precautions must be used when administering potassium iodide (SSKI)?

9. Expectorants liquefy mucus by stimulating the secretion of natural lubricant fluids from the serous glands.

10. Antitussives suppress the cough center in the brain.

11. Mucolytic agents reduce stickiness and viscosity of pulmonary secretions by acting directly on the mucus plugs to cause dissolution.

12. Bronchodilators relax the smooth muscle of the tracheobronchial tree allowing increased opening of the bronchioles and alveolar ducts, which decreases resistance to airflow into the alveolar sacs.

13. Corticosteroids are the most effective anti-inflammatory agents. Other agents are leukotriene modifiers and cromolyn.

14. See textbook, pp. 482-483.

15. See textbook, p. 479; p. 482.

16. A person with a respiratory disease should consume a well-balanced diet to maintain near-normal weight. Patients with dyspnea should be encouraged to eat small servings throughout day, take small bites, and eat slowly. Pulmocare, a nutritional supplement may be prescribed. Patients should avoid foods known to increase production of mucus (e.g., milk, chocolate). If the patient requires oxygen, it should be administered via nasal cannula during mealtime. If certain foods exacerbate respiratory conditions, they should be avoided.

17. Good hygiene; influenza and pneumococcal vaccinations. Seek medical attention at earliest signs of suspected infection.

18. See textbook, p. 485.

19. See textbook, pp. 484-486.

20. Sits upright and leans forward from the waist, resting the elbows on the knees. When hospitalized, will be placed in a high-Fowler's position.

21. See pp. 484-486, Patient Education and Health Promotion.

22. Guaifenesin (Robitussin) enhances the output of respiratory tract fluid. This increased flow of secretions decreases mucus viscosity and promotes ciliary action. A combination of ciliary action and coughing then expels the phlegm from the pulmonary system.

24. When should SSKI not be administered?

25. What types of respiratory diseases may be treated with mucolytic agents [e.g., acetylcysteine (Mucomyst)]?

26. The patient receiving medication by inhalation should be placed in what position?

27. The patient who has received a medication by inhalation should be instructed to exhale through _____ lips.

28. What patient teaching should be performed for a patient taking an expectorant?

29. What is the desired action for giving saline solution by nebulizer?

30. What classes of antitussive agents are available?

31. What are the major drawbacks to using an opiate antitussive?

32. In what type of patient must great caution be exercised if an opiate antitussive is to be administered?

33. Give one example of an antitussive agent.

34. What premedication assessments should be made prior to administering an antitussive agent, potassium iodide, saline solutions, mucolytic agent, expectorant, anticholinergic bronchodilating agent, xanthine derivative bronchodilating agent, respiratory anti-inflammatory agent, antileukotriene agents, beta-adrenergic bronchodilating agents, miscellaneous anti-inflammatory agents, and immunomodulators?

35. What are the four components of asthma therapy?

36. Review the premedication assessments associated with acetylcysteine (Mucomyst) therapy.

23. Potassium iodide (SSKI) should be diluted in water, milk, or fruit juice. The medication should be taken with food to minimize gastric irritation.

24. Do *not* give to a patient allergic to iodine or one who has hyperthyroidism, hyperkalemia, or experiences a skin eruption after taking the medication. Patients who are pregnant or those who take potassium-sparing diuretics should not take this medication.

25. Chronic emphysema, emphysema with bronchitis, asthmatic bronchitis, and pneumonia.

26. Sitting

27. Pursed

28. Teach the patient the difference between a productive and nonproductive cough, as well as measures to combat nonproductive coughs.

29. Hydration of viscous mucus.

30. Opiate and nonopiate cough suppressants.

31. Codeine may cause dependence (rarely), respiratory depression, bronchial constriction, central nervous system (CNS) depression, and constipation.

32. Patients with preexisting pulmonary distress; people already taking sedative/hypnotics, CNS depressants, or psychotropic agents; people using alcohol.

33. Codeine

34. Antitussive agent, p. 488; potassium iodide, p. 487; saline solutions, p. 487; mucolytic agents, p. 489; expectorants, p. 486; anticholinergic bronchodilating agents, pp. 492-493; xanthine derivative bronchodilating agents, p. 493; respiratory anti-inflammatory agents, p. 494; antileukotriene agents, pp. 496-497; beta-adrenergic bronchodilating agents, p. 490, miscellaneous anti-inflammatory agents, pp. 498-499, immunomodulators, p. 497.

35. Patient education, environmental control, comprehensive pharmacologic therapy, and objective monitoring via regular use of a peak flow meter.

37. Discuss the use of beta-adrenergic broncho-dilating agents in the treatment of lower respiratory disease.

38. Name two anticholinergic bronchodilating agents.

39. Patients taking ipratropium bromide (Atrovent) should be assessed for what pre-existing ophthalmic condition?

40. How do sympathomimetic (adrenergic) agents act and what assessments should be made for patients taking these medications?

41. Which drugs are classified as xanthine derivatives?

42. What is the mechanism of action of the xanthine-derivative bronchodilating agents?

43. What is the therapeutic outcome associated with xanthine-derivative bronchodilator therapy?

44. How can dosages of theophylline (Theo-Dur) be measured?

45. Describe the clinical uses of montelukast (Singulair), and zafirlukast (Accolate).

46. Describe premedication assessments for omalizumab (Xolair).

47. What is the action of cromolyn sodium (Intal)?

36. See textbook, p. 489.

37. These drugs are used to reverse airway constriction caused by acute and chronic bronchial asthma, bronchitis, and emphysema.

38. Ipratropium bromide (Atrovent) and tiotropium bromide (Spiriva).

39. Closed-angle glaucoma

40. Adrenergic agents stimulate beta$_2$ receptors, causing bronchodilation. Many of the drugs also stimulate beta$_1$ receptors in the heart. Always monitor patients taking adrenergic agents for changes in cardiac function (e.g., hypertension, tachycardia), CNS stimulation (exhibited as insomnia, nervousness, anxiety, tremors), and gastrointestinal (GI) disturbances.

41. Aminophylline, theophylline (Theo-Dur), dyphylline (Lufyllin)

42. These medications act directly on the smooth muscle of the tracheobronchial tree to dilate the bronchi, thus increasing airflow in and out of the alveolar sacs.

43. Easier breathing with less effort.

44. Theophylline levels can be monitored by a blood test. Adult: 10–20 mcg/mL.

45. See textbook, p. 496.

46. See textbook, p. 497.

47. It is a mast cell stabilizer that inhibits the release of histamine and other mediators of inflammation, making it an indirect anti-inflammatory agent. It must be administered before the body receives a stimulus to release histamine, such as an antigen that initiates an antigen-antibody allergic reaction.

Drugs Used to Treat Lower Respiratory Disease

Learning Activities

FILL-IN-THE-BLANK

Finish each of the following statements using the correct term.

1. _____ is the movement of air in and out of the lungs; _____ is the process by which oxygen passes across the alveolar membrane to the blood in the capillaries, and carbon dioxide passes from the blood to the alveolar sacs.

2. Respiratory diseases are divided into two types: _____ and _____.

3. _____ _____ is a condition in which chronic irritation causes inflammation and edema with excessive mucus secretion leading to airflow obstruction.

4. The _____ liquefy mucus by stimulating the secretion of natural lubricant fluids from the serous glands.

5. _____ agents reduce the stickiness and viscosity of pulmonary secretions by acting directly on the mucus plugs to cause dissolution.

6. _____-_____ respirations is a cyclic breathing pattern in which periods of deep breathing alternate with periods of apnea.

7. _____ agents play an important role in the treatment of asthma to reduce inflammation.

8. The _____ measures the ratio of actual oxygen content of hemoglobin compared with the hemoglobin's oxygen-carrying capacity.

9. _____ is an inflammatory disease of the bronchi and bronchioles. There are intermittent periods of acute, reversible airflow obstruction (bronchoconstriction) caused by bronchiolar inflammation and overresponsiveness to a variety of stimuli.

10. A(n) _____ is an instrument used to measure volumes of air during inhalation and exhalation.

11. Guaifenesin (Robitussin Cough Gels) is a drug known as a(n) _____.

12. This drug may produce a goiter when used over an extended length of time in children such as those with cystic fibrosis: _____ _____.

13. _____ is a medicine that acts by dissolving mucus by disrupting the chemical bonds.

14. _____ (drug class) therapy requires a period of up to 4 weeks of therapy for maximum benefits on obstructive lung disease.

15. _____ agents must NOT be considered as the primary treatment for an acute episode of asthma.

16. The _____ (drug class) relax the smooth muscle of the tracheobronchial tree.

MATCHING

Match the generic drug name with its corresponding brand name. Each option will be used only once.

_____ 17. guaifenesin

_____ 18. acetylcysteine

_____ 19. albuterol

_____ 20. metaproterenol

_____ 21. ipratropium bromide

_____ 22. montelukast

_____ 23. zafirlukast

_____ 24. omalizumab

_____ 25. cromolyn sodium

_____ 26. arformoterol

a. Xolair
b. Singulair
c. Intal
d. Accolate
e. Proventil
f. Robitussin
g. Mucomyst
h. Alupent
i. Atrovent
j. Brovana

TRUE OR FALSE

Write "T" for true and "F" for false for each statement. Correct all false statements.

_____ 27. Stimulation of the smooth muscles of the tracheobronchial tree by the cholinergic nerves causes bronchial constriction and increased mucus secretion.

_____ 28. Asthma is a constrictive disease of the bronchi and bronchioles.

_____ 29. Emphysema is a disease of alveolar destruction with fibrosis.

_____ 30. Antitussives act by suppressing the cough center located in the trachea.

_____ 31. Fingernail clubbing is a flattening or an increase in the angle between the fingernail and the nail base of the fingers.

_____ 32. Central cyanosis indicates a general lack of oxygen in the hemoglobin.

_____ 33. Molds are often asthma triggers.

_____ 34. Tiotropium bromide (Spiriva) is a rescue medications used for the treatment of patients with chronic obstructive pulmonary disease.

_____ 35. There is no acceptable role for the use of steroids in the treatment of patients with chronic obstructive pulmonary disease.

Drugs Used to Treat Lower Respiratory Disease

Practice Questions for the NCLEX® Examination

_____ 1. Which statement does the nurse include when teaching a patient about potassium iodide (SSKI)?
   1. "Do not use salt substitutes high in potassium because of potential dangerous effects from hyperkalemia."
   2. "Limit your intake of protein to prevent complications."
   3. "Maintain a maximum fluid intake of four 8-ounce glasses of fluid daily."
   4. "Double your intake of calcium products to prevent hypocalcemia."

_____ 2. Which drug is an effective cough suppressant and the standard against which other antitussive agents are compared?
   1. Dextromethorphan (Delsym)
   2. Acetylcysteine (Mucomyst)
   3. Guaifenesin (Robitussin)
   4. Codeine

_____ 3. A patient who has been prescribed acetylcysteine (Mucomyst) for the treatment of pneumonia wishes to know how the medication works. What does the nurse tell the patient?
   1. "It hydrates the mucus and reduces its viscosity."
   2. "It dissolves chemical bonds within the mucus itself, causing it to separate and liquefy, thereby reducing viscosity."
   3. "It produces bronchodilation by relaxing bronchial smooth muscle."
   4. "It reduces bronchial inflammation."

_____ 4. Which beta-adrenergic bronchodilating agents are useful in the treatment of acute bronchospasm? *(Select all that apply.)*
   1. Levalbuterol (Xopenex)
   2. Salmeterol (Serevet)
   3. Albuterol (Proventil)
   4. Formoterol fumarate (Foradil)
   5. Pirbuterol acetate (Maxair)

_____ 5. Which condition is most likely to cause complications associated with beta-adrenergic bronchodilator therapy?
   1. Diabetes mellitus
   2. Asthma
   3. Pneumonia
   4. An allergy to eggs

_____ 6. The nurse is teaching a patient how to administer 2 puffs of ipratropium bromide (Atrovent) via inhalation. The patient performs a return demonstration. Which action by the patient indicates further teaching is needed?
   1. The patient encloses the mouthpiece with the lips.
   2. The patient washes the mouthpiece with hot water.
   3. The patient inhales slowly through the mouthpiece and simultaneously presses the canister once.
   4. The patient waits 5 seconds and repeats the second inhalation.

_____ 7. Which statements about the use of zafirlukast (Accolate) with other medications
are true? *(Select all that apply.)*
1. Aspirin significantly decreases the
activity of zafirlukast.
2. Zafirlukast increases the activity of
warfarin (Coumadin).
3. Theophylline (Theo-Dur) decreases
the activity of zafirlukast.
4. Erythromycin (Eryc) decreases the
activity of zafirlukast.
5. Zafirlukast enhances the activity of
immunomodulator agents.

_____ 8. The nurse is teaching a patient about the
proper use of cromolyn sodium (Intal)
for treatment of asthma. Which statement by the patient indicates a need for
further teaching?
1. "I will take the cromolyn sodium 10
to 60 minutes before exercising."
2. "I will drink plenty of water after
taking the cromolyn capsule by
mouth so it is absorbed."
3. "I will not use cromolyn sodium for
immediate relief of asthma symptoms."
4. "I will not receive full therapeutic
benefit from cromolyn sodium therapy for 2 to 4 weeks of continuous
use."

_____ 9. Which statement does the nurse include
when teaching a patient about proper
administration of a bronchodilator and
steroid via metered-dose inhaler for
treatment of chronic obstructive pulmonary disease?
1. "Inhale halfway, then take your medicine through the inhaler."
2. "Take your steroid first, then take the
bronchodilator."
3. "Hold your breath for about 2 seconds during inhalation of the medication."
4. "Rinse your mouth with water and
spit it out after you take your steroid
by inhalation."

_____ 10. Children with cystic fibrosis who are on
long-term therapy with SSKI potassium
iodide should be assessed for the development of which condition?
1. Goiter
2. Edema
3. Tremor
4. Tachycardia

_____ 11. The patient who is taking a beta-
adrenergic bronchodilator should report
which serious adverse effects? *(Select all
that apply.)*
1. Escalation of tension
2. Tremors
3. Palpitations
4. Dizziness
5. Bronchospasm

_____ 12. Which is the most common adverse effect of long-term inhaled corticosteroid
therapy for obstructive airway disease?
1. Liver dysfunction
2. Abdominal pain
3. Thrush
4. Constipation

13. A patient is ordered dyphylline (Dilor) 500 mg
IM. The medication is available as 250 mg/
mL. How many mL does the nurse administer?
_____ mL

14. A patient is ordered terbutaline
(Brethine) 0.25 mg subcutaneously stat.
The medication is available as 1 mg/mL.
How much of the medication does the
nurse administer?
1. 0.25 cc
2. 0.5 cc
3. 1 mL
4. 1.5 mL

15. A patient is ordered diphenhydramine (Diphen)
25 mg. The medication is available as 12.5 mg/
5 mL syrup. How many mL does the nurse administer? _____ mL

Drugs Used to Treat Oral Disorders

Review Sheet

The QUESTION column and the ANSWER column have been offset so that you can cover the answers while reading the questions, allowing you to assess your knowledge.

Question	Answer
1. Summarize the major goals of treatment and drug therapy used for cold sores.	
2. Summarize the major goals of treatment and drug therapy used for canker sores.	1. The goals of treatment are to control discomfort, allow healing, prevent spread to others, and prevent complications. The cold sore should be kept moist to prevent drying. Dosasanol (Abreva) is the only FDA-approved product clinically proven to shorten healing time as well as the duration of symptoms. Local anesthetics can temporarily relieve the pain and itching and prevent drying of the lesion. Topical oral analgesics may also provide significant pain relief. Protection from the sun can help those who have cold sores that are stimulated from exposure to the sun. Secondary infections can be treated with topical antibiotic ointment.
3. Summarize the major goals of treatment and drug therapy used for mucositis. Describe how a pretreatment oral mucosal assessment is completed for patients scheduled to undergo chemotherapy.	2. The goals of treatment are similar to those for cold sores. See text for details.
4. Summarize the major goals of treatment and drug therapy for xerostomia.	3. Prevention is key in treatment of mucositis. Basic oral hygiene should be performed. See text for details on the pretreatment assessment and treatment of patients with mucositis.
5. Explain how to perform an oral assessment.	4. Xerostomia is treated by changing the medicines that cause dry mouth or with artificial saliva. Patients with xerostomia should be seen on a regular basis by a dentist. Commercially available saliva substitutes are often used.
6. Summarize the use of various types of mouthwashes.	5. See text for details.

7. When lidocaine, a local anesthetic, is used as an oral spray or as a viscous solution, what precautions should be taught to the patient?

8. Describe the World Health Organization Oral Mucositis Scale.

6. The most common mouthwashes are the fluoride-containing mouthwashes used to prevent dental caries. Medicinal mouthwashes are used to reduce plaque accumulation and gingivitis. Some mouthwashes such as Peridex are antibacterial agents used to treat oral mucositis. See text for more details on these agents.

7. Do not smoke, eat, or drink for at least 30 minutes after use. Test ability to swallow before taking oral foods or drink. These products decrease normal sensations in the mouth; test temperature of foods or drinks before ingesting to prevent accidental burning of the oral mucosa.

8. See textbook, Box 32-1.

Student Name

Drugs Used to Treat Oral Disorders

chapter

32

Learning Activities

FILL-IN-THE-BLANK

Finish each of the following statements using the correct term.

1. The medical term used to describe lack of saliva is _____.

2. Canker sores are also known as _____ _____ _____.

3. The most common form of candidiasis is often referred to as _____.

4. Candidiasis is a fungal infection caused by _____ _____.

5. If plaque is not removed within 24 hours, it begins to calcify, forming calculus or _____.

6. _____ is the general term used to describe a painful inflammation of the mucous membranes of the mouth.

7. _____ is the whitish-yellow substance that builds up on teeth and gum lines around the teeth.

TRUE OR FALSE

Write "T" for true and "F" for false for each statement. Correct all false statements.

_____ 8. Antibiotics are the standard treatment used for candidiasis.

_____ 9. Tartar is the primary cause of most tooth, gum, and periodontal disease.

_____ 10. *Halitosis* is the term used to describe very foul mouth odor.

_____ 11. Docosanol (Abreva) is the treatment of choice for canker sores.

_____ 12. Sucralfate (Carafate) suspensions applied topically have been reported to provide effective pain relief for patients with mucositis.

Copyright © 2010, 2007, 2004, 2001, 1997 by Mosby, Inc., an affiliate of Elsevier Inc. All rights reserved.

213

Drugs Used to Treat Oral Disorders

chapter

32

Practice Questions for the NCLEX® Examination

_____ 1. How many days after receiving chemotherapy is a patient most at risk for the
development of mucositis?
1. 6
2. 10
3. 12
4. 16

_____ 2. The nurse is teaching a patient who is
receiving radiation therapy to the neck
about dietary habits. Which statement by
the patient indicates a need for further
teaching?
1. "I will eat hot soup with every
meal."
2. "I will avoid alcohol."
3. "I will use bland gravy and sauces
on my foods."
4. "I will avoid the use of spicy foods."

_____ 3. Which action is most effective in providing a patient with relief of symptoms
caused by mucositis?
1. Applying amlexanox (Aphthasol)
before meals
2. Using commercially prepared
mouthwashes with alcohol
3. Avoiding exposure to the sun
4. Using 1 tablespoon of salt or hy-
drogen peroxide, or 1/2 teaspoon
of baking soda in 8 oz of water as a
mouthwash

_____ 4. Which statement does the nurse include
when teaching a patient how to care for a
cold sore?
1. "Avoid exposure of the cold sore to
any type of soap solution."
2. "Keep the cold sore dry to aid in
healing."
3. "Cold sores are caused by bacteria,
so take your antibiotics."
4. "Avoid the use of highly astringent
products such as zinc sulfate in the
area of the cold sore."

_____ 5. A patient has severe grade 3 mucositis as determined by the World Health
Organization Oral Mucositis Scale.
Which medications may be ordered for
the patient to treat oral mucositis? (Select
all that apply.)
1. Recombinant human keratinocyte
growth factor (Kepivance)
2. Milk of magnesia
3. Sucralfate suspension
4. Viscous lidocaine 2%
5. Docosanol (Abreva)

_____ 6. At 1230, a patient with mucositis reports
mouth pain and asks the nurse for a dose
of lidocaine hydrochloride. The nurse
determines the patient finished eating
lunch at 1200. The nurse administers the
medication at what time?
1. 1230
2. 1300
3. 1330
4. 1400

_____ 7. A patient with mucositis and a candidiasis infection is ordered nystatin liquid
at 1000. For the nystatin to be most effective, the patient's mouth should be
cleansed at what time?
1. 0900
2. 0930
3. 1000
4. 1030

8. A patient is ordered nystatin 500,000 units tid.
Nystatin is available as 100,000 units/mL. How
many mL of the medication does the nurse administer? _____ mL

Drugs Used to Treat Gastroesophageal Reflux and Peptic Ulcer Diseases

Review Sheet

The QUESTION column and the ANSWER column have been offset so that you can cover the answers while reading the questions, allowing you to assess your knowledge.

Question	Answer
1. What is the difference between gastroesophageal reflux disease (GERD) and peptic ulcer disease (PUD)?	
2. What are the major treatment goals for GERD and PUD?	1. GERD is more commonly referred to as *heartburn*. It is caused by the reflux of gastric secretions, primarily pepsin and hydrochloric acid, up into the esophagus. PUD is actually several stomach disorders that result from an imbalance between acidic stomach contents and the body's normal defense barriers, causing ulcerations in the GI tract.
3. What premedication assessments should be made prior to beginning antacid therapy?	2. The major treatment goals for GERD and PUD are to relieve symptoms, promote healing, and prevent recurrence.
4. What effect does the administration of an antacid have on the pH of the gastric secretions?	3. Prior to antacid therapy, check for any abnormal renal function. If present, avoid magnesium-containing products. Check bowel pattern for diarrhea or constipation. Record any gastric pain or symptoms present. If patient is pregnant or has edema, heart failure, hypertension, or salt restrictions, ensure that a low-sodium antacid is prescribed. Schedule other prescribed medications 1 hour before or 2 hours after antacids are to be administered.
5. Are antacids alkaline or acidic?	4. Antacids buffer the hydrogen ion concentration, reducing the acidity of the gastric secretions and raising the pH of the gastric contents to neutralize gastric secretions.
6. Describe effect(s) of the following active ingredients of antacids: simethicone, alginic acid, bismuth, aluminum hydroxide, magnesium oxide or hydroxide, magnesium trisilicate, and calcium carbonate.	5. Mildly alkaline.

7. What ingredients in an antacid may produce constipation?

8. What ingredients in antacids may cause diarrhea?

9. What ingredient(s) in antacids should not be administered to patients with renal disease?

10. The absorption of which antibiotics are inhibited by antacids?

11. Because antacids alter the absorption rate of digoxin and iron compounds, what dosing schedule should be used to administer antacids when these medicines are also ordered?

12. In order to obtain the most rapid onset of action, should an antacid be administered in a liquid or a tablet form?

13. Are antacid tablets recommended for the treatment of PUD?

14. Describe the action of histamine (H_2) receptor antagonists for the treatment of gastrointestinal disorders.

15. What premedication assessments should be performed for H_2 receptor antagonists?

16. When should the H_2 antagonist agents cimetidine (Tagamet), famotidine (Pepcid), nizatidine (Axid), or ranitidine (Zantac) be administered in relation to food intake?

17. If antacid therapy is continued concurrently with the use of H_2 receptor antagonists, what scheduling for the antacid should be used?

18. List the actions and uses of misoprostol (Cytotec).

6. Simethicone is a defoaming agent that breaks up as bubbles in the stomach, reducing stomach distention and heartburn. Alginic acid produces a highly viscous solution of sodium alginate that floats on top of the gastric contents. Bismuth compounds have little acid-neutralizing capacity and are therefore poor antacids. Aluminum hydroxide, magnesium oxide or hydroxide, magnesium trisilicate, and calcium carbonate all buffer gastric acidity.

7. Calcium carbonate or aluminum hydroxide products may cause constipation.

8. Magnesium

9. Patients with renal failure should not use large quantities of antacids containing magnesium.

10. Tetracycline antibiotics, ciprofloxacin, and ketoconazole

11. Administer 1 hour before or 2 to 3 hours after the antacid.

12. Liquid form

13. Tablets do not contain enough antacid to be effective for treatment of peptic ulcers. Antacid tablets should be used only for the patient with occasional indigestion or heartburn.

14. The H_2 antagonists (e.g., cimetidine, famotidine, nizatidine, ranitidine) act by blocking H_2 receptors, resulting in a decrease in the volume of acid secreted. The pH of the stomach rises as a result of a reduction in acid.

15. Perform a baseline assessment of the patient's mental status for comparison with subsequent mental status evaluations to detect CNS alterations that may occur, particularly with cimetidine therapy.

16. Cimetidine (Tagamet), famotidine (Pepcid), and ranitidine (Zantac) are administered with food. Nizatidine (Axid) is administered with or without food.

17. Antacids should be administered 1 hour before or 2 hours after the H_2 antagonist dose.

19. What premedication assessments should be performed before misoprostol (Cytotec) therapy?

20. Cite the most common adverse effect of misoprostol (Cytotec) therapy and its management.

21. What is the more common name for the substituted benzimidazoles?

22. What is the action of the proton pump inhibitors?

23. What are proton pump inhibitors used to treat?

24. What is the ending on the generic name of all proton pump inhibitors?

25. What is the action of metoclopramide (Reglan)?

18. Misoprostol is a synthetic prostaglandin E. Prostaglandins are normally present in the GI tract to inhibit gastric acid and pepsin secretion to protect the stomach and duodenal lining against ulceration. Misoprostol is used to prevent and treat gastric ulcers caused by NSAIDs, including aspirin. Whereas prostaglandin inhibition is effective in reducing pain and inflammation, especially in arthritis, prostaglandin inhibition in the stomach makes the patient more predisposed to peptic ulcers.

19. Determine if the patient is pregnant. This drug is a uterine stimulant and may induce a miscarriage. Check pattern of bowel elimination. Misoprostol may induce diarrhea.

20. Diarrhea is the most common adverse effect associated with misoprostol (Cytotec) therapy. It is dose-related and usually develops after approximately 2 weeks of therapy. The diarrhea often resolves after about 8 days, but a few patients require discontinuation of the drug. Diarrhea can be minimized by taking misoprostol with meals and at bedtime and by avoiding magnesium-containing antacids. The patient should be encouraged to include sufficient roughage in the diet.

21. Substituted benzimidazoles are more commonly known as *proton pump inhibitors*.

22. Proton pump inhibitors inhibit gastric acid secretion.

23. Proton pump inhibitors are used to treat severe esophagitis, GERD, gastric and duodenal ulcers, and hypersecretory disorders, such as Zollinger-Ellison syndrome. They may also be used in combination with antibiotics (e.g., ampicillin, amoxicillin, clarithromycin) to eradicate *Helicobacter pylori*, a common cause of PUD.

24. All generic names of proton pump inhibitors end in "-prazole."

25. Metoclopramide is a gastric stimulant; as an antiemetic it blocks dopamine in the chemoreceptor trigger zone. It increases stomach contractions, relaxes the pyloric valve, and increases peristalsis in GI tract resulting in increased rate of gastric emptying and intestinal transit.

Drugs Used to Treat Gastroesophageal Reflux and Peptic Ulcer Diseases

chapter

33

Learning Activities

FILL-IN-THE-BLANK

Finish each of the following statements using the correct term.

1. Normal pH of the stomach ranges from _____ to _____ depending on the presence of food and medications.

2. Infection of the mucous wall of the stomach by _____ _____ is one of the causes of peptic ulcer disease.

3. The proton pump inhibitors used in the treatment of peptic ulcer disease block the formation of _____ acid, reducing irritation of the gastric mucosa.

4. The three types of secretory cells lining portions of the stomach include the _____, _____, and _____ cells.

5. _____ is a medication which coats the gastric ulcer crater to protect it from gastric acid secretions.

6. Hypersecretion of gastric acid after taking calcium compounds and sodium bicarbonate is called _____ _____.

MATCHING

Match the generic drug name with its corresponding brand name. Each option will be used only once.

_____ 7. dicyclomine

_____ 8. pantoprazole

_____ 9. omeprazole

_____ 10. lansoprazole

_____ 11. esomeprazole

_____ 12. nizatidine

_____ 13. famotidine

_____ 14. cimetidine

a. Axid
b. Prevacid
c. Tagamet
d. Bentyl
e. Prilosec
f. Nexium
g. Protonix
h. Pepcid

TRUE OR FALSE

Write "T" for true and "F" for false for each statement. Correct all false statements.

_____ 15. The parietal cells secrete intrinsic factor needed for absorption of vitamin C.

_____ 16. The enzyme amylase digests fats, and the enzyme lipase digests carbohydrates.

_____ 17. The pain associated with peptic ulcer disease is most often noted when the stomach is empty, such as at night or between meals, and is relieved by food or antacids.

_____ 18. The antispasmodic agents used in the treatment of gastroesophageal reflux and peptic ulcer disease reduce the secretion of saliva, hydrochloric acid, pepsin, bile, and other enzymatic fluids necessary for digestion and decrease GI motility and secretions.

_____ 19. Prokinetic agents are used to treat gastroesophageal reflux disease.

_____ 20. Antacid tablets are effective in treating PUD.

_____ 21. Patients with renal failure may develop hypermagnesemia if magnesium-containing antacids are taken.

_____ 22. The pH of the stomach decreases when the hydrochloric acid content is reduced.

_____ 23. Smoking causes an increase in hydrochloric acid secretion.

_____ 24. Antacids containing magnesium may be dangerous to patients with renal disease.

Drugs Used to Treat Gastroesophageal Reflux and Peptic Ulcer Diseases

chapter

33

Practice Questions for the NCLEX® Examination

_____ 1. Which statement does the nurse include when teaching a patient about antacid therapy for the treatment of peptic ulcer disease?
1. "Antacids take at least 6 weeks to become effective."
2. "Antacid tablets do not contain enough antacid to be effective in treating this disease."
3. "Excessive use of magnesium antacids results in constipation."
4. "A common complaint of patients using large quantities of calcium carbonate antacids is diarrhea."

_____ 2. The nurse administered digoxin (Lanoxin) 0.125 mg PO daily at 0900. When reviewing the patient's chart at 0915, the nurse finds a new order for one tablet of Riopan three times a day. At what time does the nurse start the Riopan therapy?
1. 0930
2. 0945
3. 1030
4. 1130

_____ 3. A patient with a history of chronic renal failure is on high-dose cimetidine (Tagamet) therapy for the treatment of a duodenal ulcer. It is most important for the nurse to assess the patient for which adverse effect of this therapy?
1. Dizziness
2. Disorientation
3. Constipation
4. Diarrhea

_____ 4. The nurse is teaching a patient about misoprostol (Cytotec) therapy. Which statement made by the patient indicates a need for further teaching?
1. "To minimize diarrhea associated with this therapy, I will take magnesium-containing antacids."
2. "I will not discontinue the therapy without first consulting my health care provider."
3. "To minimize diarrhea associated with this therapy, I will take it with meals and at bedtime."
4. "I understand that I should tell my primary health care provider if I am pregnant or become pregnant while on this therapy."

_____ 5. Which assessment finding in a patient taking pantoprazole (Protonix) does the nurse report to the health care provider?
1. Diarrhea
2. Muscle pain
3. Persistent vesicular rash
4. Fatigue

_____ 6. Before starting a patient on metoclopramide (Reglan) therapy, the nurse assesses the patient for which factor?
1. Allergy to penicillins
2. History of asthma
3. History of epilepsy
4. Allergy to shellfish

_____ 7. Patients older than 65 years of age with ulcer disease usually present with which symptoms? *(Select all that apply.)*
1. Anorexia
2. Weight gain
3. Headache
4. Vague abdominal discomfort
5. Burning in the epigastric region

_____ 8. When teaching a patient about the use of antacids for the treatment of gastrointestinal disorders, which statements does the nurse include? *(Select all that apply.)*
   1. "Maalox is an example of a low-sodium antacid."
   2. "Use of an antacid with large amounts of magnesium usually results in constipation."
   3. "Calcium carbonate and sodium bicarbonate may cause rebound hyper-acidity."
   4. "Patients with renal failure should not use large quantities of antacids containing magnesium."
   5. "Antacid tablets should be used only for patients with occasional indigestion or heartburn."

9. A patient is ordered metoclopramide (Reglan) 50 mg added to 50 mL of normal saline IV piggyback as a one-time order to infuse over 30 minutes. The medication is available in a 30-mL single-dose vial of metoclopramide 5 mg/mL. How many mL of the medication does the nurse inject into the 50 mL of normal saline? _____ mL

10. A patient is ordered metoclopramide (Reglan) 15 mg PO 1 hour before each meal and at bedtime. How many mg of the medication will the patient receive in a 24-hour period? _____ mg

_____ 11. A patient is ordered Maalox Plus 30 mL PO 30 minutes after meals and at bedtime. The medication is available in a 1 fluid ounce container. How many containers are needed for a 24-hour period?
   1. 1
   2. 2
   3. 3
   4. 4

12. A patient is ordered ranitidine (Zantac) 300 mg PO at bedtime. The medication is available in 75-mg tablets. How many tablets does the nurse administer? _____ tablet(s)

Drugs Used to Treat Nausea and Vomiting

Review Sheet

The QUESTION column and the ANSWER column have been offset so that you can cover the answers while reading the questions, allowing you to assess your knowledge.

Question

1. What is an antiemetic?

2. What seven classes of drugs are used to treat nausea and vomiting?

3. What is the mechanism of action for the seven drug classes used to treat nausea and vomiting?

4. Name the most widely used antiemetic in the dopamine antagonist class used to treat nausea and vomiting associated with anesthesia and surgery, radiation therapy, and cancer chemotherapy.

5. What is the action of metoclopramide (Reglan) on the gastrointestinal tract that makes it useful as an antiemetic?

6. When is ondansetron (Zofran) administered in relation to chemotherapy?

7. What drugs are recommended for nausea and vomiting associated with pregnancy?

8. What herbal medicine is used by some cultures to treat pregnancy-induced nausea and vomiting?

9. What are the usual nursing implementations used for an adult and for an infant experiencing nausea and vomiting?

Answer

1. A medication used to prevent nausea and vomiting.

2. Dopamine antagonists, serotonin antagonists, anticholinergic agents, corticosteroids, benzodiazepines, cannabinoids, and neurokinin-1 receptor antagonists

3. See sections labeled "Action" for each drug class.

4. Prochlorperazine (Compazine)

5. Metoclopramide (Reglan) is an antagonist of both dopamine and serotonin receptors. In addition to acting on receptors in the brain, it also acts on similar receptors in the GI tract, thus making it particularly useful in treating nausea and vomiting associated with GI cancers, gastritis, peptic ulcer, radiation sickness, and migraine. Metoclopramide stimulates motility of the upper GI tract without stimulating gastric, biliary, or pancreatic secretion. It also accelerates gastric emptying and intestinal transit.

6. Ondansetron (Zofran) is administered 30 minutes before chemotherapy followed by 8 mg 8 hours later.

7. Administration of meclizine (Antivert), cyclizine (Marezine), or dimenhydrinate (Dramamine) is recommended first for nausea and vomiting associated with pregnancy.

8. Ginger

10. What are the usual premedication assessments performed by the nurse before administration of antiemetic drug therapy?

11. Define *postoperative nausea and vomiting (PONV), motion sickness, hyperemesis gravidarum, psychogenic vomiting, chemotherapy-induced nausea and vomiting (CINV), anticipatory nausea and vomiting, delayed emesis,* and *radiation-induced nausea and vomiting (RINV).*

12. Summarize drug therapy for the treatment of postoperative nausea and vomiting, motion sickness, nausea and vomiting in pregnancy, psychogenic vomiting, anticipatory nausea and vomiting, chemotherapy-induced nausea and vomiting, delayed emesis, and radiation-induced nausea and vomiting.

9. See textbook, pp. 528-529.

10. See textbook, pp. 527-528.

11. See textbook, pp. 524-526.

12. See textbook, pp. 526-527.

Drugs Used to Treat Nausea and Vomiting

Learning Activities

FILL-IN-THE-BLANK

Finish each of the following statements using the correct term.

1. _____ is the involuntary labored, spasmodic contractions of the abdominal and respiratory muscles without the expulsion of gastric contents.

2. Nausea and vomiting associated with motion are thought to result from stimulation of the _____ system of the ear, with subsequent transmission of this stimulus to the vestibular network located near the vomiting center.

3. A pregnant woman with severe persistent vomiting that interferes with nutrition, fluid, and electrolyte balance may be experiencing _____ _____, a condition in which starvation, dehydration, and acidosis are superimposed on the vomiting syndrome.

4. Most agents used to reduce nausea and vomiting from motion sickness are chemically related to _____.

5. In many cultures, the herb _____ is used to treat pregnancy-induced nausea and vomiting.

6. Drugs used to treat nausea and vomiting are referred to as _____ agents.

MATCHING

Match the generic drug name to its corresponding brand name. Each option will be used only once.

_____ 7. prochlorperazine

_____ 8. granisetron

_____ 9. trimethobenzamide

_____ 10. ondansetron

_____ 11. meclizine

_____ 12. nabilone

_____ 13. aprepitant

_____ 14. diphenhydramine

_____ 15. lorazepam

a. Tigan
b. Kytril
c. Antivert
d. Compazine
e. Zofran
f. Ativan
g. Cesamet
h. Emend
i. Benadryl

TRUE OR FALSE

Write "T" for true and "F" for false for each statement. Correct all false statements.

_____ 16. There are several physiologic mechanisms of nausea and vomiting, but none are well-understood.

_____ 17. Pain not treated with appropriate analgesia induces nausea and vomiting.

_____ 18. Older adults between the ages of 60–70 years have the highest incidence of postoperative nausea and vomiting based on age groups.

_____ 19. Patients under nitrous oxide anesthesia have a higher incidence of nausea and vomiting than do those under halothane, enflurane, or isoflurane.

_____ 20. Antiemetic agents are generally more effective if administered before the onset of nausea, rather than after it has started.

_____ 21. Adverse effects associated with the use of dopamine antagonists in the treatment of nausea and vomiting include symptoms of dystonia, parkinsonism, and tardive dyskinesia.

_____ 22. Dysphoric effects results from use of cannabinoids for the treatment of nausea and vomiting include depressed mood, hallucinations, dreaming or fantasizing, distortion of perception, paranoid reactions, and elation.

_____ 23. Patients receiving warfarin therapy should be instructed to have an INR check approximately 7 to 10 days after aprepitant (Emend) therapy because co-administration with aprepitant results in decreased metabolism of warfarin and increased INR.

_____ 24. Patients receiving anticholinergic agents for the treatment of nausea and vomiting must be placed on fluid restrictions.

Drugs Used to Treat Nausea and Vomiting

Practice Questions for the NCLEX® Examination

_____ 1. Which statement about phenothiazine therapy for the treatment of nausea and vomiting is true?
1. Phenothiazines often cause hypertension.
2. Phenothiazines are safe to use in patients with seizure disorders.
3. A rash is a common side effect of phenothiazine therapy and does not need to be reported to the primary care provider.
4. Phenothiazines may suppress the cough reflex.

_____ 2. A patient is ordered 200 mg of trimethobenzamide (Tigan) IM. What does the nurse do next?
1. Assesses the patient for allergy to benzocaine or local anesthetics
2. Uses a one-half inch needle to administer this medication
3. Injects into the deltoid region
4. Injects into the vastus lateralis

_____ 3. A patient with a history of motion sickness is scheduled to be transported to another health care facility located about 90 minutes away. The primary care provider has ordered dimenhydrinate (Dramamine) 100 mg by mouth for the patient. The patient is scheduled to depart at 0900. When does the nurse administer the medication for it to be most effective?
1. 0700
2. 0730
3. 0830
4. 0900

_____ 4. Which agents used to treat nausea and vomiting are considered a Schedule III controlled substance?
1. Cannabinoids
2. Anticholinergics
3. Dopamine antagonists
4. Serotonin antagonists

_____ 5. A patient is having involuntary, labored, spasmodic contractions of the abdominal and respiratory muscles without the expulsion of gastric contents. What is the patient experiencing?
1. Constipation
2. Retching
3. Vomiting
4. Diarrhea

_____ 6. Which signs/symptoms are adverse effects of anticholinergic agents used for the treatment of motion sickness? (Select all that apply.)
1. Diarrhea
2. Urinary retention
3. Blurred vision
4. Dry mouth
5. Rhinorrhea

_____ 7. What does management of a patient with postoperative nausea and vomiting (PONV) include? (Select all that apply.)
1. Restricted fluids
2. Supplemental oxygen
3. Acupuncture
4. Transcutaneous electrical nerve stimulation (TENS)
5. Benzodiazepines

_____ 8. A patient is ordered ondansetron (Zofran) 8 mg PO 30 minutes before the start of chemotherapy. The medication is available as 4 mg/5 mL. How many mL of ondansetron does the nurse administer?
1. 8
2. 10
3. 12
4. 14

9. A patient is ordered prochlorperazine (Compazine) 5 mg IM stat. The medication is available as 5 mg/mL. How many mL of the medication does the nurse administer? _____ mL

10. A patient is ordered trimethobenzamide (Tigan) 200 mg IM. The medication is available as 100 mg/mL. How many mL of the medication does the nurse administer? _____ mL

Drugs Used to Treat Constipation and Diarrhea

Review Sheet

The QUESTION column and the ANSWER column have been offset so that you can cover the answers while reading the questions, allowing you to assess your knowledge.

Question	Answer

1. What is the mechanism of action of:
  a. stimulant laxatives?
  b. osmotic laxatives?
  c. lubricant laxatives?
  d. bulk-producing laxatives?
  e. fecal softeners?
  f. opioid antagonists?	

2. What is the onset of action for:
  a. stimulant laxatives?
  b. osmotic laxatives?
  c. lubricant laxatives?
  d. bulk-producing laxatives?
  e. fecal softeners?
  f. opioid antagonists?
	1. a. Direct action on the intestine causing irritation that promotes peristalsis and evacuation.
	  b. Hypertonic compounds that draw water into the intestine from surrounding tissues. The accumulated water affects stool consistency and distends the bowel.
	  c. Lubricate intestinal wall and soften the stool allowing a smooth passage of fecal contents. Peristalsis does not appear to be increased.
	  d. Cause water to be retained in stool, thus increasing bulk that stimulates peristalsis.
	  e. Draw water into stool causing it to soften. No stimulation of peristalsis.
	  f. Mu-opioid receptor antagonist that binds to opioid receptors in the GI tract inhibiting the constipation-producing effects of opioid drugs. Methylnaltrexone does not cross the blood-brain barrier; it does not interfere with the analgesic effects of the opioids.

3. When administering fecal softeners, what factors must be considered to promote the action of these laxative agents?	2. a. 6–10 hours orally; 60–90 minutes rectally
	  b. 1–3 hours
	  c. 6–8 hours
	  d. 12–24 hours, up to 72 hours
	  e. up to 72 hours
	  f. 4 hours after subcutaneous administration

4. Differentiate between the action of systemic and local antidiarrheal agents.	3. Adequate fluid intake is essential.

5. What premedication assessments should be performed before administration of an anti-diarrheal agent?

6. The ingredients of laxative products frequently cause adverse effects and may be contraindicated in patients with what types of conditions?

7. What are the benefits of polyethylene glycol-electrolyte solution as an osmotic laxative?

8. Describe treatment for opioid-induced constipation in patients with advanced illness who are receiving palliative care when response to laxative therapy has not been adequate.

9. Examine Table 35-1 to identify the names and types of laxatives commonly prescribed and Table 35-2 for antidiarrheal agents prescribed.

4. Systemic: Decrease peristalsis and GI motility via the autonomic nervous system, allowing the mucosal lining to absorb nutrients, water, and electrolytes and leaving a formed stool from the residue remaining in the colon. Local: Adsorb excess water to cause a formed stool and to adsorb irritants or bacteria that cause diarrhea.

5. Take medication history and examine for drugs that may be contributing to the diarrhea (such as antacids containing magnesium or laxative products, antibiotics, or products containing large quantities of sorbitol), and review for precipitating factors. Patients with infection-based diarrhea should not receive antidiarrheal agents.

6. Patients with severe pain or discomfort; those who have nausea, vomiting, or fever; patients with a preexisting condition (diabetes mellitus, abdominal surgery); those taking medicines that cause constipation (iron, aluminum antacids, antispasmodics, muscle relaxants); patients who have used other laxatives without success; and laxative abusers.

7. Polyethylene glycol-electrolyte solution is a relatively new approach to osmotic laxative therapy. It pulls electrolytes and water into the solution in the lumen of the bowel and exchanges sodium ions to replace those removed from the body. The result is a diarrhea that cleanses the bowel for colonoscopy and barium enema x-ray examination with no significant dehydration or loss of electrolytes.

8. Methylnaltrexone, an opioid antagonist has been used to treat this condition. It is a mu-opioid receptor antagonist that binds to opioid receptors in the GI tract inhibiting the constipation-producing effects of opioid drugs. It does not cross the blood-brain barrier, therefore it does not interfere with the analgesic effects of opioids.

9. See textbook, pp. 546-548.

Drugs Used to Treat Constipation and Diarrhea

Learning Activities

FILL-IN-THE-BLANK

Finish each of the following statements using the correct term.

1. _____ is the infrequent, incomplete, or painful elimination of feces.

2. _____ is an increase in the frequency or fluid content of bowel movements.

3. Patients with deficiencies of digestive enzymes such as _____ or _____ have difficulty digesting certain foods and diarrhea usually develops because of irritation from undigested food.

4. When drugs such as _____ or _____ are used regularly for pain control in patients, it is imperative that the individual know what stool softeners should be initiated as long as constipating medicines are being taken.

5. _____ and _____ laxatives may be used in geriatric and pregnant patients because there is little cramping accompanying their use.

6. _____, an opioid antagonist, is used for the treatment of opioid-induced constipation in patients with advanced illness who are receiving palliative care, when response to laxative therapy has not been adequate.

MATCHING

Match the generic drug name with its corresponding brand name. Each option will be used only once.

_____ 7. diphenoxylate with atropine

_____ 8. opium

_____ 9. bismuth subsalicylate

_____ 10. difenoxin with atropine

_____ 11. attapulgite

_____ 12. *Lactobacillus acidophilus*

a. Motofen
b. Pepto-Bismol
c. Paregoric
d. Lomotil
e. Lactinex
f. Parepectolin

Match each laxative product with its method of action.

_____ 13. Citrate of Magnesia

_____ 14. X-Prep

_____ 15. Metamucil

_____ 16. Kondremul

_____ 17. MiraLax

a. Stimulant
b. Osmotic
c. Bulk-forming
d. Lubricant
e. Saline

TRUE OR FALSE

Write "T" for true and "F" for false for each statement. Correct all false statements.

_____ 18. Anemia can be one of the diseases that contributes to the development of constipation.

_____ 19. Habitual constipation leads to an increased incidence of hemorrhoids.

_____ 20. Using laxatives or enemas daily should be avoided because they decrease the muscular tone and mucus production of the rectum and may result in water and electrolyte imbalance.

_____ 21. Daily bowel movements are necessary for good health.

_____ 22. Diarrhea is a symptom and not a disease.

Drugs Used to Treat Constipation and Diarrhea

chapter

35

Practice Questions for the NCLEX® Examination

_____ 1. A pregnant patient who is at 30 weeks gestation reports to her primary care provider that she is extremely constipated and in need of assistance. Which type of laxative is most likely to be ordered for this patient?
   1. Stimulant
   2. Saline
   3. Bulk-forming
   4. Polyethylene glycol-electrolyte solution

_____ 2. Of the following patients, which is most likely to benefit from the effects of a laxative?
   1. 27-year-old who has colitis
   2. 49-year-old diagnosed with appendicitis
   3. 34-year-old paraplegic
   4. 65-year-old with gastritis

_____ 3. Which medication is a 55-year-old patient recovering from a recent myocardial infarction likely receive to prevent constipation or straining at stool?
   1. Stool softener
   2. Saline laxative
   3. Stimulant laxative
   4. Bulk-forming laxative

_____ 4. A patient experiencing diarrhea with extreme pain would likely receive which drug to inhibit peristalsis and assist with the pain the patient is experiencing?
   1. Diphenoxylate with atropine (Lomotil)
   2. Opium (Paregoric)
   3. Loperamide (Imodium)
   4. Difenoxin with atropine (Motofen)

_____ 5. Which antidiarrheal agent has the potential to cause a hypertensive crisis when administered with a monoamine oxidase inhibitor?
   1. Bismuth subsalicylate (Pepto-Bismol)
   2. Lactobacillus acidophilus (Lactinex)
   3. Loperamide (Imodium)
   4. Diphenoxylate with atropine (Lomotil)

_____ 6. Which statements about bulk-forming laxatives are true? _(Select all that apply.)_
   1. They are generally considered to be the drug of choice for people who are incapacitated and need a laxative regularly.
   2. They may be used in the treatment of patients with irritable bowel syndrome.
   3. They are used to treat certain types of diarrhea.
   4. Adequate volumes of water must be taken with bulk-forming laxatives.
   5. They are used to relieve acute constipation.

_____ 7. Which statement does the nurse include when teaching a patient about the use of osmotic laxatives?
   1. "These agents usually work within 8 to 12 hours."
   2. "These agents should be used only intermittently because chronic use may cause loss of normal bowel function."
   3. "Osmotic laxatives work by making the stool softer."
   4. "Osmotic laxatives restore normal intestinal flora."

8. A patient is ordered 2 mg opium (Paregoric) PO daily at 0900. The medication is available as 2 mg/5 mL. How many mL of the medication does the nurse administer at 0900? _____ mL

9. A patient is ordered diphenoxylate with atropine (Lomotil) 5 mg four times daily. The medication is available in 2.5-mg tablets. How many tablets does the nurse administer in a 24-hour period? _____ tablet(s)

10. A patient is ordered loperamide (Imodium) 4 mg PO for acute diarrhea. The medication is available as 2-mg tablets. How many tablets does the nurse administer? _____ tablet(s)

Drugs Used to Treat Diabetes Mellitus

chapter

36

Review Sheet

The QUESTION column and the ANSWER column have been offset so that you can cover the answers while reading the questions, allowing you to assess your knowledge.

Question	Answer
1. Diabetes mellitus is a group of diseases characterized by _____.	
2. Summarize type 1 diabetes mellitus.	1. Diabetes mellitus is a group of diseases characterized by hyperglycemia (fasting plasma glucose [FPG] >125 mg/dL) and abnormalities in fat, carbohydrate, and protein metabolism which lead to microvascular, macrovascular, and neuropathic complications.
3. Summarize type 2 diabetes mellitus.	2. Type 1 diabetes mellitus, formerly known as *insulin-dependent diabetes mellitus* (IDDM), affects 5% to 10% of the population. It is caused by an autoimmune destruction of the beta cells in the pancreas. It occurs more frequently in juveniles, but patients can become symptomatic for the first time at any age. The onset of this form of diabetes usually has a rapid progression of symptoms characterized by polydipsia, polyphagia, polyuria, increased frequency of infections, loss of weight and strength, irritability, and often ketosis. Since there is no insulin secretion from the pancreas, the patient requires administration of exogenous insulin.
4. Name some other types of diabetes that are a part of other diseases having features not generally associated with the diabetic state.	3. Type 2 diabetes mellitus, formerly known as *non-insulin–dependent diabetes mellitus* (NIDDM), represents about 90% of the diabetic population. It is characterized by a decrease in beta cell activity, insulin resistance, or an increase in glucose production by the liver. Over time, the beta cells of the pancreas fail and exogenous insulin may be required. Most people with type 2 diabetes mellitus also have metabolic syndrome, also known as *insulin resistance syndrome* and *syndrome X*. The onset of type 2 diabetes mellitus is usually more insidious than that of type 1 diabetes mellitus. The pancreas still maintains some capability to produce and secrete insulin.

5. Summarize gestational diabetes mellitus.

6. What is impaired glucose tolerance (IGT) or impaired fasting glucose (IFG)?

7. "Polydipsia" is _____.

8. "Polyuria" is _____.
9. What are the symptoms of neuropathies?
10. What is the immediate goal for treatment of diabetes mellitus?

11. Describe the intensive therapy for diabetes management.

12. Name the groups of oral antidiabetic agents.

13. Describe incretin-based therapy.

14. Describe the criteria used to diagnose diabetes mellitus.
15. Describe the recommendations for exercise for people with impaired glucose tolerance.
16. What are the usual causes of hypoglycemia?
17. When should ketone testing of the urine be performed?

18. What is the difference between the glycosylated hemoglobin and fructosamine tests to measure glucose?

4. Pheochromocytoma, acromegaly, and Cushing's syndrome. Others include malnutrition, infection, drugs and chemicals that induce hyperglycemia, defects in insulin receptors, and certain genetic syndromes.
5. Gestational diabetes mellitus occurs when women have abnormal glucose tolerance during pregnancy.
6. IGT or IFG is used to describe those patients who are often euglycemic in their daily living, but develop hyperglycemia when challenged with an oral glucose tolerance test. This intermediate state between normal glucose homeostasis and diabetes is now known as *prediabetes*.
7. Increased thirst
8. Increased frequency of urination
9. Numbness and tingling of extremities (paresthesia), loss of sensations, postural hypotension, impotence, and difficulty controlling urination
10. The primary treatment goal of type 1 and type 2 diabetes is normalization of blood glucose levels.
    Unrestricted diets and activities are not possible. Dietary treatment of diabetes using medical nutrition therapy (MNT) and exercise constitutes the basis for management of most patients, especially those with the type 2 form of the disease.
11. Intensive therapy describes a comprehensive program of diabetes care that includes self-monitoring of blood glucose four or more times daily, medical nutritional therapy, exercise, and for those patients with type 1 diabetes, three or more insulin injections daily or use of an insulin pump for continuous insulin infusion.
12. Secretogogues, biguanide, thiazolidinediones, alpha-glucosidase inhibitors, and incretin-based therapy
13. See textbook, p. 579.

14. See Table 36-2 for criteria for the diagnosis of diabetes mellitus.
15. See textbook, p. 558.
16. Too much insulin, insufficient food intake to cover insulin taken, imbalances from diarrhea and vomiting, or excessive exercise without additional carbohydrate intake are common causes of hypoglycemia.
17. When serum glucose is 240 mg/dL or above, test for the presence of ketones.

19. What signs and symptoms result from peripheral vascular disease?

20. What types of visual complications are people with diabetes mellitus more susceptible to?

21. How often should people with diabetes mellitus have an eye exam?

22. How can complications of diabetes affecting the kidneys be identified?

23. What is the source of endogenous insulin? What are the primary animal sources of exogenous insulins?

24. What methods are used to produce human exogenous insulin?

25. Is insulin required for glucose transport into the brain or liver tissue?

26. Why can't insulin be administered orally?

27. Differentiate among *onset, peak,* and *duration* in relation to insulin therapy.

28. What are the most rapid-acting forms of insulin manufactured today?

29. Do short-acting, intermediate-acting, and long-acting insulins differ in terms of onset, peak, and duration of action?

30. How far in advance of a meal should a rapid-acting insulin be administered?

31. How far in advance of a meal should a short-acting insulin be administered?

32. Examine Table 36-6 in the textbook and identify compatibility of insulin combinations.

33. What are the major advantages of insulin glargine and detemir?

18. The glycosylated hemoglobin measures glucose control over the previous 8–10 weeks, while the fructosamine test measures the amount of glucose bonded to the protein fructosamine over the previous 1–3 weeks. Each has a benefit in measuring glucose control.

19. Cyanosis or reddish-blue discoloration in the hands, feet, and legs. Pallor and coolness in the feet and legs. Ulcerations may develop. When any circulatory impairment is found, pedal and radial pulses should be checked at least every 4 hours.

20. Blurred vision may occur with hyperglycemia. With advanced diabetes mellitus, there are changes in small blood vessels in the eyes (microangiopathies). Retinal hemorrhages, degeneration of retinal vascular tissue, cataracts, and blindness may also occur.

21. Regular eye exams to detect changes in the eye should be performed at least annually and more often as deemed appropriate by the health care provider.

22. Presence of proteinuria, elevated serum creatinine, and blood urea nitrogen. People with diabetes mellitus are more likely to have urinary tract infections.

23. Endogenous insulin is produced by the beta cells of the pancreas. Synthetic insulin is the primary source of insulin for recently diagnosed diabetics. Beef and pork pancreas are the primary animal sources of exogenous insulin, but fish and sheep pancreas have been used as well.

24. Most common source of human insulin production is with recombinant DNA.

25. No

26. Insulin is destroyed by the proteolytic enzymes in the gastrointestinal tract.

27. Onset is the time required for the initial effect of insulin to occur. Peak is the time of the maximum effect of insulin. Duration is the length of time insulin remains active.

28. The most rapid-acting insulins are the insulin analogs, new synthetic forms called lispro, aspart, and glulisine.

29. Yes. See Table 36-5.

30. Rapid-acting insulins should be administered 10–15 minutes before a meal.

31. Short-acting insulins should be administered 30 minutes before a meal.

32. See Table 36-6.

34. How should insulin be stored?

35. What does "U-100" mean?

36. What kind of syringe is used to measure U-100 insulin?

37. What is the only type of insulin used intravenously?

38. Why is it important to teach the patient to rotate insulin sites within one area before proceeding to the next area on a rotation schedule?

39. What effect does the long-term use of one injection site have on insulin absorption?

40. With increased activity and exercise, what adjustment may be required in the insulin dose?

41. When are patients who are receiving rapid-acting, short-acting, intermediate-acting, or long-acting insulin most likely to develop hypoglycemia if the dose is excessive or meals are not taken as planned?

42. When are blood or urine tests for glucose performed in relation to meals and insulin administration?

33. Insulin glargine and detemir are biosynthetic long-acting insulins. They are absorbed from the subcutaneous tissue in a uniform manner without large fluctuations in insulin levels, reducing the possibility of hypoglycemic reactions. Either product is usually injected in the evening to serve as a 24-hour basal source of insulin for the body.

34. It is recommended that insulin be neither allowed to freeze nor heated above a temperature of 98° F. A general rule of thumb is that the bottle of insulin should be stored in the refrigerator (not the freezer) until opened. Because patients find it uncomfortable to inject cold insulin, the bottle may then be kept at room temperature until gone. It is recommended that once an insulin vial is opened, it should be discarded in 30 days. Even though the insulin has not "gone bad," there is concern that the contents are no longer sterile and that the vial may become a reservoir for infection, especially in patients who reuse needles. At sustained temperatures above room temperature, insulins lose potency rapidly.

35. U-100 means 100 units of insulin are contained in 1 mL of solution.

36. An insulin syringe calibrated in 100 units has been available for years; however, because U-100 = 100 units in 1 mL, a tuberculin syringe could also be used to accurately measure the dosage.

37. Regular insulin

38. To prevent hypertrophy or atrophy of subcutaneous tissue

39. Absorption is prolonged and control of glucose may require an increase in the insulin dose. If switching from an injection site that has been used repeatedly to one used infrequently, the dose of insulin may need to be decreased to prevent hypoglycemia. Each patient's reactions are somewhat variable, but patients may become hypoglycemic. A snack may be required to cover the action of the insulin, or the insulin dose could be reduced if the increased activity can be anticipated.

40. Because of risk of hypoglycemia, the insulin dose could be reduced if increased activity can be anticipated.

41. If the patient injects insulin at 7 AM, rapid-acting insulin may induce hypoglycemia within 1–3 hours; short-acting insulin: occurs before lunch; intermediate-acting insulin: between 3 PM and supper; and long-acting insulin: between 2 AM and breakfast.

43. Differentiate between the symptoms of hypoglycemia and hyperglycemia.

44. What are the treatments for hypoglycemia and hyperglycemia?

45. If uncertain whether a patient is hypoglycemic or hyperglycemic, what action should be taken?

46. Why do allergic reactions to insulins occur?

47. What complications are associated with diabetes mellitus?

48. Describe the procedure for mixing two insulins in the same syringe.

49. What effect does the administration of beta-adrenergic blocking agents concurrent with insulin have on symptoms of hypoglycemia?

42. 1/2 hour before meals and at bedtime

43. Hypoglycemia: rapid onset, nervousness, tremors, headache, apprehension, sweating, hunger, double or blurred vision, lack of coordination, unconsciousness. Hyperglycemia: gradual onset, increased thirst, headache, nausea and vomiting, rapid pulse, shallow respirations, acetone odor on breath, unconsciousness.

44. Hypoglycemia: If conscious and able to swallow: 2–4 oz fruit juice with 2 teaspoons sugar or honey added, or 1 cup skim milk, 4 oz nondiet soft drink, or piece of candy (not chocolate), or frosting added. If unable to swallow: 20–50 mL glucose 50% IV. Hyperglycemia: Hospitalize the patient, identify the cause, hydrate the patient and give insulin IV; stabilize electrolytes, especially potassium. See also drug monograph for glucagon.

45. Treat for hypoglycemia.

46. Allergy may be caused by a protein from the animal source of insulin (e.g., pork, beef) or from the protein modifiers used to extend the duration of insulin (e.g., isophane). An acute reaction with a rash over the entire body is a rare, but possible, symptom of an anaphylactic reaction that must be treated with antihistamines, epinephrine, and steroids. Allergic reactions can be minimized by changing to an insulin without protein modifiers or to insulins derived from biosynthetic (nonanimal) sources; by using unscented alcohol swabs. Local irritation can be minimized by using disposable syringes and needles and by checking the patient's injection technique.

47. Microvascular complications are those that arise from destruction of capillaries in eyes, kidneys, and peripheral tissues. Macrovascular complications are those associated with atherosclerosis of middle to large arteries such as those in the heart and brain. Comorbid diseases that often arise include hypertension; cardiovascular disease leading to myocardial infarction and stroke; retinopathy leading to blindness; renal disease leading to end-stage renal disease and the need for dialysis; peripheral arterial disease leading to nonhealing ulcers, infections, and lower extremity amputations; neuropathies with sexual dysfunction, bladder incontinence, paresthesias, and gastroparesis; and periodontal disease with loss of teeth.

48. See the text for details.

50. What drug class does the drug metformin (Glucophage) belong to and what is its mechanism of action?

51. For what type of allergy should you check the chart and the patient before initiating therapy with a sulfonylurea oral hypoglycemic agent?

52. What is the effect of sulfonylurea hypoglycemic agents combined with ethanol on blood glucose levels?

53. What are the therapeutic outcomes expected from a biguanide oral antidiabetic agent, sulfonylurea oral hypoglycemic agents, meglitinide oral hypoglycemic agents, thiazolidinedione oral antidiabetic agents, alpha-glucosidase inhibitor agents, incretin-mimetic agents, and amylinomimetic agents?

54. What adverse effects can be expected with acarbose (Precose) and miglitol (Glyset)?

55. What affect can acarbose (Precose) and miglitol (Glyset) have on digoxin absorption?

56. What is the action of glucagon?

57. Name an incretin-mimetic agent.

58. Discuss the use and action of DPP-4 inhibitor therapy in the treatment of diabetes mellitus.

59. Name a drug in the DPP-4 inhibitor class.

49. Beta-adrenergic blocking agents mask the signs of hypoglycemia.

50. Metformin (Glucophage) represents a class of oral antidiabetic agents known as the *biguanides*. Metformin decreases hepatic glucose production by inhibiting glucogenolysis and gluconeogensis, reduces absorption of glucose from the small intestine, and increases insulin sensitivity improving glucose uptake in peripheral muscle and adipose cells. It may also stimulate glucose metabolism by anaerobic glycolysis. The net result is a significant decrease in fasting and postprandial blood glucose and hemoglobin A_{1c} concentrations. Insulin must be present for metformin to be active, and therefore is not effective in type 1 diabetes.

51. Sulfonamides. The patient who is allergic to sulfonamides may also be allergic to sulfonylureas.

52. Hypoglycemia. Also may result in an Antabuse-like reaction manifested by facial flushing, pounding headache, breathlessness, and nausea.

53. More appropriate control of FPG and glycosylated hemoglobin concentration with fewer long-term complications from poorly controlled type 2 diabetes

54. Abdominal cramps, diarrhea, flatulence. Resolves with continued use of acarbose or miglitol.

55. These drugs may inhibit digoxin absorption.

56. Glucagon breaks down stored glycogen to glucose to be used as an energy source.

57. Exenatide (Byetta) is an incretin-mimetic agent.

58. See textbook, p. 581.

59. Sitagliptin (Januvia)

Drugs Used to Treat Diabetes Mellitus

chapter

36

Learning Activities

FILL-IN-THE-BLANK

Finish each of the following statements using the correct term.

1. The category of diabetes mellitus reserved for women who show abnormal glucose tolerance during pregnancy is called _____ diabetes mellitus.

2. _____ is a hormone produced in the beta cells of the pancreas and is a key regulator of metabolism.

3. The most rapidly acting insulins are the insulin analogs, new synthetic forms called _____, _____, and _____.

4. _____ insulin is the only dosage form of insulin that is approved to be injected by both intravenous and subcutaneous routes of administration.

5. _____ is a hormone secreted by the alpha cells of the pancreas that breaks down stored glycogen to glucose, resulting in elevated blood glucose levels.

6. The _____ are nonsulfonylurea oral hypoglycemic agents that lower blood glucose by stimulating the release of insulin from the beta cells of the pancreas.

7. Insulin is required to transport glucose into skeletal and heart muscle and fat. It is not required for glucose transport into the _____.

8. _____ of the skin can be prevented by rotating the insulin injection sites.

MATCHING

Match the generic drug name with its corresponding brand name. Each option will be used only once.

_____ 9. tolbutamide

_____ 10. chlorpropamide

_____ 11. pramlintide

_____ 12. glyburide

_____ 13. sitagliptin

_____ 14. exenatide

_____ 15. rosiglitazone

_____ 16. repaglinide

a. Prandin
b. Glynase
c. Orinase
d. Avandia
e. Januvia
f. Symlin
g. Diabinese
h. Byetta

TRUE OR FALSE

Write "T" for true and "F" for false for each statement. Correct all false statements.

_____ 17. Diabetes mellitus is a group of diseases characterized by hyperglycemia resulting from defects in insulin secretion, insulin action, or both.

_____ 18. Type 2 diabetes mellitus was formerly known as *insulin dependent diabetes mellitus* (IDDM).

_____ 19. Type 1 diabetes mellitus occurs only in juveniles.

_____ 20. In Type 2 diabetes mellitus, the pancreas is not able to produce or secrete any insulin.

_____ 21. Insulin is not required for glucose transport into the brain tissue.

_____ 22. Insulin must always be stored in the refrigerator.

_____ 23. Rotation of injection sites of subcutaneous insulin is important to avoid atrophy or hypertrophy of subcutaneous fat tissue.

_____ 24. Sitagliptin (Januvia) is a DPP-4 inhibitor used to reduce elevated fasting and postprandial hyperglycemia in patients with type 2 diabetes mellitus who are taking metformin and who have not achieved adequate glycemic control.

_____ 25. Exenatide (Byetta) is used to reduce blood sugar in patients with type 1 diabetes mellitus.

Drugs Used to Treat Diabetes Mellitus

chapter **36**

Practice Questions for the NCLEX® Examination

_____ 1. The nurse administers 4 units of lispro insulin to a patient at 0800. At what time is the patient most at risk for the development of hypoglycemia?
   1. 1000
   2. 1200
   3. 1400
   4. 1600

_____ 2. The nurse is teaching a patient about insulin administration. Which statement made by the patient indicates a need for further teaching?
   1. "I will keep insulin I am using at room temperature."
   2. "I will freeze unopened insulin bottles until I need to use them."
   3. "I will roll the NPH insulin bottle between my hands before administration."
   4. "I do not need to roll the Regular insulin in my hands before administration."

_____ 3. Which drug when taken with insulin is most likely to induce hypoglycemia, and/or mask many of the symptoms of hypoglycemia?
   1. Opioids
   2. Calcium channel blockers
   3. Nonsteroidal anti-inflammatory agents
   4. Beta-adrenergic blocking agents

_____ 4. Which statement about metformin (Glucophage) is true?
   1. Metformin stimulates the release of insulin from the pancreas.
   2. Metformin will not cause hypoglycemia.
   3. Patients taking metformin are at high risk for rapid weight gain.
   4. Patients taking metformin require bloodwork to assess a rapid rise in triglycerides as a result of this therapy.

_____ 5. Which of the following is most likely to benefit from treatment with sulfonylurea oral hypoglycemic agents?
   1. Patient with type 1 diabetes mellitus
   2. Patient with type 2 diabetes mellitus that is not controlled by diet and exercise
   3. 18-month-old infant newly diagnosed with diabetes
   4. Patient on a current regimen of 60 units of NPH insulin a day

_____ 6. Which drug acts to lower blood glucose by increasing the sensitivity of muscle and fat tissue to insulin, allowing more glucose to enter the cells in the presence of insulin for metabolism?
   1. Meglitinide oral hypoglycemic agents
   2. Sulfonylurea oral hypoglycemic agents
   3. Biguanide oral antidiabetic agents
   4. Thiazolidinedione oral antidiabetic agents

_____ 7. It is important for the nurse to inform female patients with diabetes that an alternative method of birth control should be used when taking which oral hypoglycemic agent?
   1. Meglitinides
   2. Sulfonylureas
   3. Biguanides
   4. Thiazolidinediones

_____ 8. What are common adverse effects associated with acarbose (Precose) therapy? *(Select all that apply.)*
   1. Hypoglycemia
   2. Abdominal cramps
   3. Jaundice
   4. Flatulence
   5. Diarrhea

_____ 9. Which statements does the nurse include when teaching health promotion activities to a patient with type 2 diabetes mellitus? *(Select all that apply.)*
   1. "If you feel sick, cut your insulin dose by half."
   2. "If your blood glucose is greater than 240 mg/dL, you should test your urine for ketones."
   3. "Notify your primary health care provider immediately if you are unable to keep anything down."
   4. "Extra insulin is often needed to meet the demands of illness, so be aware of the development of hyperglycemia which is common in patients with acute illness, injury, or surgery."
   5. "Store unused insulin in the freezer."

_____ 10. Which statements about biosynthetic long-acting insulins glargine (Lantus) and detemir (Levemir) are true? *(Select all that apply.)*
   1. They have a very high risk of hypoglycemic reactions because of large fluctuations in insulin levels.
   2. These drugs are always administered first thing in the morning.
   3. They provide a 24-hour basal source of insulin for the body.
   4. Neither insulin glargine or detemir should be mixed with other insulins.
   5. Both medications are administered via an insulin pump.

_____ 11. Which insulins are long-acting insulins? *(Select all that apply.)*
   1. Apidra (glulisine)
   2. Humalog (lispro)
   3. Lantus (glargine)
   4. Levemir (detemir)
   5. Novolog (aspart)

12. The physician orders 20 units of 70/30 insulin. How many units of regular insulin does the patient receive? _____ units

13. A patient is ordered Novolin R Regular U-100 insulin 12 units with Novolin N NPH U-100 insulin 40 units subcutaneously before breakfast. How many total units of insulin does the patient receive? _____ units

14. A patient is ordered pioglitazone (Actos) 45 mg PO once daily in the morning. The medication is available in 30-mg tablets. How many tablets does the nurse administer? _____ tablet(s)

Drugs Used to Treat Thyroid Disease

Review Sheet

The QUESTION column and the ANSWER column have been offset so that you can cover the answers while reading the questions, allowing you to assess your knowledge.

Question	Answer
1. What glands regulate the function of the thyroid gland?	
2. What body functions are regulated by the thyroid gland?	1. Hypothalamus and anterior pituitary gland.
3. What is another name for myxedema?	2. Growth and maturation; carbohydrate, protein, and lipid metabolism; thermal regulation; cardiovascular function; lactation; and reproduction are all processes affected by thyroid function.
4. Excessive thyroid secretion results in what conditions?	3. Hypothyroidism in adult patients
5. What is a normal thyroid state called?	4. Hyperthyroidism, also known as *thyrotoxicosis*.
6. Thyroid replacement hormones are used to replace what hormones secreted by the thyroid gland?	5. Euthyroid state.
7. What focused assessment should be performed by the nurse when a patient has hypothyroid or hyperthyroid disorders?	6. Liothyronine (T_3) and levothyroxine (T_4)
8. If a patient has hypothyroidism, what change in his or her weight over the past few months could be anticipated?	7. See textbook, pp. 585-586.
9. A patient with hyperthyroidism may require what dietary changes?	8. Weight gain
10. What type of environment does a patient with hypothyroidism or hyperthyroidism need?	9. Increase in calories to meet metabolic needs—as much as 4000 to 5000 calories daily.
11. List the thyroid hormone replacement products' brand names and ingredients.	10. Hypothyroidism = warm environment; hyperthyroidism = cool environment
12. Of the thyroid products available, which has the most rapid onset of action?	11. Levothyroxine (T_4)—(Synthroid, Levoxyl) Liothyronine (T_3)—(Cytomel) Liotrix (T_3, T_4)—(Thyrolar) Thyroid USP
13. Are thyroid replacement hormones given to a patient with hypothyroidism or hyperthyroidism?	12. Liothyronine (T_3) (Cytomel)
14. List the signs and symptoms of hypothyroidism and hyperthyroidism.	13. Hypothyroidism

15. What are the three products available to treat hyperthyroidism?
16. State the action of propylthiouracil (PTU, Propacil) and methimazole (Tapazole).
17. Describe the desired therapeutic outcome(s) for antithyroid medications.

18. What are the adverse effects to assess when propylthiouracil (PTU) or methimazole (Tapazole) are administered?

19. What laboratory studies should be performed at periodic intervals for people taking propylthiouracil (PTU, Propacil)?
20. Would a patient with hyperthyroidism be more likely to require a smaller or larger dose of a digitalis glycoside?

14. See textbook, pp. 584-585.

15. Radioactive iodine (^{131}I), propylthiouracil (PTU, Propacil), and methimazole (Tapazole)

16. Propylthiouracil (PTU, Propacil) and methimazole (Tapazole) block the synthesis of T_3 and T_4 in the thyroid gland; the drugs do not destroy T_3 and T_4 already produced.

17. The primary therapeutic outcome expected from propylthiouracil (Propacil) or methimazole (Tapazole) is a gradual return to normal thyroid metabolic function.

18. Skin eruptions, pruritus, headaches, salivary or lymph node enlargement, sore throat, purpura, jaundice, and progressive weakness.

19. RBC, WBC, and differential counts

20. A larger dose

Drugs Used to Treat Thyroid Disease

Learning Activities

FILL-IN-THE-BLANK

Finish each of the following statements using the correct term.

1. _____ is a hypothyroidism that occurs during adult life.

2. Excessive formation of thyroid hormones and their secretion into the circulatory system causes hyperthyroidism, also known as _____.

3. Thyroid gland function is regulated by the _____ and the _____-_____ gland.

4. The historical name for congenital hypothyroidism is _____.

5. The characteristic eye changes of patients with hyperthyroidism including edema of the tissues around the eyeballs are referred to as _____.

MATCHING

Match the generic drug name with its corresponding brand name. Each option will be used only once.

_____ 6. levothyroxine

_____ 7. liotrix

_____ 8. liothyronine

a. Thyrolar
b. Synthroid
c. Cytomel

TRUE OR FALSE

Write "T" for true and "F" for false for each statement. Correct all false statements.

_____ 9. A patient diagnosed with hypothyroidism will have high serum levels of circulating T_3 and T_4 hormones.

_____ 10. The thyroid gland is a large, reddish, ductless gland in front of and on either side of the trachea.

_____ 11. The thyroid hormones are triiodothyronine and thyroxine.

_____ 12. Congenital hypothyroidism is a very common disorder found today.

_____ 13. Myxedema may be caused by excessive use of antithyroid drugs used to treat hyperthyroidism.

_____ 14. Hyperthyroidism is a condition caused by excessive production of thyroid hormone.

_____ 15. Thyroid replacement hormones block the release of T_3 and T_4 in the body, thereby making the hormones available for metabolic functioning.

_____ 16. Baseline premedication assessments prior to initiation of thyroid replacement hormones are vital signs, weight, bowel elimination pattern, and laboratory studies to identify thyroid hormone levels.

_____ 17. The hypothyroid patient will be hyperactive.

_____ 18. The resting pulse rate of a hyperthyroid patient upon awakening will be low.

_____ 19. A patient with hypothyroidism would show dramatic weight loss as one symptom.

Drugs Used to Treat Thyroid Disease

Practice Questions for the NCLEX® Examination

_____ 1. Which manifestation does the nurse expect to find upon assessing a patient who has been diagnosed with hyperthyroidism?
1. Cardiac enlargement
2. Constipation
3. Subnormal body temperature
4. Puffy face

_____ 2. A patient is receiving insulin, warfarin (Coumadin), digoxin (Lanoxin), and estrogen therapy. The patient has now been ordered thyroid replacement therapy. With the addition of this therapy, the nurse anticipates that the patient will be affected in which way?
1. The patient will most likely require a decreased dosage of the warfarin.
2. The patient will be at high risk for the development of hyperglycemia.
3. The patient will most likely require an increased dosage of digoxin.
4. The patient may require a decreased dosage of thyroid hormone because of the estrogen therapy.

_____ 3. Which statements about iodine-131 (^{131}I) are true? *(Select all that apply.)*
1. It is administered intravenously.
2. It has no color.
3. It is radioactive.
4. It is used to treat hypothyroidism.
5. It destroys hyperactive thyroid tissue with essentially no damage to other tissue.

_____ 4. The nurse has been teaching a patient diagnosed with hyperthyroidism about proper nutritional habits to follow. Which patient statement indicates a need for further teaching?
1. "I will limit my fluid intake to three 8-ounce glasses of water a day."
2. "I will eat a high-calorie diet, about 4000 to 5000 calories a day."
3. "I will drink uncaffeinated cola."
4. "I will avoid chocolate."

_____ 5. A patient who has undergone a thyroidectomy is at greatest risk for the development of which electrolyte disturbance?
1. Hyponatremia
2. Hypokalemia
3. Hypochloremia
4. Hypocalcemia

_____ 6. In assessing a patient with myxedema, the nurse expects to find which manifestations? *(Select all that apply.)*
1. Subnormal body temperature
2. Puffy face
3. Dry skin
4. Decreased blood pressure
5. Thin skin

_____ 7. Which medications interact with propylthiouracil (Propacil)? *(Select all that apply.)*
1. Acetaminophen (Tylenol)
2. Warfarin (Coumadin)
3. Digoxin (Lanoxin)
4. Furosemide (Lasix)
5. Ibuprofen (Motrin)

8. A patient is prescribed methimazole (Tapazole) 15 mg PO daily at 1000. The medication is available in 5-mg tablets. How many tablets does the nurse administer? _____ tablet(s)

9. A patient is ordered liothyronine sodium (Cytomel) 25 mcg daily at 1000. The medication is available as 25 mcg per tablet. How many tablets does the nurse administer?
_____ tablet(s)

_____ 10. When administering iodine-131 (^{131}I) to a patient, what actions does the nurse take? *(Select all that apply.)*
   1. Adds the medication to water and has the patient swallow it
   2. Wears latex gloves when administering the drug
   3. Avoids spilling the medication
   4. Changes the patient's bedding after each dose
   5. Maintains hazardous medication precautions when working with the drug

Corticosteroids

Review Sheet

The QUESTION column and the ANSWER column have been offset so that you can cover the answers while reading the questions, allowing you to assess your knowledge.

Question	Answer
1. Define *corticosteroids*.	
2. For what types of illnesses are glucocorticoids frequently prescribed?	1. Hormones secreted by the adrenal cortex of the adrenal gland.
3. What endogenous hormone is known as a glucocorticoid?	2. To treat diseases or disorders that are inflammatory or allergic in nature. Glucocorticoids have anti-inflammatory, antiallergenic, and immunosuppressant activity. They may also be used to reduce nausea and vomiting associated with chemotherapy.
4. Do exogenous corticosteroids cure disease?	3. Cortisol
5. What adverse effects may be observed with the administration of glucocorticoids?	4. Exogenous corticosteroids do not cure disease unless the adrenal glands have been surgically removed and corticosteroids are used for replacement therapy. Usually, steroids provide relief of symptoms without treating the underlying disease.
6. What time of day is best to administer glucocorticoids?	5. Hyperglycemia, glycosuria (corticosteroids stimulate formation of glucose while decreasing use of glucose by the body); electrolyte imbalances and fluid accumulation due to mineralocorticoid effects that cause sodium and water retention and potassium and hydrogen excretion; increased susceptibility to infection; peptic ulcer formation by decreasing the protective secretions of the gastric mucosa; delayed wound healing because of protein breakdown; visual changes, cataracts; osteoporosis—inhibits bone formation and growth; see textbook, p. 599.
7. Why do corticosteroids and diuretics produce or enhance hypokalemia when given simultaneously?	6. Between 6 AM and 9 AM to minimize suppression of normal adrenal function.
8. Why must patients taking corticosteroids be cautioned to avoid contact with people with infections?	7. Diuretics (except potassium-sparing diuretics) and corticosteroids cause the loss of potassium.

9. What instructions should be given to a patient taking corticosteroids?

10. What baseline assessments should be completed for patients taking any type of corticosteroids?

11. Review the signs and symptoms of Addison's disease and Cushing's disease and contrast these with the signs and symptoms of adrenocortical excess and deficiency.

12. What effect do glucocorticoids have on blood glucose levels?

13. What type of health teaching should be done for a patient receiving steroid therapy?

14. What is the major glucocorticoid secreted by the adrenal cortex?

15. Why is an alternate-day schedule for administration of corticosteroids used?

16. What effect do corticosteroids have on potassium balance?

17. What is the main function of the mineralocorticoids?

8. Corticosteroids diminish the production of antibodies, resulting in a suppressed immune system, making the patient susceptible to infection. The anti-inflammatory properties of these drugs also mask the presence of infection. Even the slightest signs and symptoms of an infection may indicate the presence of a major infection.

9. See textbook, p. 596.

10. Daily weight; blood pressure in supine and sitting position; intake and output for hospitalized patients; electrolyte studies, especially sodium and potassium; check mental status; blood glucose; signs and symptoms of infection; signs and symptoms of ulcers.

11. See a general medical-surgical nursing text.

12. Hyperglycemia

13. An identification bracelet should be worn by the patient at all times. If the patient has been on long-term therapy, he or she should not suddenly discontinue drug therapy. See textbook for specific drug therapy prescribed by reviewing the drug monograph.

14. Cortisol

15. Alternate-day schedule, between 6 AM and 9 AM, minimizes suppression of normal adrenal function. Also administer with meals to minimize gastric irritation.

16. Enhance loss of potassium. Be especially alert when diuretics such as furosemide (Lasix), thiazides, bumetanide (Bumex), and other non-potassium–sparing diuretics are prescribed concurrently.

17. The mineralocorticoids (fludrocortisone [Florinef] and aldosterone) maintain fluid and electrolyte balance and are used to treat adrenal insufficiency caused by hypopituitarism or Addison's disease.

Corticosteroids

Learning Activities

FILL-IN-THE-BLANK

Fill in each of the following statements using the correct term.

1. The mineralocorticoids consist of
    _____ and _____.

2. _____ are hormones secreted by the adrenal cortex of the adrenal gland.

3. The two most common electrolyte disturbances associated with corticosteroid therapy are _____ and
    _____.

4. The major glucocorticoid of the adrenal cortex is _____.

5. Glucocorticoids are most frequently prescribed because of their _____ and
    _____ properties.

MATCHING

Match the generic drug name with its corresponding brand name. Each option will be used only once.

_____ 6. desoximetasone

_____ 7. prednisolone

_____ 8. dexamethasone

_____ 9. methylprednisolone

_____ 10. betamethasone

a. Prelone
b. Solu-Medrol
c. Celestone
d. Topicort
e. Decadron

TRUE OR FALSE

Write "T" for true and "F" for false for each statement. Correct all false statements.

_____ 11. The glucocorticoids maintain fluid and electrolyte balance.

_____ 12. Mineralocorticoids regulate carbohydrate, fat, and protein metabolism.

_____ 13. Patients receiving corticosteroid therapy have higher incidence of peptic ulcer disease.

_____ 14. Corticosteroid therapy may induce hyperglycemia, particularly in prediabetic or diabetic patients.

_____ 15. Corticosteroids are secreted from the adrenal medulla.

_____ 16. Psychotic behavior may be seen during corticosteroid therapy.

_____ 17. Glucocorticoids taken for long-term therapy may produce cataracts.

_____ 18. Corticosteroid therapy does not mask the signs and symptoms of infection.

_____ 19. To minimize suppression of normal adrenal function, corticosteroids may be administered on alternate days.

_____ 20. Corticosteroids should not be discontinued abruptly.

_____ 21. Glucocorticoids should be administered between 6 PM and 9 PM to maintain normal adrenal function.

_____ 22. The major glucocorticoid secreted by the adrenal cortex is cortisol.

Corticosteroids

Practice Questions for the NCLEX® Examination

_____ 1. What is the priority assessment for the nurse to make when caring for a patient on fludrocortisone (Florinef) therapy for Addison's disease?
1. Allergy
2. Hyponatremia
3. Hypokalemia
4. Hypotension

_____ 2. The nurse has been teaching a patient with an exacerbation of rheumatoid arthritis about the use of glucocorticoids. Which statement by the patient indicates a need for further instruction?
1. "This drug has cured my disease."
2. "This drug is relieving the inflammation associated with rheumatoid arthritis."
3. "My fingers will not change back to normal shape due to this drug treatment."
4. "I must be aware that I am more susceptible to infections when taking these drugs."

_____ 3. A patient is ordered once-daily therapy with methylprednisolone (SoluMedrol) for treatment of systemic lupus erythematosus. The nurse instructs the patient to take the medication at what time?
1. 0800
2. 1200
3. 1400
4. 1600

_____ 4. When caring for children on long-term glucocorticoid therapy, what is the priority monitoring parameter for the nurse to assess?
1. Weight
2. Skeletal growth
3. Urinary output
4. Cognitive development

_____ 5. The nurse assesses the eyes of patients receiving long-term therapy with glucocorticoids because they are at highest risk for the development of which condition?
1. Presbyopia
2. Glaucoma
3. Cataracts
4. Retinal detachment

_____ 6. Patients taking corticosteroid therapy are instructed to report which symptoms to the health care provider? *(Select all that apply.)*
1. Dyspnea
2. Dry cough
3. Worsening fatigue
4. Angina
5. Edema of the feet and ankles

_____ 7. Which statements does the nurse include when teaching patients about corticosteroid therapy? *(Select all that apply.)*
1. "A high-sodium diet is needed when taking corticosteroids."
2. "A low-potassium diet is needed when taking corticosteroids."
3. "Take the corticosteroid before 9:00 AM."
4. "Take the medication with food."
5. "Most of the calories consumed should come from fats."

_____ 8. The nurse is assessing a patient taking glucocorticoids for the treatment of rheumatoid arthritis. Which findings are indications that the medication is exerting its desired effect? *(Select all that apply.)*
1. Relief of pain
2. Elevated sedimentation rates
3. Normalization of preexisting joint deformities
4. Increased energy
5. Relief of swelling

9. A patient is prescribed 15 mg of prednisone (Deltasone). The medication is available as an oral solution 5 mg/5 mL. How many mL does the nurse administer? _____ mL

10. An order reads Solu-Medrol 100 mg IV every 6 hours. The medication label reads 500 mg of powdered Solu-Medrol for IM or IV injection. Directions on the label state "Reconstitute with 8 mL of bacteriostatic water." After reconstituting the Solu-Medrol, how many mg/mL of Solu-Medrol are there? _____ mg/mL

To administer 100 mg, the nurse draws up how many mL from the medication vial to administer the ordered 100 mg? _____ mL

_____ 11. Glucocorticoids must be used with caution in patients with which disorders? *(Select all that apply.)*
1. Type 1 diabetes mellitus
2. Type 2 diabetes mellitus
3. Upper respiratory infections
4. Severe hay fever
5. Mental disturbances

Gonadal Hormones

Review Sheet

The QUESTION column and the ANSWER column have been offset so that you can cover the answers while reading the questions, allowing you to assess your knowledge.

Question

1. What is another name for the male sex hormones?

2. What male characteristics are attributed to androgens?

3. When androgens are given to females, what effects can be anticipated?

4. Describe the effect of the administration of testosterone to boys before completion of bone growth.

5. When would androgens be prescribed for postmenopausal women?

6. Review the uses and effects of estrogens on the body systems.

7. Describe the relationship between hormone replacement therapy in women and the development of cardiovascular disease.

8. What are the common and serious adverse effects of estrogen therapy?

9. What are progestins used to treat?

10. What are androgens used to treat?

Answer

1. Androgens; testosterone is the primary hormone.

2. Normal growth and development of male sex organs and secondary sex characteristics (e.g., growth and maturation of prostate, seminal vesicles, penis, and scrotum; development and distribution of male hair on the body; deepening of the voice).

3. Masculinization, if given in sufficient doses (e.g., deepening voice, hirsutism, acne, menstrual irregularity); electrolyte imbalance of Na^+, K^+, Cl^-, and Ca^{++}; gastric irritation.

4. May cause premature closure of the epiphyseal line, inhibiting normal bone growth.

5. Androgens are used for palliation of breast cancer in postmenopausal women with certain cell types of cancer. They suppress cancer cell growth.

6. See textbook, pp. 602-603.

7. Results of a recent controlled study, the Women's Health Initiative (WHI), indicate that hormone replacement therapy is associated with a small increase in the risk for cardiovascular disease.

8. Common adverse effects are weight gain, edema, breast tenderness, nausea. Serious adverse effects are hypertension, hyperglycemia, thrombophlebitis, and breakthrough vaginal bleeding.

9. Progestins are used to treat secondary amenorrhea, breakthrough uterine bleeding, and endometriosis. They may also be used in combination with estrogens as oral contraceptives.

11. What premedication assessments should be performed prior to therapy with estrogens, progestins, and androgens?

12. What serious adverse effect can androgen therapy have on calcium levels in patients being treated for breast cancer?

13. Identify common estrogen, progestin, and androgen medications.

10. Androgens are used to treat hypogonadism, eunuchism, androgen deficiency, and palliation of breast cancer in postmenopausal women with certain cell types of cancer. Androgens may treat wasting syndrome associated with AIDS.

11. See textbook: estrogens, p. 603; progestins, p. 605; androgens, p. 606.

12. Hypercalcemia

13. Examine Tables 39-1, 39-2, and 39-3.

Gonadal Hormones

Learning Activities

FILL-IN-THE-BLANK

Finish each of the following statements using the correct term.

1. In addition to producing sperm, the testes produce _____, the male sex hormone.

2. _____ are other steroid hormones that produce masculinizing effects.

3. _____ is the female hormone that is thought to be associated mainly with body changes that favor the implantation of the fertilized ovum, continuation of pregnancy, and preparation of the breasts for lactation.

4. The gonads are called the _____ in males, and the _____ in females.

5. Androgen therapy in females produces _____.

MATCHING

Match the generic drug name with its corresponding brand name. Each option will be used only once.

_____ 6. estradiol

_____ 7. norethindrone

_____ 8. testosterone pellets

_____ 9. conjugated estrogens

_____ 10. fluoxymesterone

a. Aygestin
b. Estrace
c. Premarin
d. Testopel
e. Androxy

TRUE OR FALSE

Write "T" for true and "F" for false for each statement. Correct all false statements.

_____ 11. Patients with diabetes mellitus who receive gonadal hormones may experience alterations in the blood glucose levels.

_____ 12. The use of estrogens during early pregnancy is contraindicated.

_____ 13. Male children receiving androgens must have the effects of the drug monitored by periodic x-ray of long bones.

_____ 14. Estrogens are used to slow the disease progression (and minimize discomfort) in patients with advanced prostatic cancer.

_____ 15. Progestins may be used to treat wasting syndrome associated with AIDS.

Gonadal Hormones

chapter

39

Practice Questions for the NCLEX® Examination

_____ 1. Patients taking androgen therapy are most likely to develop which electrolyte imbalance?
   1. Hyperkalemia
   2. Hypernatremia
   3. Hypocalcemia
   4. Hypochloremia

_____ 2. What are indications of androgen overdose in male patients? *(Select all that apply.)*
   1. Gynecomastia
   2. Hypertension
   3. Excessive sexual stimulation
   4. Priapism
   5. Deepening of the voice

_____ 3. What conditions is progestin therapy used to treat? *(Select all that apply.)*
   1. Severe acne
   2. Breakthrough uterine bleeding
   3. Secondary amenorrhea
   4. Endometriosis
   5. Hot flash symptoms of menopause

_____ 4. A patient taking concurrent phenytoin (Dilantin) and conjugated estrogen (Premarin) is taught to recognize which signs that indicate phenytoin toxicity? *(Select all that apply.)*
   1. Headache
   2. Nystagmus
   3. Sedation
   4. Lethargy
   5. Edema

_____ 5. The nurse is teaching a patient about the adverse effects of estrogen therapy. Which statement by the patient indicates a need for further teaching?
   1. "Weight gain is a common adverse effect of estrogen therapy."
   2. "Breast tenderness is to be expected when I start this drug."

   3. "Low blood pressure is a common side effect of estrogen therapy."
   4. "If I experience any breakthrough bleeding between my menstrual periods, I will notify my primary care provider immediately."

_____ 6. What are the therapeutic uses for estrogen therapy? *(Select all that apply.)*
   1. To relieve hot flash symptoms of menopause
   2. To treat acne in males
   3. To treat advanced prostate cancer
   4. To treat osteoporosis
   5. To provide contraception

_____ 7. While assessing a patient on estrogen therapy, which adverse effect does the nurse report to the health care provider?
   1. Breakthrough bleeding
   2. Weight gain
   3. Breast tenderness
   4. Nausea

_____ 8. A patient is ordered testosterone USP in a gel base (Transdermal System) 5 mg every 24 hours. The nurse teaches the patient to rotate the application sites for the patch to which areas of the body? *(Select all that apply.)*
   1. Hips
   2. Abdomen
   3. Thighs
   4. Buttocks
   5. Scrotum

9. A patient is ordered 10 mg of progesterone IM for amenorrhea. The medication is available as 50 mg/mL. How many mL of the medication does the nurse administer? _____ mL

10. A patient is ordered estradiol (Estrace) 2 mg PO daily. The medication is available as 0.5 mg per tablet. How many tablets will the patient receive in one week? _____ tablets

Drugs Used in Obstetrics

Review Sheet

The QUESTION column and the ANSWER column have been offset so that you can cover the answers while reading the questions, allowing you to assess your knowledge.

Question	**Answer**
1. Identify the factors that need to be assessed during prenatal management of a pregnant woman and during and following normal labor and delivery.	
2. Describe nursing assessments and interventions needed for the pregnant patient experiencing potential obstetrical complications [e.g., infection; hyperemesis gravidarum; miscarriage; abortion; premature rupture of membranes (PROM), gestational diabetes, pregnancy-induced hypertension (PIH); intrauterine fetal death, and hemolysis, elevated liver enzymes, and low platelet count syndrome (HELLP)].	1. See textbook, pp. 610-614.
3. How is preterm labor defined?	2. See textbook, pp. 611-612.
4. What is the fetal fibronectin test?	3. See textbook, p. 612.
5. State the methods and time parameters of each approach to the termination of a pregnancy.	4. A fetal fibronectin test may be ordered to assess the presence of preterm labor in patients whose presenting symptoms are questionable, so that early interventions can be initiated when indicated to prevent preterm delivery. This test is for women with intact membranes and cervical dilatation of less than 3 cm.
6. Cite the recommended times of administration for RhoGAM (human) and rubella vaccine in relation to pregnancy.	5. Before 12 weeks gestation: dilatation and evacuation (D&E); 12–20 weeks gestation: saline or prostaglandin administered intra-amniotically, intramuscularly, or by vaginal suppository; intrauterine fetal death after 20 weeks gestation: prostaglandin suppositories with or without oxytocin augmentation.

7. Describe the nursing assessments and interventions used for PIH.

6. *Previous immunization.* Although there is no need to administer RhoGAM to a woman who is already sensitized to the Rh factor, the risk is no more than that when given to a woman who is not sensitized. When in doubt, administer RhoGAM.

Before administration:
1. *Never* administer the IGIM full dose or microdose products intravenously. (The IGIV full dose product may be administered intramuscularly or intravenously.)
2. *Never* administer to a neonate.
3. *Never* administer to an Rh-negative patient who has been previously sensitized to the Rh antigen.
4. *Confirm* that the mother is Rh negative.

Pregnancy. Postpartum prophylaxis—one standard dose vial of IGIM intramuscularly or one standard dose vial of IGIV intramuscularly or intravenously. Additional vials may be necessary if there was unusually large fetal-maternal hemorrhage.

Antepartum prophylaxis—one standard dose vial IM at about 28 weeks gestational age. This must be followed by another vial administered within 72 hours of delivery. After amniocentesis, miscarriage, abortion, or ectopic pregnancy—less than 13 weeks of gestation: one microdose vial IM within 72 hours; 13 or more weeks of gestation: one standard dose vial IM within 72 hours.

Transfusion accident—Rh-negative, premenopausal women who receive Rh-positive red cells by transfusion: one standard dose vial IM for each 15 mL of transfused packed red cells.

Idiopathic thrombocytopenic purpura—

Before administration:
1. *Confirm* that the mother is Rh positive.
2. *Follow* manufacturer's instructions on dilution and administration of Rho[D] IGIV.

IV—Initial dose: 250 units/kg as a single injection. Additional doses are dependent upon response. Rubella vaccine should be given to a patient whose rubella titer is low, immediately after pregnancy.

8. State the purpose of administering glucocorticoids to certain women in preterm labor.

7. Take vital signs at regularly scheduled intervals and compare with baseline readings. Report elevations of systolic pressure of 30 mm Hg or more above the previous readings, or systolic blood pressure of 140 mm Hg or more, or diastolic pressure of 90 mm Hg or more. Edema may be present: monitor intake and output (I&O) and check state of hydration. Intake of 1000 mL more than the output over the preceding 24 hours is generally allowed. Perform assessment of edema: daily weights, report a weight gain of 2 or more pounds in any 1-week period. Discourage the heavy use of salt. Monitor urine for the presence of protein. Electrolyte studies should be done at regular intervals. Hematocrit will become elevated as the patient becomes dehydrated. Information from the serum estriols and L/S ratio give indications of fetal maturity. Seizure precautions: monitor for drowsiness, hyperreflexia, visual disturbances, or severe pain. Report any of these symptoms immediately. Give prescribed medications (e.g., sedatives, antihypertensives, anticonvulsants). Observe for complications (e.g., started labor, pulmonary edema, heart failure).

9. Summarize the care needs of the pregnant woman during normal labor and delivery.

10. Identify the name, dosage, route of administration, and correct time for administering uterine stimulants.

11. Describe the normal sequence of changes in the appearance of lochia during the postpartum period.

12. Summarize the immediate nursing care needs of the neonate following delivery.

13. Discuss the rationale for inspection of the placenta and cord following delivery of the newborn.

14. Summarize the Centers for Disease Control recommendations for prophylaxis of ophthalmia neonatorum.

15. Identify assessment data essential in detecting postpartum hemorrhage.

16. State the drug actions and nursing assessments needed to monitor therapeutic response and development of common and serious adverse effects from uterine stimulants, uterine relaxants, clomiphene citrate (Clomid), RhoGAM, erythromycin ophthalmic ointment, and phytonadione (vitamin K).

17. List premedication assessments needed prior to an oxytocin (Pitocin) infusion.

8. Glucocorticoids are administered IM to the woman in preterm labor to accelerate fetal lung maturation and to minimize hyaline membrane disease.

9. See textbook, p. 616, for summary of normal labor and delivery needs.

10. See textbook, pp. 619-624.

11. Blood-red immediately after delivery, progressing to a more watery or pinkish color.

12. See text discussion: Immediate Neonatal Care, pp. 616-617.

13. Verify presence of one vein and two arteries in the cord and inspect the placenta to be certain it is intact and no fragments or pieces have been retained.

14. See textbook, p. 617, for acceptable agents that prevent gonococcal ophthalmia neonatorum and chlamydial ophthalmia neonatorum.

15. Fundus height and firmness, lochia color and amount, as well as vital signs.

16. See individual drug monographs for details.

18. What are signs and symptoms of fetal distress?

19. If fetal distress occurs during oxytocin (Pitocin) therapy, what actions should be taken immediately?

20. State the primary clinical indications for use of uterine stimulants.

21. Describe specific nursing concerns and appropriate nursing actions when uterine stimulants are administered for induction of labor, augmentation of labor, and postpartum atony and hemorrhage.

22. Explain the limitations of the use of oxytocin for the purpose of initiating a therapeutic abortion.

23. Review the procedure for insertion of vaginal suppositories.

24. Differentiate among the uses and actions on the uterus of dinoprostone (Prepidil), misoprostol (Cytotec), ergonovine maleate (Ergotrate maleate) and methylergonovine maleate (Methergine), and oxytocin (Pitocin).

17. Maternal vital signs, especially blood pressure and pulse rate; mother's hydration status including urine output and I&O. (This will form baseline data for subsequent monitoring during drug therapy.) Monitor characteristics of uterine contractions (e.g., frequency, rate, duration, and intensity); report duration over 90 seconds. Monitor fetal heart rate and rhythm. Perform reflex testing as specified in drug monograph. Check amount and characteristics of vaginal discharge.

18. See textbook, p. 623.

19. Slow oxytocin infusion to lowest rate in accordance with hospital policy. Turn mother to left lateral position, administer O_2 by mask or nasal cannula, call the health care provider immediately.

20. Four primary clinical uses: (1) induction or augmentation of labor; (2) control of postpartum atony and hemorrhage; (3) control of postsurgical hemorrhage (e.g., cesarean section); and (4) induction of therapeutic abortion.

21. Induction of labor: check vital signs every 15 minutes, use an infusion pump, monitor contractions (e.g., frequency, duration, and intensity), and fetal heart tones. Monitor for fetal distress (fetal heart rate of 160 bpm followed by bradycardia below 120 bpm). If fetal distress occurs, reduce oxytocin infusion to the slowest rate, turn mother to left lateral position, and administer oxygen. Monitor I&O of all patients receiving oxytocin and report accumulation of water by the body, known as "water intoxication."

22. Uterine smooth muscle is not very responsive to oxytocin stimulation until late in the third trimester.

23. See Administration of Vaginal Medications in Chapter 8.

25. Compare the effects of methylergonovine maleate and ergonovine maleate on lactation.

24. Dinoprostone (Prepidil): uterine smooth muscle stimulant. Used during pregnancy to increase the frequency and strength of uterine contractions and produce cervical softening and dilatation. Used to expel uterine contents in cases of intrauterine fetal death, benign hydatidiform mole, missed spontaneous miscarriage, and second trimester abortion.

    Misoprostol (Cytotec): synthetic prostaglandin E used to induce uterine contractions in the pregnant uterus.

    Ergonovine maleate (Ergotrate maleate), methylergonovine maleate (Methergine): both stimulate contractions of the uterus. They cannot be used for induction of labor because they cause sudden, intense uterine activity. Used in postpartum patients to control bleeding and maintain uterine firmness.

    Oxytocin (Pitocin): stimulates smooth muscle of the uterus, blood vessels, and mammary glands. Can be used during the third trimester to initiate labor. Drug of choice to induce labor at term or to augment uterine contractions during first and second stages of labor.

26. Identify specific actions, dosage and administration, and nursing assessments needed during the use of oxytocin (Pitocin) therapy.

27. What is the effect of oxytocin (Pitocin) on fluid balance?

25. Do not use ergonovine in patients who wish to breastfeed. Methylergonovine may be used as an alternative because it will not inhibit stimulation of milk production by prolactin.

26. Observe the rate of infusion of oxytocin and the fetal monitor for measurement of contractions. Assess for nausea, vomiting, fetal distress, hypertension or hypotension, seizure activity, and water intoxication.

27. Oxytocin can alter fluid balance by stimulating antidiuretic hormone, causing the body to accumulate water. Signs and symptoms include drowsiness, listlessness, headache, confusion, oliguria, edema, and in extreme cases, seizures.

28. Compare the effects of uterine stimulants and uterine relaxants on the pregnant uterus.

28. Uterine stimulants increase uterine activity. Uterine relaxants are used to delay or prevent labor and delivery in selected patients.

29. Review the effects of adrenergic agents on $beta_1$ and $beta_2$ receptors and identify the relationship of these actions to the serious adverse effects when adrenergic agents are used to inhibit preterm labor.

30. What are the effects of adrenergic agents on serum glucose and electrolyte balance?

29. Adrenergic or sympathetic control
    $Beta_1$: increase rate and force of heart contractions.
    $Beta_2$: relaxation of smooth muscles in bronchi, uterus, gastrointestinal tract, and peripheral vascular area. Monitor for tachycardia and hypotension.

30. May cause hyperglycemia because of stimulation of the sympathetic system, resulting in an increase in glycogenolysis. Continuous, long-term infusions of terbutaline may also cause hypokalemia. Monitor serum electrolytes periodically.

31. Describe specific assessments needed before and during the use of terbutaline sulfate (Brethine).

32. What are the baseline laboratory studies needed before the initiation of terbutaline sulfate (Brethine) therapy?

33. Describe the potential effects of terbutaline sulfate (Brethine) on the neonate.

34. For what clinical condition is clomiphene citrate (Clomid) used?

35. Identify the preliminary screening needed before initiation of clomiphene citrate therapy.

36. What safety precautions are needed in the event that visual disturbances occur with the use of clomiphene citrate (Clomid)?

37. At what specific time during the menstrual cycle can ovulation be anticipated with the use of clomiphene citrate (Clomid)?

38. What is the action of magnesium sulfate on the central nervous system?

39. At what level of concentration in the blood does magnesium sulfate depress the central nervous system and block peripheral nerve transmission, producing anticonvulsant effects and smooth muscle relaxation?

40. Prepare a list of assessments that should be implemented during the administration of magnesium sulfate to detect toxicity.

41. Explain the rationale for monitoring urine output during magnesium sulfate therapy.

42. What reflexes are the primary monitoring parameters for magnesium sulfate therapy?

43. Identify treatment for magnesium sulfate toxicity.

44. Describe specific procedures and precautions needed during the intravenous administration of magnesium sulfate.

45. What nursing assessments are needed for infants born to mothers receiving magnesium sulfate?

31. Obtain baseline vital signs and weight. Monitor maternal and fetal heart rates. Perform baseline mental status assessment (e.g., alertness, orientation, anxiety level, muscle strength, tremors). Monitor diabetic patients for hyperglycemia.

32. Serum glucose, chloride, sodium, potassium, hematocrit, and carbon dioxide before initiation of therapy

33. Neonatal adverse effects include hyperglycemia followed by hypoglycemia, hypotension, hypocalcemia, and paralytic ileus.

34. It is used to induce ovulation in women who are not ovulating because of reduced circulating estrogen levels.

35. A complete physical exam to rule out other pathologic causes for lack of ovulation should be performed, as well as tests to rule out possible pregnancy.

36. See a health care provider for an eye exam. Avoid tasks requiring visual acuity (e.g., driving or operating power machinery). Visual disturbances usually subside in a few days to weeks following discontinuation of the medication.

37. Usually 6–10 days after the last dose of medication

38. It depresses the central nervous system (CNS) and blocks peripheral nerve transmission, causing muscle relaxation.

39. Blood concentrations of greater than 4 mEq/L.

40. Deep tendon reflexes: Patellar reflex qh (IV), or before every dose (IM). Hourly urine output: report output of less than 30 mL/hour or less than 100 mL/4 hours. Vital signs: take every 15–30 minutes. Respirations must be at least 16/minute before further doses are administered. If blood pressure drops, do not administer another dose. Fetal distress: do not administer. Mental status: check orientation and alertness before initiating therapy.

41. With reduced urine output, toxicity is more likely to occur.

42. The presence or absence of patellar reflex, biceps reflex, or radial reflex are primarily monitoring parameters for magnesium sulfate therapy

43. Administer calcium gluconate 10%. Stop magnesium infusion.

44. Use an infusion pump. Periodic neurologic exam, I&O, fetal assessment, vital signs.

46. What emergency supplies should be available in the immediate vicinity during magnesium sulfate therapy?

47. What are the action and purpose of administration of RhoGAM?

48. Identify the specific dosage, administration precautions, and proper timing of the administration of RhoGAM.

49. State the appropriate treatment of fever, arthralgia, and generalized aches and pains that can be anticipated following RhoGAM administration.

50. What is the purpose of erythromycin ophthalmic ointment (Ilotycin)?

51. Describe the specific procedures used to instill erythromycin ophthalmic ointment (Ilotycin).

52. What are the causative organisms of ophthalmia neonatorum?

53. Explain the rationale for administering phytonadione (vitamin K) to the neonate.

54. What is the preferred site for intramuscular administration of vitamin K to a neonate?

55. Review the anatomical structures associated with the administration of intramuscular medications in an infant.

56. What are the serious adverse effects associated with phytonadione (vitamin K) therapy?

45. Infants born of mothers who receive magnesium sulfate must be monitored for hypotension, hyporeflexia, and respiratory depression.

46. Calcium gluconate 10% solution ready for IV administration. Ambu bag, in case of respiratory depression. Discontinue the IV infusion.

47. It is used to prevent Rh immunization of the Rh– patient exposed to Rh+ blood as a result of a transfusion accident, during termination of pregnancy, or as a result of a delivery of an Rh+ infant. Action: prevents Rh hemolytic disease in subsequent delivery. Also used in the treatment of idiopathic thrombocytopenic purpura.

48. See drug monograph, pp. 628-629.

49. Use acetaminophen, not aspirin or other anti-inflammatory agents.

50. Erythromycin ophthalmic ointment (Ilotycin) is used prophylactically to prevent ophthalmia neonatorum caused by *Neisseria gonorrhoeae* or *Chlamydia trachomatis*.

51. See Dosage and Administration, textbook p. 630.

52. *Neisseria gonorrhoeae* or *Chlamydia trachomatis*

53. Vitamin K is a fat-soluble vitamin necessary for the production of the blood-clotting factors in the liver. Vitamin K is absorbed from the diet and is normally produced by the bacterial flora in the gastrointestinal tract, from which it is absorbed and transported to the liver for clotting factor production. Newborns have not yet colonized the colon with bacteria and are often deficient in vitamin K. They may be deficient in these clotting factors and are therefore more susceptible to hemorrhagic disease in the first 5–8 days after birth.

55. Lateral aspect of the thigh

55. See Parenteral Medications and Administration: Intradermal, Subcutaneous, and Intramuscular Routes in Chapter 11.

56. Petechiae, generalized ecchymoses, or bleeding from the umbilical stump, circumcision site, nose, or gastrointestinal tract

Drugs Used in Obstetrics

chapter

40

Learning Activities

FILL-IN-THE-BLANK

Finish each of the following statements using the correct term.

1. _____ _____ is the term used to describe persistent severe vomiting associated with pregnancy.
2. The health status of the neonate is estimated at 1 minute and 5 minutes after delivery using the _____ rating system.
3. An Rh-negative mother may receive Rho(D) immune globulin within _____ hours of the completion of the pregnancy.
4. On delivery, the breasts secrete a thin, yellow fluid called _____.
5. _____ is a hormone produced in the hypothalamus and stored in the pituitary that when released, it stimulates the smooth muscle of the uterus, blood vessels, and the mammary glands.
6. Oxytocin (Pitocin) infusions should be monitored by both a _____ (an instrument that measures uterine contractions) and a fetal heart monitor.
7. Normal fetal heart rate is between _____ to _____ beats per minute.
8. _____ is the most common electrolyte imbalance associated with terbutaline sulfate therapy.
9. RhoGAM is given to an Rh-_____ mother.
10. An adverse effect of _____ is water intoxication.

MATCHING

Match the generic drug name with its corresponding brand name. Each option will be used only once.

_____ 11. methylergonovine maleate
_____ 12. oxytocin
_____ 13. terbutaline sulfate
_____ 14. clomiphene citrate
_____ 15. erythromycin ophthalmic ointment
_____ 16. dinoprostone
_____ 17. misoprostol

a. Pitocin
b. Clomid
c. Methergine
d. Ilotycin
e. Brethine
f. Cytotec
g. Prepidil

TRUE OR FALSE

Write "T" for true and "F" for false for each statement. Correct all false statements.

_____ 18. Treatment of preterm labor often includes administration of uterine relaxants such as terbutaline sulfate (Brethine) and magnesium sulfate.
_____ 19. It is a legal requirement that every newborn infant's eyes be treated prophylactically for *Neisseria gonorrhoeae*.
_____ 20. In general, oxytocin (Pitocin) should not be used to hasten labor.
_____ 21. Temperature elevations to approximately 38° C (100.6° F) occurring within 15–45 minutes and continuing for up to 6 hours are common adverse effects of dinoprostone (Prepidil) therapy.
_____ 22. Methylergonovine maleate (Methergine) therapy plays an active role in cervical softening and dilation unrelated to uterine muscle stimulation.
_____ 23. Methylergonovine maleate (Methergine) is used for the induction of labor.
_____ 24. Ergonovine maleate (Ergotrate) should not be used in patients who wish to breastfeed.
_____ 25. Oxytocin (Pitocin) is the drug of choice for inducing labor at term and for augmenting uterine contractions during the first and second stages of labor.

Drugs Used in Obstetrics

Practice Questions for the NCLEX® Examination

_____ 1. A patient at 36 weeks gestation is ordered to receive dinoprostone (Prepadil) transvaginally to continue cervical ripening. Which practice does the nurse follow when administering this medication?
1. Places dinoprostone in the anterior fornix of the vagina
2. Removes the dinoprostone at the onset of labor
3. Warms the dinoprostone to body temperature before insertion
4. Has the patient remain supine for 15 minutes after insertion of the dinoprostone and then has her ambulate

_____ 2. The nurse assesses a patient receiving an infusion of oxytocin (Pitocin) to induce labor and determines the infant is in distress. Which actions does the nurse take? *(Select all that apply.)*
1. Turns the patient to the right lateral position
2. Notifies the health care provider immediately
3. Reduces the oxytocin infusion to the slowest possible rate according to hospital policy
4. Administers oxygen by nasal cannula or face mask
5. Administers a bolus of magnesium sulfate

_____ 3. Which activity does the nurse perform when administering oxytocin (Pitocin) for the induction of labor?
1. Positions the patient in the lithotomy position for ease of insertion
2. Prepares the patient for general anesthesia
3. Sets up an IV pole to administer the oxytocin via gravity drip
4. Administers oxytocin via a constant infusion pump to control the rate of administration

_____ 4. When working with patients receiving oxytocin (Pitocin) therapy, the nurse must assess for the development of water intoxication because oxytocin therapy causes which effect?
1. Extreme thirst in patients
2. Hypocalcemia
3. Stimulation of antidiuretic hormone
4. Hypertension

_____ 5. The nurse is assessing a postpartum patient who has received oxytocin (Pitocin) therapy. It is most important for the nurse to determine if the patient received _____ during the labor process.
1. Antibiotics
2. A local anesthetic containing epinephrine
3. A Foley catheter
4. Solid food

_____ 6. What are neonatal adverse effects of terbutaline sulfate (Brethine)? *(Select all that apply.)*
1. Paralytic ileus
2. Hypoglycemia
3. Hyperglycemia
4. Hyperkalemia
5. Hypercalcemia

_____ 7. A patient is receiving magnesium sulfate to inhibit preterm labor. Which drug does the nurse have readily available if magnesium intoxication should occur?
1. Atropine
2. Epinephrine
3. Calcium gluconate
4. Potassium chloride

_____ 8. A patient has been ordered Rho(D) immune globulin after delivery. Which action does the nurse take?
1. Confirms that the mother is Rh negative
2. Administers the Rho(D) immune globulin to the mother and neonate
3. Ensures that the mother is not allergic to eggs
4. Administers IGIM full-dose intravenously to the mother

_____ 9. When administering erythromycin ophthalmic ointment to a neonate, what does the nurse do?
1. Administers the ointment from the outside of the eye in towards the nose
2. Instills a ribbon of the ointment along the upper conjunctival surface
3. Administers the ointment within 2 hours of birth
4. Irrigates the eyes after instillation

_____ 10. The nurse administers phytonadione (vitamin K) via which route?
1. Intravenous
2. Intramuscular
3. Subcutaneous
4. Oral

_____ 11. Which are clinical indications for the use of uterine stimulants? _(Select all that apply.)_
1. Induction of labor
2. Control of postpartum atony and hemorrhage
3. Control of postsurgical hemorrhage, as in cesarean birth
4. Induction of therapeutic abortion
5. Suppression of milk production for non-nursing mothers

_____ 12. What are neonatal adverse effects of magnesium sulfate therapy? _(Select all that apply.)_
1. Hyperglycemia
2. Hypotension
3. Hyporeflexia
4. Respiratory depression
5. Hyperkalemia

13. A patient is ordered clomiphene citrate (Clomid) 50 mg daily PO for 5 days. The medication is available in 50-mg tablets. How many tablets will the patient have remaining after 2 days of therapy? _____ tablet(s)

14. A patient is ordered 10 units of oxytocin (Pitocin) IM after delivery of the placenta. The medication is available as 10 units/mL. How many mL does the nurse administer? _____ mL

15. A patient is ordered misoprostol (Cytotec) 200 mcg four times daily. The medication is available as 100 mcg per tablet. How many tablets will the patient receive in a 24-hour period? _____ tablet(s)

Drugs Used in Men's and Women's Health

Review Sheet

The QUESTION column and the ANSWER column have been offset so that you can cover the answers while reading the questions, allowing you to assess your knowledge.

Question	Answer
1. Define *leukorrhea*.	
2. What types of infection are known to develop in the mouth, gastrointestinal tract, or vagina with the use of broad-spectrum antibiotics?	1. Leukorrhea is an abnormal, usually whitish, vaginal discharge.
3. List the diseases collectively known as sexually transmitted diseases (STDs).	2. *C. albicans* and others, listed in Table 41-2.
4. Identify the components of a female and/or male reproductive history.	3. See Box 41-1, p. 633.
5. Describe the medication history necessary for a comprehensive men's and women's health assessment.	4. See textbook, pp. 632-635.
6. List laboratory studies used to detect infection in the male or female reproductive system.	5. See textbook, p. 635.
7. Identify basic hygiene measures that should be taught to men and women.	6. See textbook, p. 635.
8. Explain in detail the proper method of applying vaginal medications topically or intravaginally and discuss medication regimens used for both partners in a sexual relationship.	7. See textbook, p. 636.
9. How is a psychosocial assessment that focuses on obtaining data related to STDs completed?	8. See Patient Education and Health Promotion, Medications, textbook, p. 637.
10. Discuss the action of oral contraceptives.	9. See textbook, p. 635.
11. What is the primary purpose of the extended- and continuous-cycle oral contraceptives?	10. See textbook, pp. 637-638.

12. What is the relationship between cigarette smoking and use of oral contraceptives?

13. Discuss the major adverse effects of and contraindications for the use of oral contraceptives.

14. Develop a specific education plan for teaching patients about oral contraceptives.

15. What medications, when combined with oral contraceptive therapy, require the use of an alternate form of contraceptive therapy?

16. What herbal product may reduce the effectiveness of oral contraceptives?

17. Explain how the transdermal contraceptive, ethinyl estradiol/norelgestromin (Ortho-Evra) is applied and the patient teaching that should be done regarding its use.

18. What drugs are contained in the vaginal ring (NuvaRing)?

19. Describe the procedure for insertion of the NuvaRing.

20. Explain the health teaching that should be initiated when the NuvaRing is prescribed.

21. What serious adverse effects must be reported with the use of the NuvaRing?

22. Differentiate between the symptoms of obstructive and irritative benign prostatic hypertrophy (BPH).

23. Describe the medical treatment of BPH.

11. A primary purpose for these contraceptives is to shorten the duration of menses, decreasing the frequency to four times per year, or completely eliminating menses. Other advantages include a lower cumulative dose of hormones taken compared with oral contraceptives cycled monthly, and the alleviation of symptoms of coexisting medical conditions that may be exacerbated during menses.

12. Cigarette smoking increases the risk of serious adverse cardiovascular effects in people who both smoke and use combination oral contraceptives. This risk increases with age and heavy smoking and is quite significant in women older than 35 years of age. Women who use oral contraceptives are strongly encouraged not to smoke.

13. Diseases that may be aggravated by oral contraceptive therapy include hypertension, gallbladder disease, diabetes mellitus, severe varicose veins, seizure disorders, oligomenorrhea or amenorrhea, and rheumatic heart disease. Adverse effects common with oral contraceptive therapy are nausea, headache, weight gain, spotting, depression, fatigue, chloasma, yeast infections, vaginal itching or discharge, and changes in libido.

14. See textbook, Nursing Process for Oral Contraceptives: Instructions for Using Combination Oral Contraceptives, pp. 638-641.

15. See textbook, pp. 643-644.

16. St. John's wort

17. See textbook, pp. 645-646. Patients should be advised that in November 2005, the FDA issued a cautionary note about greater exposure to estrogens from the patch compared to taking a similar oral contraceptive tablet product. In general, increased estrogen exposure may increase the risk of blood clots.

18. Ethinyl estradiol (an estrogen) and norelestromin (a progestin) are contained in the NuvaRing.

19. See textbook, pp. 646-647.

20. See textbook, pp. 646-647.

21. Vaginal discharge, breakthrough bleeding, yeast infection, blurred vision, severe headaches, dizziness, leg pain, chest pain, shortness of breath, or acute abdominal pain.

22. See Table 41-6, p. 648.

24. What is androgenetic alopecia? How is it treated?

23. Alpha$_1$-adrenergic blocking agents are used to reduce mild to moderate urinary obstruction manifestations in men with BPH. They produce a 20% to 30% increase in urine flow rate in up to 50% of men with urinary symptoms. The antiandrogen agents dutasteride (Avodart) and finasteride (Proscar) are used to reduce DHT levels which reduce the hyperplastic cell growth associated with prostatic hyperplasia. It is used to treat the symptoms associated with BPH, reduce the risks associated with urinary retention, and minimize the need for surgery associated with BPH.

25. What premedication assessments should be made prior to administering alpha$_1$-adrenergic blocking agents and antiandrogen agents?

24. Androgenetic alopecia is male pattern baldness. Finasteride (Propecia) is used to treat androgenetic alopecia.

26. Define *erectile dysfunction* and differentiate among vascular, neurologic, and psychologic causative factors.

25. See textbook, pp. 649-651.

27. Why is it important to check for a history of cardiovascular disease before initiating phosphodiesterase inhibitor therapy?

26. See textbook, p. 651.

28. What phosphodiesterase inhibitor has been approved for once-daily dosing?

27. Phosphodiesterase inhibitor therapy can cause fatal interactions with nitroglycerin or isosorbide use.

28. Tadalafil (Cialis)

Drugs Used in Men's and Women's Health

Learning Activities

FILL-IN-THE-BLANK

Finish each of the following statements using the correct term.

1. _____ is an excessive whitish vaginal discharge that may occur at any age affecting almost all females at some time in their lives.

2. _____ is manifested by irregular periods, infrequent periods, and spotting between periods.

3. St. John's wort may _____ the liver's metabolism of oral contraceptive hormones, possibly resulting in a _____ in contraceptive effect.

4. _____ is an antiandrogen agent used to treat androgenetic alopecia.

5. _____ is an erection that will not go away.

MATCHING

Match the generic drug name with its corresponding brand name. Each option will be used only once.

_____ 6. tadalafil

_____ 7. sildenafil

_____ 8. dutasteride

_____ 9. finasteride

_____ 10. norelgestromin-ethinyl estradiol

a. Ortho Evra
b. Viagra
c. Cialis
d. Proscar
e. Avodart

TRUE OR FALSE

Write "T" for true and "F" for false for each statement. Correct all false statements.

_____ 11. The consistent use of male latex condoms significantly reduces the risk of HIV infection in men and women and of gonorrhea in men, but male condoms may be less effective in protecting against STDs that are transmitted by skin-to-skin contact because the infected areas may not be covered by the condom.

_____ 12. The reporting requirements to the health department of individual cases of syphilis, gonorrhea, and chlamydia vary from state to state.

_____ 13. Many of the adverse effects of combination-type contraceptives are caused by the estrogen component of the tablet.

_____ 14. Because of a possibility of birth defects, oral contraceptives should be discontinued for one month before attempting pregnancy.

_____ 15. There is a higher incidence of ectopic pregnancy with the minipill when compared to other oral contraceptives because the minipill does not inhibit ovulation in all women.

_____ 16. Erectile dysfunction is an inevitable outcome of aging.

Drugs Used in Men's and Women's Health

chapter **41**

Practice Questions for the NCLEX® Examination

_____ 1. The nurse teaches a patient that after inserting a vaginal medication (cream or suppository) she should remain in a recumbent position for at least how many minutes to allow time for drug absorption?
1. 5
2. 10
3. 20
4. 30

_____ 2. The nurse has provided teaching for a patient on oral contraceptives. Which statement by the patient indicates the teaching has been effective?
1. "I will start the first pill on the first day my period begins."
2. "I will use another form of birth control during the first month."
3. "If I miss one pill, I will take two pills as soon as I remember and two the next day."
4. "I will take one pill in the morning one day, and the next day I will take the pill in the evening to rotate times the pill is taken."

_____ 3. In teaching a patient about the use of norelgestromin-ethinyl estradiol transdermal system (Ortho Evra), which statements does the nurse include? (_Select all that apply._)
1. "Trim the patch to best fit the area where you wish to apply it."
2. "Do not place the patch on your breast."
3. "Avoid lotions or creams in the areas of the skin where the patch is applied because the patch may not adhere properly."
4. "If the patch is partially detached for less than 24 hours, try to reapply it in the same place or replace it with a new patch immediately."
5. "Apply the patch to the buttock, abdomen, upper outer arm, or upper torso."

_____ 4. When teaching a patient about dutasteride (Avodart) therapy, which statement does the nurse include?
1. "If there is no improvement of symptoms after two weeks of treatment, the dutasteride will be discontinued."
2. "Men treated with dutasteride should not donate blood until at least six months after stopping therapy."
3. "Dutasteride is used to treat male pattern baldness."
4. "Dutasteride will cause an increase in serum prostate specific antigen (PSA) levels."

_____ 5. When providing teaching for a patient regarding oral contraceptive therapy, which statement does the nurse include?
   1. "Cigarette smoking increases the risk of serious adverse cardiovascular effects in women who both smoke and use combination oral contraceptives."
   2. "If you miss one pill, take two pills at the regularly scheduled time."
   3. "If you miss one pill, start another form of birth control immediately."
   4. "Discontinue use of the pill for one month before attempting pregnancy."

_____ 6. Which statement about sildenafil (Viagra) therapy is true?
   1. If a patient is taking sildenafil, he should not take nitroglycerin therapy for the treatment of angina.
   2. Nitrates from food sources react with sildenafil.
   3. Higher doses of sildenafil therapy may be necessary with concurrent use of cimetidine.
   4. Sildenafil therapy often causes patients to develop glaucoma.

_____ 7. The nurse is teaching a patient about tadalafil (Cialis) therapy. Which statement made by the patient indicates teaching has been successful?
   1. "This drug is an aphrodisiac."
   2. "I will take this medication three times a day on a regular basis."
   3. "I can expect the medication to work within 30 minutes."
   4. "If I develop chest pain, I will take nitroglycerin."

_____ 8. Which information does the nurse include when teaching a patient about the use of the norelgestromin-ethinyl estradiol transdermal system (Ortho Evra)? _(Select all that apply.)_
   1. "A new patch should be applied on the same day of the week."
   2. "Apply the first patch during the first 24 hours of the menstrual period or on the first Sunday after menses begins."
   3. "If the patch is detached for less than 24 hours, apply a new patch to the same location."
   4. "If two consecutive periods are missed, a pregnancy test is in order."
   5. "Contraceptive therapy should be discontinued if pregnancy is confirmed."

9. A patient is ordered dutasteride (Adovart) 0.5 mg PO daily. The medication is available as 1/2 mg per capsule. How many capsules does the nurse administer? _____ capsule(s)

10. A patient is ordered sildenafil citrate (Revatio) 20 mg PO three times a day. The medication is available as 20 mg per tablet. How many tablets will the patient receive in a 24-hour period? _____ tablet(s)

Drugs Used to Treat Disorders of the Urinary System

Review Sheet

The QUESTION column and the ANSWER column have been offset so that you can cover the answers while reading the questions, allowing you to assess your knowledge.

Question	Answer
1. Differentiate among pyelonephritis, cystitis, prostatitis, and urethritis.	
2. Identify the components of an assessment of the urinary tract.	1. Pyelonephritis is kidney infection, cystitis is bladder infection, prostatitis is prostate gland infection, and urethritis is infection of the urethra.
3. Why is the use of strict aseptic technique needed with indwelling catheters?	2. See textbook, p. 656.
4. In older adults, what is a common sign of a UTI?	3. To prevent urinary tract infections (UTIs).
5. Study Table 42-1 to identify details found on a routine urinalysis report.	4. New confusion in an older adult patient may be the only sign of a UTI.
6. What measures should be taught to prevent UTIs?	5. See Table 42-1, textbook p. 657.
7. Should a urine specimen for bacterial culture and sensitivity be collected before or after starting antimicrobial therapy?	6. Personal hygiene measures—wiping front to back in females, keeping perineal area clean, avoiding nylon underwear and constrictive clothing in perineal area, avoiding scented bubble bath products and colored toilet paper, washing the perineal area immediately before and after intercourse, and urinating after intercourse.
8. What health teaching should be completed when a patient has a UTI?	7. A urine specimen for culture and sensitivity should be collected before administering the first dose of an antimicrobial agent.
9. What are the actions of urinary antimicrobial agents?	8. Force fluids, 2000 mL or more per day. Continue medication for the entire course of treatment, even if symptoms have subsided fairly rapidly. Return for urine culture when scheduled. Have patient report perineal itching, vaginal discharge, or breakdown of tissue. Teach the patient ways to prevent future infections.
10. What criteria are used to select a urinary antimicrobial agent?	9. Urinary antimicrobial agents are substances that are secreted and concentrated in the urine in sufficient amounts to have an antiseptic effect on the urine and the urinary tract.
11. What is the mechanism of action of fosfomycin (Monurol)?	10. Identification of the specific pathogen by gram stain or urine culture and sensitivity.

12. What are the desired therapeutic outcomes of therapy with quinolone antibiotics?

13. Why are some urinary antimicrobial agents prescribed to be taken after the urine culture is sterile?

14. What drug class is approved for one-dose treatment of UTIs?

15. Identify premedication assessments used for quinolone therapy.

16. How is fosfomycin (Monurol) administered?

17. What are the major advantages of norfloxacin (Noroxin) over other quinolones cinoxacin and nalidixic acid (NegGram) for the treatment of UTIs?

18. What type of deficiency precludes the use of nalidixic acid (NegGram)?

19. Why must the urine be acidic during the administration of methenamine mandelate (Mandelamine)?

20. Urine pH should be maintained below what value for optimal results from methenamine mandelate (Mandelamine) therapy?

21. How is urinary tract acidification accomplished for methenamine mandelate (Mandelamine) therapy?

22. When a patient is on methenamine mandelate (Mandelamine) therapy, what drugs should not be administered because they cause alkalinization of the urine?

23. What color change in the urine may occur with nitrofurantoin (Macrodantin) therapy?

24. Which urinary drug class of urinary antimicrobial agent is most likely to cause photosensitivity?

25. Name two medicines that may be used in nonobstructive urinary retention (e.g., postoperatively, during postpartum period).

26. What drug should be readily available for treatment of serious adverse effects of bethanechol chloride (Urecholine)?

27. What is oxybutynin chloride (Ditropan) used to treat?

11. Fosfomycin (Monurol) inhibits bacterial cell wall synthesis and reduces adherence of bacteria to epithelial cells of urinary tract.

12. Resolution of the urinary tract infection

13. To prevent recurrence of a urinary tract infection

14. Fosfomycin antibiotics (Monurol)

15. See textbook, p. 660.

16. Empty entire contents of single-dose packet into 90–120 mL (3–4 oz) of water (not hot), stir to dissolve, and ingest immediately. Fosfomycin (Monurol) may be taken with or without food.

17. Norfloxacin (Noroxin) has an advantage over other quinolones because it has a much broader spectrum of activity against gram-positive and gram-negative microorganisms. It also can be administered orally to patients.

18. When using nalidixic acid (NegGram), the nurse should assess for history of glucose-6-phosphate dehydrogenase deficiency, and if present, withhold the drug and contact the health care provider.

19. For methenamine mandelate (Mandelamine) to be effective, it must be converted to formaldehyde to suppress the growth of bacteria. The urine has to be acidic for this reaction to occur. Therefore, the patient may have vitamin C prescribed simultaneously for this purpose.

20. When the pH is above 5.5, methenamine mandelate (Mandelamine) is less likely to be converted to formaldehyde. Therefore, pH needs to be maintained at 5.5 or below.

21. Ascorbic acid (vitamin C) is often prescribed to help maintain the acidity of the urine.

22. Acetazolamide and sodium bicarbonate produce alkaline urine, preventing the conversion of methenamine mandelate (Mandelamine) to formaldehyde, thereby inactivating the medication.

23. The urine may become tinted yellow to rust-brown but this should not be a cause for alarm.

24. Quinolone antibiotics

25. Bethanechol chloride (Urecholine) and neostigmine (Prostigmin)

26. Atropine sulfate

28. Name a urinary analgesic and describe its action.
29. What changes in urine color can often occur following the administration of phenazopyridine hydrochloride (Pyridium)?
30. What are the three primary symptoms of overactive bladder syndrome?

31. What class of drugs are used to treat overactive bladder syndrome?
32. What is the action of the anticholinergic agents used in the treatment of overactive bladder syndrome?

27. Oxybutynin chloride (Ditropan) is a bladder antispasmodic.
28. Phenazopyridine hydrochloride (Pyridium) acts as a local anesthetic on the mucosa of the ureters and bladder, reducing spasm.
29. The color of the urine will become reddish orange, but the patient should be informed that this is no cause for alarm.
30. Frequency, urgency, and urinary incontinence
31. Anticholinergic agents are the drugs of choice.

32. The anticholinergic agents are also known as *urinary antispasmodic agents*. They block the cholinergic receptors of the detrusor muscle of the bladder causing relaxation. They decrease involuntary contractions of the detrusor muscle and improve bladder volume capacity.

Drugs Used to Treat Disorders of the Urinary System

Learning Activities

FILL-IN-THE-BLANK

Finish each of the following statements using the correct term.

1. The normal amount of protein expected in a urinalysis is _____ to _____.

2. Oxybutynin chloride (Ditropan) is a(n) _____ agent that acts directly on the smooth muscle of the bladder.

3. _____ is the first antibiotic agent to be approved as a single-dose treatment for urinary tract infections.

4. Patients taking phenazopyridine hydrochloride (Pyridium) should be cautioned that their urine will become _____ in color.

5. The organism _____ accounts for about 80% of noninstitutionally acquired uncomplicated urinary tract infections.

6. In the presence of acidic urine, methenamine mandelate (Mandelamine) forms _____.

7. In order for methenamine mandelate (Mandelamine) to be active, the urine must be at a pH of _____ or below.

8. Oxybutynin chloride (Ditropan) is used to treat bladder _____.

MATCHING

Match the generic drug name with its corresponding brand name. Each option will be used only once.

_____ 9. fosfomycin

_____ 10. bethanechol chloride

_____ 11. phenazopyridine hydrochloride

_____ 12. oxybutynin

_____ 13. tolterodine

_____ 14. fesoterodine

_____ 15. nitrofurantoin

a. Ditropan
b. Urecholine
c. Detrol
d. Pyridium
e. Monurol
f. Macrodantin
g. Toviaz

TRUE OR FALSE

Write "T" for true and "F" for false for each statement. Correct all false statements.

_____ 16. The incidence of urinary tract infections in women is approximately 10 times higher than in men.

_____ 17. Patients with pyelonephritis have an infection of the bladder.

_____ 18. Phenazopyridine hydrochloride (Pyridium) relieves burning, pain, urgency, and frequency associated with urinary tract infections.

_____ 19. Nitrofurantoin (Macrodantin) is an antibiotic that is not effective against microorganisms in the blood or in tissues outside the urinary tract.

_____ 20. Urinary tract infections are second only to upper respiratory infections as a cause of morbidity from infection.

Drugs Used to Treat Disorders of the Urinary System

Practice Questions for the NCLEX® Examination

_____ 1. Which statement does the nurse include when teaching a patient about fosfomycin (Monurol) therapy?
1. "This medication will treat bladder and kidney infections."
2. "If you should experience nausea after taking the fosfomycin, notify your health care provider at once."
3. "Dissolve the fosfomycin in 3–4 ounces of water and drink immediately."
4. "To consume the fosfomycin, sprinkle the contents of the packet on dry toast or cereal and take it in its dry form."

_____ 2. A patient with a history of diabetes mellitus requiring use of Clinitest is prescribed sucralfate (Carafate) and warfarin (Coumadin) therapy. The health care provider has just ordered nalidixic acid (NegGram) for the treatment of a urinary tract infection which the patient has developed. When working with this patient, what will the nurse do?
1. Administer the sucralfate with the nalidixic acid.
2. Encourage the patient to drink 8–12 8 oz glasses of water daily.
3. Be aware that nalidixic acid may produce false-negative Clinitest results.
4. Assess for clotting problems, because the nalidixic acid will most likely decrease the anticoagulant effects of warfarin.

_____ 3. Of the following patients, which is the best candidate for tolterodine (Detrol) therapy?
1. 45-year-old with a history of ulcerative colitis
2. 73-year-old with prostatitis
3. 60-year-old with narrow-angle glaucoma
4. 50-year-old with asthma

_____ 4. A patient is experiencing burning, frequency, pain, and urgency associated with a urinary tract infection. The nurse expects the health care provider to order which medication to treat these symptoms?
1. Phenazopyridine hydrochloride (Pyridium)
2. Oxybutynin chloride (Ditropan)
3. Methenamine mandelate (Mandelamine)
4. Nitrofurantoin (Macrodantin)

_____ 5. A postpartum patient who had a complicated vaginal delivery of a baby 9 hours ago is unable to void despite multiple nonpharmacologic interventions by the nurse. The nurse expects the health care provider to order which drug to facilitate bladder tone and urination?
1. Bethanechol chloride (Urecholine)
2. Neostigmine (Prostigmin)
3. Oxybutynin chloride (Ditropan)
4. Tolterodine (Detrol)

_____ 6. Of the following patients, which are considered to have a urinary tract infection? *(Select all that apply.)*
1. Male with pyelonephritis
2. Female diagnosed with cystitis
3. Male with prostatitis
4. 4-year-old male with urethritis
5. Female with vaginitis

_____ 7. Which statements about phenazopyridine hydrochloride (Pyridium) for the treatment of patients with urinary tract infections are correct? *(Select all that apply.)*
1. Pyridium produces a local anesthetic effect on the mucosa of the ureters and bladder.
2. Pyridium is most effective against gram-negative bacterial urinary tract infections.
3. Pyridium relieves burning, pain, urgency, and frequency associated with urinary tract infections.
4. Pyridium reduces bladder spasms.
5. Pyridium causes the color of urine to become reddish-orange.

_____ 8. Oxybutin chloride (Ditropan) should be avoided for use in patients who have which conditions? *(Select all that apply.)*
1. Allergy to penicillin
2. Glaucoma
3. Myasthenia gravis
4. Ulcerative colitis
5. Prostatitis

_____ 9. Which statements about methenamine mandelate (Mandelamine) are correct? *(Select all that apply.)*
1. Tablets should not be crushed, as this will allow the formation of formaldehyde in the stomach.
2. It should not be administered with sodium bicarbonate.
3. It will become inactive if administered with ascorbic acid (vitamin C).
4. It should not be discontinued if nausea, vomiting, and belching develop without first consulting the health care provider.
5. It is used in patients susceptible to chronic, recurrent urinary tract infections.

_____ 10. Which statements does the nurse include when teaching a patient about overactive bladder syndrome (OAB)? *(Select all that apply.)*
1. "The first line of pharmacologic treatment of OAB is the anticholinergic agents."
2. "OAB cannot be cured."
3. "Patients with OAB should be instructed to avoid caffeine."
4. "The goals of therapy for OAB are to decrease frequency by increasing voided volume, decrease urgency, and reduce incidents of urinary urge incontinence."
5. "A chronic infection is the cause of OAB."

_____ 11. A patient is ordered trospium (Sanctura) 20 mg PO bid. In the facility, breakfast and dinner are served at 0800 and 1700. At what times does the nurse administer the trospium?
1. 0700 and 1600
2. 0730 and 1630
3. 0800 and 1700
4. 0830 and 1730

12. A patient is prescribed 5 mg of oxybutynin (Ditropan) PO tid. The medication is available in syrup form, 5 mg/5 mL. How many mL of the medication does the nurse administer?
_____ mL

Drugs Used to Treat Glaucoma and Other Eye Disorders

Review Sheet

The QUESTION column and the ANSWER column have been offset so that you can cover the answers while reading the questions, allowing you to assess your knowledge.

Question	Answer
1. Identify the major structures of the eye (e.g., cornea, pupil, iris, canal of Schlemm).	
2. Define: *miosis, mydriasis, cycloplegia, intraocular pressure*, and *glaucoma*.	1. Refer to the textbook for a review of the basic structure and function of the eye. In particular, examine the location of the canal of Schlemm, Fig. 43-3. Note that dilation of the iris could result in a blockage of the canal of Schlemm.
3. Explain the normal drainage system of the eye.	2. Miosis: contraction of the iris sphincter muscle causing narrowing of the pupil of the eye. Mydriasis: contraction of the dilator muscle and relaxation of the sphincter muscle causing dilation of the pupil of the eye. Cycloplegia: paralysis of the ciliary muscles. Intraocular pressure (IOP) results from the excessive production of the aqueous humor or from decreased fluid outflow. Glaucoma: an eye disorder characterized by an increase in the IOP.
4. Explain the cause, symptoms, and precipitating factors associated with acute closed-angle glaucoma.	3. Aqueous humor flows between the lens and the iris into the anterior chamber of the eye. It drains through channels located near the junction of the cornea and the sclera through meshwork into the canal of Schlemm and then into the venous system of the eye.
5. What is the principal treatment of acute closed-angle glaucoma?	4. Acute closed-angle glaucoma occurs when there is a sudden increase in IOP caused by a mechanical obstruction of the trabecular network in the iridocorneal angle. This occurs in patients who have narrow anterior chamber angles. Symptoms develop gradually and appear intermittently for short periods, especially when the pupil is dilated. Symptoms include blurred vision, halos around white lights, frontal headache, and eye pain. Patients often associate the symptoms with stress or fatigue. An attack can be precipitated by administration of a mydriatic agent such as atropine or scopolamine for eye examination.

6. Explain open-angle glaucoma.

5. Acute angle-closure glaucoma requires immediate treatment with the administration of miotic agents to relieve the pressure of the iris against the trabecular network and allow drainage of the aqueous humor. Mannitol may be administered to draw aqueous humor from the eye, and acetazolamide may be administered to reduce formation of aqueous humor. Analgesics and antiemetics may be administered if pain and vomiting persist. Surgery is then required to correct the abnormality.

7. What is the principal treatment of open-angle glaucoma?

6. Open-angle glaucoma develops insidiously over the years as pathologic changes at the iridocorneal angle prevent the outflow of aqueous humor through the trabecular network to Schlemm's canal and into the veins of the eye.

8. Identify the normal IOP reading when taken with a tonometer.

7. Historically, miotic agents (e.g., pilocarpine) have been most commonly used to increase outflow of aqueous humor; recently beta-adrenergic blocking agents (e.g., timolol maleate) have become the initial drugs of choice. Other agents used are sympathomimetic agents (e.g., brimonidine), the carbonic anhydrase inhibitors (e.g., acetazolamide), and the cholinesterase inhibitors (e.g., echothiophate iodide).

9. Compare the mechanisms of action of drugs used to lower IOP.

8. 10–21 mm Hg

10. Describe the actions of drugs known as *mydriatic agents* and *miotic agents*.

9. Osmotic agents elevate osmotic pressure of the plasma, causing fluid from the extravascular spaces to be drawn into the blood, thereby reducing IOP.

   Carbonic anhydrase inhibitors inhibit the enzyme carbonic anhydrase resulting in a decrease of aqueous humor production, thereby lowering IOP.

   Cholinergic agents produce contraction of the iris (miosis) and ciliary body musculature (accommodation), thereby permitting outflow of aqueous humor by widening the filtration angle, thus decreasing IOP.

   Cholinesterase inhibitors prevent the metabolism of acetylcholine, the cholinergic neurotransmitter within the eye. This results in increased cholinergic activity, which results in decreased IOP and miosis.

   Adrenergic agents have several uses in ophthalmology. These agents cause pupil dilation, increased outflow of aqueous humor, vasoconstriction, relaxation of ciliary muscle, and decreased formation of aqueous humor.

   Beta-adrenergic blocking agents are thought to reduce production of aqueous humor.

   Prostaglandin agonists increase outflow of aqueous humor, thus reducing IOP.

11. What is the action of osmotic agents on the eye?

10. Mydriatic agents dilate the pupil and miotic agents constrict the pupil.

12. What are the serious adverse effects from the use of osmotic agents?

13. Osmotic agents may produce circulatory overload. What types of assessments will the nurse perform? What findings will the nurse report to the primary care provider?

14. List nursing responsibilities for the IV administration of mannitol (Osmitrol).

15. Before administering a carbonic anhydrase inhibitor, what should the nurse assess the patient for?

16. What are cholinergic agents used for? What are the advantages of these agents?

17. List and describe common and serious adverse effects of cholinergic agents.

11. Osmotic agents elevate the osmotic pressure of the plasma, causing fluid from the extravascular space to be drawn into the blood. The effect on the eye is reduction of volume of intraocular fluid, which produces a decrease in IOP.

12. Thirst, nausea, dehydration, electrolyte imbalance (potassium, sodium, and chloride), headache, and circulatory overload.

13. Patients taking osmotic agents should be assessed at regularly scheduled intervals for signs and symptoms of fluid overload, pulmonary edema, or heart failure. The nurse should perform lung assessments and report the development of crackles and increasing dyspnea, frothy sputum, or cough.

14. An in-line filter should be used because mannitol has a tendency to crystallize. Do not administer if crystals are present. The nurse should follow directions in the literature accompanying the medication for a warm bath to dissolve the crystals, and then cool the solution before administration. The IV site should be assessed at regular intervals for any signs of infiltration. Tissue necrosis may occur from infiltration into the surrounding tissue. If infiltration occurs, the nurse should stop the IV, report, and then elevate the extremity and follow hospital protocol for extravasation. Veins in the lower extremities should not be used because this may cause phlebitis or thromboembolism.

15. The nurse should assess whether the patient is pregnant; if pregnancy is suspected, the medication should be withheld and the primary care provider should be notified. The patient should also be assessed for an allergy to sulfonamide antibiotics. If the patient has an allergy to sulfonamide antibiotics, the medication should be withheld and the primary care provider should be notified. The nurse should also ensure that contact lenses have been removed before instillation of the drops, and that baseline lab studies have been drawn and general assessment data has been recorded. The patient should be assessed for signs of gastric symptoms before initiating drug therapy and if present, the medication should be administered with milk or food.

16. Cholinergic agents lower IOP in patients with glaucoma by widening the filtration angle, which permits outflow of aqueous humor. They may also be used to counter the effects of mydriatic and cycloplegic agents after surgery or ophthalmoscopic examinations. They are effective in many cases of chronic glaucoma. The advantages of these agents include: adverse effects are less severe and less frequent than those of anticholinesterase agents; they provide better control of IOP with fewer fluctuations in pressure.

18. Explain how the systemic effects of cholinergic agents can be prevented.

19. What is the action of cholinesterase inhibitors?

20. What do indications of overdose or excessive administration of cholinesterase inhibitors include? If these symptoms become severe, what medication should be administered?

21. What actions should be taken when cholinesterase inhibitors are used by farmers handling insecticides and pesticides?

22. What are the actions of adrenergic agents?

23. Adrenergic agents should be used with caution in patients who have which conditions or disorders?

24. What are the beta-adrenergic blocking agents used for in ophthalmology and what is their mechanism of action?

25. What are the advantages of using beta-adrenergic blocking agents to reduce IOP compared to anticholinergic agents?

26. What is the action of a prostaglandin agonist on the eye?

27. Explain the precautions for instilling ophthalmic prostaglandin agonist medications to a person who wears contacts.

28. What are the effects of prostaglandin agonists on the eye pigment and other structures of the eye?

17. Common adverse effects of cholinergic agents include reduced visual acuity, conjunctival irritation, erythema, headache, pain, and discomfort. Serious adverse effects include signs of systemic toxicity manifested by diaphoresis, salivation, abdominal discomfort, diarrhea, bronchospasm, muscle tremors, hypotension, dysrhythmia, and bradycardia. These symptoms are indications of excessive administration. The health care provider should be notified for dosage adjustment. The adverse effects themselves usually do not need to be treated because they will resolve by withholding cholinergic therapy.

18. Systemic effects of cholinergic agents can be prevented by carefully blocking the inner canthus for 3–5 minutes after instilling the medication to prevent absorption via the nasolacrimal duct.

19. Cholinesterase is an enzyme that destroys acetylcholine, the cholinergic neurotransmitter. Cholinesterase inhibitors prevent the metabolism of acetylcholine within the eye. This causes increased cholinergic activity which results in decreased IOP and miosis.

20. Systemic toxicity of cholinesterase inhibitors is manifested by diaphoresis, salivation, vomiting, abdominal cramping, urinary incontinence, diarrhea, dyspnea, bronchospasm, muscle tremors, hypotension, dysrhythmias, and bradycardia. Parenteral atropine should be administered if symptoms become severe.

21. Added absorption of insecticides and pesticides may occur through the skin and respiratory tract. Respiratory masks and frequent washing and clothing changes are advisable.

22. Adrenergic agents cause pupil dilation, increased outflow of aqueous humor, vasoconstriction, relaxation of the ciliary muscle, and decrease in the formation of aqueous humor.

23. Adrenergic agents should be used with caution in patients with hypertension, diabetes mellitus, hyperthyroidism, heart disease, arteriosclerosis, or long-standing bronchial asthma.

24. The beta-adrenergic blocking agents are used to reduce elevated IOP. The exact mechanism of action is not known, but these agents are thought to reduce the production of aqueous humor.

25. Unlike anticholinergic agents, beta-adrenergic blocking agents do not produce blurred or dim vision or night blindness because IOP is reduced with little or no effect on pupil size or visual acuity.

26. Prostaglandin agonists decrease IOP by increasing outflow of aqueous humor.

27. Remove contact lenses, instill medication, and wait 15 minutes to reinsert the contact lenses.

29. What is the action of the anticholinergic agents on the eye?

30. What are the uses of the anticholinergic agents for the eye?

31. When mydriatic agents are administered, what patient reaction to bright lights is observed?

32. What specific medication is used to treat an ophthalmic fungal infection? What is the action of this drug?
33. Antifungal agents may produce what adverse effects?

34. Name the ophthalmic antiviral agents. What is the action of these agents? What are they used to treat?
35. Explain the use of antibacterial agents in the treatment of ophthalmic conditions.

36. What is the major use of corticosteroid therapy in the eye?

37. What is the effect of prolonged ocular steroid therapy?

38. Why is corticosteroid therapy not used for the treatment of infections of the eye?
39. What are the effects of the ophthalmic anti-inflammatory agents? What is their mechanism of action?

28. The prostaglandin agonists may gradually cause changes to pigmented tissues, including changes to the eye color, increasing the amount of brown pigment in the iris. The eyelids may also develop color changes. There may also be an increased growth of eyelashes.
29. Anticholinergic agents cause the smooth muscle of the ciliary body and iris to relax, producing mydriasis (extreme dilation of the pupil) and cycloplegia (paralysis of the ciliary muscle).
30. The anticholinergic agents are used to examine the interior of the eye, measure the proper strength of lenses for eyeglasses (refraction), and rest the eye in inflammatory conditions of the uveal tract.
31. The mydriasis produced allows excessive light into the eyes, causing the patient to squint. Sunglasses will help reduce the brightness.
32. Natamycin (Natacyn) is an ophthalmic antifungal agent. It alters the cell wall of the fungus to prevent it from serving as a selective barrier, therefore causing loss of fluids and electrolytes.
33. Adverse effects of antifungal agents include sensitivity to bright light, blurred vision, lacrimation, redness, and eye pain.
34. Ophthalmic antiviral agents include idoxuridine, trifluridine, and vidarabine. They act by inhibiting viral replication. Idoxuridine is particularly effective against initial herpes simplex infections. Trifluridine is used to treat recurrent infections or for patients who are intolerant of or resistant to idoxuridine or vidarabine therapy. Vidarabine is used topically as an ophthalmic ointment to treat eye infections caused by herpes simplex types 1 and 2. It may be effective in treating recurrent keratitis that is resistant to idoxuridine and trifluridine.
35. Antibacterial agents are used to treat superficial eye infections and for prophylaxis against gonorrhea infection in the eyes of newborn infants (ophthalmia neonatorum).
36. Corticosteroid therapy is used for allergic reactions of the eye and other acute, noninfectious inflammatory conditions of the sclera, cornea, and anterior uveal tract.
37. Prolonged ocular steroid therapy may cause glaucoma and cataracts.
38. Corticosteroid therapy must not be used in bacterial, fungal, or viral infections of the eye because corticosteroids decrease defense mechanisms and reduce resistance to pathologic organisms.

40. What is the desired action of an antihistamine on the eye?

41. The drug fluorescein is used for what purpose?

42. When are artificial tears used?

43. Summarize macular degeneration and its treatment.

39. The ophthalmic anti-inflammatory agents have anti-inflammatory, antipyretic, and analgesic activities on the eye. They inhibit the biosynthesis of prostaglandins that are responsible for an increase in intraocular inflammation and pressure. They also inhibit prostaglandin-mediated constriction of the iris (miosis) that is independent of cholinergic mechanisms.

40. Antihistamines are H_2 antagonists that act by inhibiting release of histamine from mast cells. They are used for relief of signs and symptoms and prevent itching associated with allergic conjunctivitis.

41. Fluorescein is used for fitting hard contact lenses and as diagnostic aid to identify foreign bodies in the eye and abraded or ulcerated areas of the cornea. It is also useful for evaluating retinal vasculature for abnormal circulation.

42. Artificial tear solutions are products made to mimic natural secretions of the eye. They provide lubrication for dry eyes and for artificial eyes. They are also used to prevent drying when a person has lost the blink reflex such as during surgery or when comatose.

43. Macular degeneration is a deterioration of the macula, a small area in the retina at the back of the eye that is required to see fine details clearly or to judge distances such as when driving an automobile. Central vision is affected by blurriness, dark areas, and distortion. Peripheral vision is usually not affected. Many older adults develop macular degeneration as part of the body's natural aging process. Treatment includes pegaptanib (Macugen) and ranibizumab (Lucentis). They are selective vascular endothelial growth factor (VEGF) antagonist. VEGF is secreted and binds to its receptors located primarily on the surface of endothelial cells of blood vessels. VEGF induces new blood vessel growth and increases vascular permeability and inflammation, all of which are thought to contribute to the progression of the wet form of age-related macular degeneration. Pegaptanib and ranibizumab are antagonists that bind to extracellular VEGF, preventing it from binding to VEGF receptors, thus preventing it from forming new blood vessels. Pegaptanib is injected into the vitreous humor of the affected eye once every six weeks, whereas ranibizumab is administered once monthly.

Student Name _____

Drugs Used to Treat Glaucoma and Other Eye Disorders

chapter

43

Learning Activities

FILL-IN-THE-BLANK

Finish each of the following statements using the correct term.

1. _____ is contraction of the iris sphincter muscle, which causes the pupil to narrow.

2. _____ is contraction of the dilator muscle and relaxation of the sphincter muscle, which causes the pupil to dilate.

3. Paralysis of the ciliary muscle is termed _____.

4. _____ is an eye disease characterized by abnormally elevated IOP, which may result from excessive production of the aqueous humor or from diminished ocular fluid outflow.

5. _____ is used in fitting hard contact lenses and as a diagnostic aid in identifying foreign bodies in the eye and abraded or ulcerated areas of the cornea.

6. Before the administration of mannitol (Osmitrol) intravenously, the nurse should check the solution for _____.

7. Carbonic anhydrase inhibitors should not be administered to a patient who is allergic to _____.

8. The _____ _____ may gradually cause changes to pigmented tissues, including change to eye color, increasing the amount of brown pigment in the iris.

MATCHING

Match the generic drug name with its corresponding brand name. Each option will be used only once.

_____ 9. ganciclovir

_____ 10. levofloxacin

_____ 11. tropicamide

_____ 12. carteolol

_____ 13. dipivefrin hydrochloride

_____ 14. acetazolamide

_____ 15. triamcinolone

_____ 16. gatifloxacin

a. Quixin
b. Ocupress
c. Diamox
d. Vitrasert
e. Mydriacyl
f. Propine
g. Zymar
h. Triesence

TRUE OR FALSE

Write "T" for true and "F" for false for each statement. Correct all false statements.

_____ 17. The lens is a transparent, gelatinous mass of fibers encased in an elastic capsule situated behind the iris.

_____ 18. The cornea, the eye's white portion, is contiguous with the iris and is nontransparent.

_____ 19. One of the greatest challenges in the care of chronic eye disorders such as glaucoma is convincing the patient of the need for long-term treatment and adherence to the therapeutic regimen.

_____ 20. Postoperative positioning of the patient after eye surgery usually requires having the patient lie on his or her back or on the nonoperative side.

_____ 21. Natamycin (Natacyn) is an antibacterial agent used to treat infections of the eye.

_____ 22. If infiltration occurs with administration of intravenous mannitol (Osmitrol), the nurse should stop the infusion, report, and then elevate the extremity and follow hospital protocol for extravasation.

Drugs Used to Treat Glaucoma and Other Eye Disorders

Practice Questions for the NCLEX® Examination

_____ 1. By which routes are osmotic agents administered to reduce IOP? *(Select all that apply.)*
   1. Intravenously
   2. Orally
   3. Topically
   4. Intramuscularly
   5. Subcutaneously

_____ 2. The nurse assesses a patient for an allergy to which factor before administering acetazolamide (Diamox)?
   1. Penicillin
   2. Eggs
   3. Sulfonamides
   4. Nuts

_____ 3. To prevent systemic effects of ophthalmic cholinergic agents, the nurse carefully blocks the inner canthus of the eye for how many minutes?
   1. 1–2
   2. 3–5
   3. 8–10
   4. 12–14

_____ 4. The patient with which disorder has the lowest risk for developing complications related to ophthalmic adrenergic agents?
   1. Mild hypertension
   2. Type I diabetes mellitus
   3. Renal failure
   4. Hyperthyroidism

_____ 5. Which statement by a patient indicates that teaching about ophthalmic antiviral agents has been effective?
   1. "I will not exceed 5 days of continuous therapy because more than that will cause ocular toxicity."
   2. "If transient tearing occurs upon instillation of the medication, I will rub my eyes to stop the tearing."
   3. "I will discontinue treatment immediately if redness of the sclera develops after instilling the medication."
   4. "I will use sunglasses to help reduce the brightness of light after instilling the medication."

_____ 6. Which statements does the nurse include when teaching a patient about health promotion after eye surgery? *(Select all that apply.)*
   1. "Avoid bending at the waist."
   2. "Avoid any straining with stool."
   3. "Report any pain not relieved by prescribed medications."
   4. "Use aseptic technique when instilling eye medications."
   5. "Cough at least 10 times every hour."

_____ 7. What are actions of adrenergic agents used in ophthalmology? *(Select all that apply.)*
   1. Increased outflow of aqueous humor
   2. Vasodilatation
   3. Constriction of the ciliary muscle
   4. Decreased formation of aqueous humor
   5. Pupil constriction

_____ 8. What are systemic adverse effects of atropine sulfate (Isopto-Atropine)? *(Select all that apply.)*
1. Bradycardia
2. Diarrhea
3. Blurred vision
4. Vasodilation
5. Dry mouth

_____ 9. A patient is ordered acetazolamide (Diamox) 500 mg for injection. The medication is available as 500 mg per vial. Preparation instructions are to reconstitute 500 mg acetazolamide with 5 mL of sterile water for injection. How many mL of acetazolamide does the nurse administer?
1. 1
2. 3
3. 4
4. 5

_____ 10. The nurse administers 1 drop of olopatadine (Patanol) to each eye of a patient and records it in the patient's medication administration record. Which documentation most accurately represents this administration?
1. "gtt OU"
2. "1 drop olopatadine (Patanol) OS"
3. "Drop X 1 olopatadine (Patanol) eyes"
4. "1 drop olopatadine (Patanol) each eye"

11. Methazolamide 100 mg is ordered bid at 0800 and 1600. The medication is available in 25-mg tablets. How many tablets does the nurse administer? _____ tablet(s)

Drugs Used for Cancer Treatment

Review Sheet

The QUESTION column and the ANSWER column have been offset so that you can cover the answers while reading the questions, allowing you to assess your knowledge.

Question	**Answer**
1. Define *cancer*.	
2. What is apoptosis?	1. Cancer is a disorder of cellular growth, lifespan, and death. It is a group of abnormal cells that generally proliferate (multiply) more rapidly than do normal cells, lose the ability to perform specialized functions, invade surrounding tissue, and develop growth in other tissues distant to the site of original growth (metastasis).
3. What are the phases of the cell cycle?	2. Normal cells have a genetically programmed lifecycle that includes cell death known as *apoptosis*. Many types of cancer cells also lose the ability to die properly as part of their normal lifecycle.
4. What are the major groups of chemotherapeutic agents currently used?	3. See textbook, pp. 688-689.
5. What are the targeted anticancer agents?	4. The major groups of chemotherapeutic agents currently used are classified as alkylating agents, antimetabolites, natural products, antineoplastic antibiotics, hormones, targeted anticancer agents, chemoprotective agents, and bone marrow stimulants.
6. What are chemoprotective agents?	5. The targeted anticancer agents have evolved from research that indicates that cell membrane receptors control cell proliferation, cell migration, angiogenesis, and cell death that are integral to the growth and spread of cancer. Targeted anticancer agents are noncytotoxic drugs that target the key pathways that provide growth and survival advantages for cancer cells. Because these pathways are relatively specific for cancer cells, theoretically, targeted agents are not associated with toxicities common with cytotoxic chemotherapy.
7. What do the bone marrow stimulants do in the treatment of cancer?	6. Chemoprotective agents help reduce the toxicity of chemotherapeutic agents to normal cells.

8. What is combination therapy?

7. Bone marrow stimulants trigger the recovery of bone marrow cells several days earlier than would be the natural course of recovery from treatment with chemotherapy which kills cancer cells and bone marrow cells. The major benefit of this earlier recovery is that the patient's immune system is able to respond to and stop infections from being so pathologic, and patients are able to be released from the isolation room several days earlier.

9. State baseline assessments needed during the initiation of cancer therapy.

8. Using both a cell cycle-specific and cell cycle-nonspecific agent at the same time for treatment of cancer

10. Cite the goals of chemotherapy and specific factors affecting the patient dosage, drug identification, drug preparation, and drug administration.

9. The type of cancer being treated; the emotional status of the patient; the understanding the patient has of the diagnosis; the patient's usual methods of coping; the patient's degree of pain, usual eating pattern, and elimination pattern.

11. State the nursing interventions needed for people experiencing adverse effects from chemotherapy.

10. Control of growth of the cancer cells is the primary goal of treatment. See other goals, textbook pp. 689, 697. Since many of the cancer drugs have similar spellings, it is imperative to check the drug name closely. Cancer drugs are given in a variety of forms: orally, intravenously, by bolus, and so forth. Therefore, the physician's order must be checked carefully. Many cancer drugs require reconstitution—follow directions precisely. When drugs are given IV, check the IV site carefully for extravasation. During oral administration, maintain an accurate record of the medication on the flow sheet and record any adverse effects experienced.

12. State the five classes of antineoplastic agents.

11. See textbook for adverse effects associated with chemotherapy. Monitor for nausea and vomiting, hydration, positioning, changes in bowel patterns, stomatitis, alopecia, neurotoxicity, musculoskeletal complaints, bone marrow depression, infection, thrombocytopenia, and activity intolerance.

12. Alkylating agents, antibiotics, antimetabolites, natural products, and hormones.

13. Define *cell cycle-specific* and *cell cycle-nonspecific antineoplastic agents*.

14. When is chemotherapy most effective?

13. The action of cell cycle-specific antineoplastic agents occurs in a specific phase of the cell's growth. Cell cycle-nonspecific antineoplastics are active throughout the cell cycle.

14. When cells of the tumor are small in number and rapidly dividing.

15. Why is it difficult to kill tumor cells in the G_0 phase?

16. What criteria are used to choose the type of chemotherapy to be administered?

15. Many chemotherapeutic agents kill cells when in the replication phase. Cells in the resting phase (G_0) of the cell cycle are not dividing and therefore are not susceptible to destruction by chemotherapeutic agents.

17. Describe the major indications for the use of trastuzumab (Herceptin).

16. Type of tumor cells, the rate of growth, and size of the tumor.

18. Discuss the three chemoprotective agents amifostine (Ethyol), dexrazoxane (Zinecard, Totect), and mesna (Mesnex). What are they primarily used for?

19. List questions that may be asked when taking a health history of the risk factors the individual has for development of cancer.

20. What are the common adverse effects to expect/report associated with chemotherapy?

21. Why is it sometimes advisable to discuss birth control and reproductive counseling prior to initiation of chemotherapy?

22. What type of oral hygiene measures should be instituted when chemotherapy is administered?

23. What are common signs and symptoms of bleeding the nurse should assess for, especially when platelet counts are decreased?

24. What is meant by "neutropenic precautions"?

25. When several courses of intravenously administered chemotherapy are planned, the antineoplastic agents are frequently administered via _____.

26. What three types of emesis are associated with antineoplastic therapy?

27. Identify whether the following agents are cell cycle-specific or cell cycle-nonspecific: alkylating agents, antimetabolites, natural products, and antineoplastic antibiotics. What is the action of hormones?

17. Trastuzumab (Herceptin) is used to treat metastatic breast cancer with HER-2-postive tumors.

18. Examine Table 44-3 for detailed discussion.

19. See textbook, p. 697.

20. It depends on the type of chemotherapy drug administered. Generally, myelosuppression, anemia, bleeding, stomatitis, diarrhea or constipation, alopecia, anorexia, nausea, and vomiting are common adverse effects associated with chemotherapy. See a medical-surgical textbook for specific interventions for each of these adverse effects. Also read Implementation and Health Promotion, pp. 702-705.

21. Reproductive abilities may be affected and agents may pass through the placental barrier, thus being potentially harmful to a fetus.

22. See Chapter 32.

23. Epistaxis, hematuria, bruises, petechiae, dark, tarry stools, "coffee ground emesis," blurred vision, excessive menstrual flow, hemoglobin, hematocrit.

24. Neutropenic precautions are designed to minimize the individual's exposure to microorganisms. Handwashing, avoiding exposure to individuals with infection, no fresh flowers or fruits and vegetables, no freestanding water (e.g., plants, flowers, humidifiers, denture cups). Avoid pets and people receiving immunizations.

25. Implantable vascular access devices

26. Acute, delayed, and anticipatory emesis (see also Chapter 34)

27. *Alkylating agents*: cell cycle-nonspecific
Antimetabolites: many are cell cycle-specific S phase
Natural products: cell cycle-specific
Antineoplastic antibiotics: act through various mechanisms to prevent replication as well as RNA synthesis. See drug class for discussion of specific antibiotic agents that are cell cycle-specific and cell cycle-nonspecific.
Hormones: alter the hormone environment of the cell

Drugs Used for Cancer Treatment

Learning Activities

FILL-IN-THE-BLANK

Finish each of the following statements using the correct term.

1. When a cancer is beyond control, the goal of treatment may be _____, or the alleviation of symptoms.

2. In cancer treatment, the _____ are a group of medicines that help reduce the toxicity of chemotherapeutic agents to normal cells.

3. The ability of a malignant tumor to invade surrounding tissue and develop growths in other tissues distant to the site of original growth is referred to as _____.

4. _____ is the phase of cellular proliferation in which the cell divides into two equal daughter cells.

5. _____ and _____ are natural derivatives of the periwinkle plant that are used in the treatment of neoplasms.

MATCHING

Match the generic drug name with its corresponding brand name. Each option will be used only once.

_____ 6. busulfan

_____ 7. bendamustine

_____ 8. streptozocin

_____ 9. bleomycin

_____ 10. epoetin alfa

_____ 11. filgrastim

_____ 12. oxaliplatin

_____ 13. decitabine

_____ 14. tamoxifen

_____ 15. vorinostat

a. Zanosar
b. Neupogen
c. Treanda
d. Procrit
e. Myleran
f. Blenoxane
g. Zolinza
h. Soltamox
i. Dacogen
j. Eloxatin

TRUE OR FALSE

Write "T" for true and "F" for false for each statement. Correct all false statements.

_____ 16. The overall goal of cancer chemotherapy is to give a dose large enough to be lethal to the cancer cells, but small enough to be tolerable for normal cells.

_____ 17. Chemotherapy is most effective when the tumor is large and the cell replication is slow.

_____ 18. Combination therapy in the treatment of cancer, using cell cycle-specific and cell cycle-nonspecific agents, is superior in therapeutic effects than the use of single-agent chemotherapy.

_____ 19. Treatment of cancer often requires a combination of surgery, radiation, chemotherapy, and immunotherapy.

_____ 20. Cell cycle-nonspecific drugs are active throughout the cell cycle and may be more effective against slowly proliferating neoplastic tissue.

Drugs Used for Cancer Treatment

Practice Questions for the NCLEX® Examination

_____ 1. A patient has severe lesions in his mouth as an adverse effect of chemotherapy. When does the nurse schedule oral hygiene measures using prescribed local anesthetic and antimicrobial solutions?
  1. In the morning when the patient awakens and before bed
  2. After each meal
  3. Once every eight hours
  4. Hourly while the patient is awake

_____ 2. Which statements about hydration and chemotherapy are correct? *(Select all that apply.)*
  1. Some chemotherapeutic agents require prehydration to prevent damage to the kidneys.
  2. Some chemotherapeutic agents require prehydration to prevent damage to the bladder.
  3. Prehydration prevents hair loss.
  4. Prehydration will prevent dehydration from vomiting in highly emotogenic chemotherapy.
  5. Malleability of the eyeballs can be used to assess the patient's hydration status.

_____ 3. The nurse is teaching a patient how to manage chemotherapy-induced diarrhea upon discharge from the outpatient cancer center. The nurse concludes that teaching was successful when the patient makes which comment?
  1. "I will decrease my fluid consumption to two 8-ounce glasses of liquid a day to keep my stool from being liquid."
  2. "I will eliminate spicy foods from my diet."
  3. "I will eat a diet high in fat to make up for lost calories."
  4. "I will eat foods low in protein to prevent diarrhea from developing."

_____ 4. The nurse is teaching a patient about measures that should be initiated to minimize the chance of infection due to chemotherapy-induced neutropenia. Which patient statement indicates that more teaching is needed?
  1. "I will wash my hands at frequent intervals."
  2. "I will avoid being around people who are known to have an infection."
  3. "I will eat fresh fruit and vegetables to be sure to get an adequate source of vitamins on a daily basis."
  4. "I will avoid being around my grandchildren when they have recently received their immunizations."

_____ 5. When teaching patients with cancer about pain relief measures, the nurse should include which information? *(Select all that apply.)*
  1. Pain is a normal response of the body to cancer; you will get used to it.
  2. Pain medications should be taken at prescribed intervals to obtain maximum relief.
  3. Start stool softeners and take them regularly to prevent constipation when morphine or codeine therapy is used.
  4. Spinal morphine may be delivered effectively via epidural or intrathecal catheters when oral and rectal forms of pain management no longer suffice.
  5. Addiction to pain medications is a major complication of cancer therapy.

_____ 6. The nurse anticipates the use of which medication to treat a patient with chemotherapy-induced anemia?
1. Sargramostim (Leukine)
2. Oprelvekin (Neumega)
3. Filgrastim (Neupogen)
4. Epoetin alfa (Epogen)

_____ 7. Which cancer chemotherapeutic antibiotic is most likely to cause cardiotoxicity?
1. Dactinomycin (Actinomycin)
2. Bleomycin (Blenoxane)
3. Doxorubicin (Adriamycin)
4. Mitomycin C (Mutamycin)

_____ 8. What information does the nurse include when teaching a patient about darbepoetin (Aranesp) therapy? _(Select all that apply.)_
1. It stimulates red blood cell production.
2. It is administered via subcutaneous injection.
3. It is used to reduce the neutropenia interval in bone marrow transplantation.
4. It is stimulates the production of clotting factors.
5. It is used to treat anemia associated with hemodialysis.

_____ 9. When teaching a group of patients who are being treated for cancer about the use of steroids in cancer therapy, which statements does the nurse include? _(Select all that apply.)_
1. "Steroids can also help reduce edema secondary to radiation therapy."
2. "Steroids can be used to restore some degree of a sense of well-being in critically ill patients."
3. "Steroids can be used as palliative therapy in temporarily suppressing fever."
4. "Steroids can be used to reduce diaphoresis."
5. "Steroids are used to help fight off infection."

10. A patient is ordered methotrexate 25 mg per day for 8 days. The medication is available in 10-mg and 15-mg tablets. How many total tablets will the patient receive in 8 days? _____ tablets

11. A patient is ordered leuprolide acetate (Lupron) 1 mg/day subcutaneously. The medication is available as 5 mg/mL. How many mL of the medication does the nurse administer? _____ mL

12. A patient is ordered mechlorethamine hydrochloride (Nitrogen mustard) 0.2 mg/kg IV once daily for one week. The patient weighs 70 kilograms. How many milligrams of the medication will the patient receive in one week? _____ mg

Drugs Used to Treat the Muscular System

Review Sheet

The QUESTION column and the ANSWER column have been offset so that you can cover the answers while reading the questions, allowing you to assess your knowledge.

Question	Answer
1. Describe the nursing assessments needed to evaluate a patient with a skeletal muscle disorder.	
2. What adjustments are usually required during the initial phase when treating an individual with muscle spasms and pain?	1. See textbook, pp. 708-709.
3. What nursing measures can be implemented to alleviate lower back pain?	2. Immobilize and elevate the affected part; range-of-motion exercises may be prescribed to prevent muscle atrophy and contractures.
4. Immediately following a muscle injury _____ packs will reduce the swelling.	3. Maintain proper body alignment; elevate the head of the bed 15–20 degrees and flex the knees slightly. Give prescribed analgesics and muscle relaxants.
5. To decrease swelling following an injury, how should the affected part be treated?	4. Ice
6. What two classes of drugs are used to relieve pain and inflammation associated with musculoskeletal disorders?	5. Elevated and immobilized
7. Describe muscle spasticity and its treatment.	6. Analgesic agents are used for pain and anti-inflammatory agents are used to reduce the inflammatory response.
8. Describe muscle spasms and their treatment.	7. *Spasticity* is defined as an upper motor neuron disorder, possibly due to a conduction interruption in the nerve pathway. It is characterized by muscle hypertonicity and involuntary jerks, which produce stiff, awkward movements. It is often a complication in patients with multiple sclerosis or cerebral palsy.
9. Compare the site of action of centrally acting and direct-acting muscle relaxants.	8. Muscle spasms are often associated with musculoskeletal trauma or inflammation. Spasms are sudden alternating contractions and relaxations or sustained contractions of muscle. Muscle spasms are treated with antispasmodic agents as well as centrally acting skeletal muscle relaxants which act within the brainstem, basal ganglia, and the spinal cord to induce muscle relaxation.

10. Both centrally acting and direct-acting skeletal muscle relaxants can produce hepatotoxicity. What are the signs and symptoms of this toxicity?

11. What premedication assessments should be made before administering centrally acting skeletal muscle relaxants?

12. Which class of muscle relaxants can cause photosensitivity?

13. What are the primary uses of baclofen?

14. Describe the signs of respiratory depression.

15. What laboratory values would be used to confirm hypoxia and hypercapnia?

16. Why are centrally acting muscle relaxants not given to people with long-term muscle spasticity?

17. What are the uses of dantrolene (Dantrium)?

18. Explain when and why neuromuscular blocking agents are administered.

19. What effect do neuromuscular blocking agents have on consciousness?

20. What effect do neuromuscular blocking agents have on salivation?

21. What nursing assessments should be made when a neuromuscular blocking agent has been administered?

9. Centrally acting muscle relaxants depress the central nervous system. Their major benefit may be their sedative effects. Direct-acting skeletal muscle relaxants act directly on the skeletal muscle producing generalized, mild weakness of skeletal muscles.

10. Anorexia, nausea, vomiting, jaundice, hepatomegaly, splenomegaly, and abnormal liver function tests (e.g., AST, ALT, LDH)

11. Baseline vital signs, mental status assessment, laboratory studies as ordered (e.g., liver function, complete blood count)

12. Direct-acting skeletal muscle relaxants

13. Baclofen is used to manage muscle spasticity resulting from multiple sclerosis, spinal cord injuries, and other spinal cord diseases.

14. Early signs: restlessness; anxiety; decreased mental alertness; headache; increase in heart rate, blood pressure, and respiratory rate. Later signs: heart rate increases; blood pressure decreases; cyanosis; use of accessory chest, abdominal, and neck muscles in respiratory effort; flaring nostrils. Changes in mental status: confusion progressing to coma.

15. Hypercapnia (elevated pCO_2), hypoxemia (decreased pO_2), and decreased oxygen saturation (SaO_2)

16. They would further reduce the functioning of the individual by reducing the overall strength of the remaining active muscle fibers.

17. Control spasticity of chronic disorders (e.g., cerebral palsy, multiple sclerosis, spinal cord injury, stroke syndrome). Dantrolene is also used to treat neuroleptic malignant syndrome and unusual reactions to neuromuscular agents used with balanced anesthesia.

18. To provide muscle relaxation during anesthesia, facilitate endotracheal intubation and prevent laryngospasm, decrease muscular activity in electroshock therapy, and aid in reducing muscle spasms associated with tetanus.

19. No effects. Unless anesthetized, the patient is fully conscious but unable to respond due to neuromuscular blockade.

20. The histamine release caused by neuromuscular blockers may produce increased salivation. In patients who are paralyzed or who have incomplete return of control over swallowing, coughing, and deep breathing, these secretions may obstruct the airway.

22. Review the drug interactions that enhance therapeutic and toxic effects of neuromuscular blocking agents and identify the three classes of drugs commonly administered that may interact with neuromuscular blocking agents.

23. Where in the patient's chart is administration of a neuromuscular blocking agent recorded?

24. Name common neuromuscular blocking agents by their generic and brand names.

25. What premedication assessments should be done prior to the administration of a neuromuscular blocking agent?

26. Explain the treatment of overdose of neuromuscular blocking agents.

21. Patent, adequate airway, check lung sounds bilaterally. Residual effects may be apparent for up to 72 hours especially in neonates and infants—watch for respiratory depression. Check cough reflex and ability to swallow. Question any antibiotic orders that prescribe aminoglycosides or tetracycline when neuromuscular blockers have been used.

22. Aminoglycoside antibiotics, beta-adrenergic blocking agents, and diuretics that cause potassium depletion.

23. Anesthesiologist's record

24. See Table 45-2.

25. See textbook, p. 714.

26. See textbook, p. 714.

Drugs Used to Treat the Muscular System

Learning Activities

FILL-IN-THE-BLANK

Finish each of the following statements using the correct term.

1. Neuromuscular blocking agents may cause patients to experience an increase in salivation due to release of _____.

2. Antibiotic orders that prescribe _____ and _____ should be questioned in patients who have received neuromuscular blockers, as these drugs may potentiate the neuromuscular blocking activity.

3. In treating patients who have over-dosed on neuromuscular blocking agents, _____ _____ is usually administered with neostigmine or pyridostigmine to block bradycardia, hypotension, and salivation induced by these agents.

4. Analgesics, sedatives, and tranquilizers, in combination with muscle relaxants, may potentiate respiratory depression. This may occur _____ hours or more after drug administration.

MATCHING

Match the generic drug name with its corresponding brand name. Each option will be used only once.

_____ 5. vecuronium bromide

_____ 6. rocuronium bromide

_____ 7. succinylcholine

_____ 8. dantrolene

_____ 9. baclofen

a. Lioresal
b. Norcuron
c. Zemuron
d. Dantrium
e. Anectine

TRUE OR FALSE

Write "T" for true and "F" for false for each statement. Correct all false statements.

_____ 10. Assessment of the patient's vital signs, mental status, and particularly respiratory function is mandatory for people receiving neuromuscular blocking agents.

_____ 11. The development of cyanosis is an early sign of respiratory complications associated with the administration of neuromuscular blocking agents.

_____ 12. In the immediate period after muscle injury, heat packs are applied to alleviate swelling, and later in the course of treatment, ice packs are used to provide comfort.

_____ 13. Immediately after muscular trauma, immobilization of the affected part will decrease muscle spasms and therefore decrease pain.

_____ 14. Patients receiving neuromuscular blocking agents usually experience a decrease in the amount of saliva produced.

Drugs Used to Treat the Muscular System

Practice Questions for the NCLEX® Examination

_____ 1. Which statements about centrally acting skeletal muscle relaxants are true? *(Select all that apply.)*
1. They directly relax the muscles by suppressing nerve conduction at the myoneural junction.
2. They produce sedation in patients receiving them.
3. They are the agents of choice for the treatment of muscle spasticity associated with cerebral or spinal cord disease.
4. They produce their therapeutic effect by depressing the central nervous system.
5. They have a direct effect on the neuromuscular junction causing relaxation.

_____ 2. Which statement by a patient taking dantrolene (Dantrium) for treatment of muscle spasticity of stroke syndrome indicates that more patient education is needed?
1. "I will avoid exposure to the sun but I can still use a tanning lamp."
2. "If I develop adverse effects from this medication, I will not discontinue treatment until I notify my health care provider."
3. "I will notify my health care provider if my skin turns yellow."
4. "I know that it might take up to a week for me to see any response to this drug."

_____ 3. Which drugs are antidotes for neuromuscular blocking agents? *(Select all that apply.)*
1. Edrophonium chloride (Tensilon)
2. Pyridostigmine bromide (Mestinon)
3. Naloxone (Narcan)
4. Neostigmine methylsulfate (Prostigmin)
5. Propranolol hydrochloride (Inderal)

_____ 4. Which description about patients receiving neuromuscular blocking agents is accurate?
1. They are at risk for the development of bronchospasm, edema, and urticaria.
2. They experience complete analgesia.
3. They have an enhanced cough reflex.
4. They experience a decrease in salivation.

_____ 5. Of the following drugs, which is considered the safest to administer to a patient who has received a neuromuscular blocking agent?
1. Halothane
2. Gentamicin
3. Propranolol
4. Insulin

_____ 6. Which statements about the effects of neuromuscular blocking agents in patients with muscular disorders are true? *(Select all that apply.)*
  1. Neuromuscular blocking agents have no effect on consciousness.
  2. Neuromuscular blocking agents have no effect on memory.
  3. Neuromuscular blocking agents have no effect on pain threshold.
  4. Pain medications are contraindicated in patients receiving neuromuscular blocking agents.
  5. The IV route is the only method for administering neuromuscular blocking agents.

_____ 7. What does immediate treatment of a musculoskeletal injury include?
  1. Application of heat
  2. Thromboembolic deterrent hose (TED)
  3. Application of ice
  4. Exercise of the affected part

_____ 8. What is the primary use of centrally acting skeletal muscle relaxants?
  1. To treat muscle spasticity
  2. To strengthen remaining active muscles
  3. To provide analgesia
  4. To relieve muscle spasms

_____ 9. A patient who has returned from abdominal surgery reports pain. The patient had received a neuromuscular blocking agent as part of the anesthesia for the surgery. What additional data is essential for the nurse to obtain before administering the prescribed analgesic?
  1. Laboratory results for CBC and electrolytes
  2. Vital signs
  3. Family history
  4. Estimated time of discharge

10. A patient is ordered methocarbamol (Robaxin) 1.5 g qid. The medication is available as 500 mg/tablet. How many tablets does the nurse administer? _____ tablet(s)

11. A patient is ordered carisoprodol (Soma) 350 mg PO qid. The medication is available as 350 mg/tablet. In a 24-hour period, how many mg of carisoprodol will the patient receive? _____ mg

12. A patient is ordered succinylcholine (Anectine) 20 mg IV stat. The medication is available as 20 mg/mL in 10-mL vials. How many mL of succinylcholine does the nurse draw up? _____ mL

Antimicrobial Agents

Review Sheet

The QUESTION column and the ANSWER column have been offset so that you can cover the answers while reading the questions, allowing you to assess your knowledge.

Question	Answer
1. What criteria are used to select an antimicrobial agent?	
2. Describe the signs and symptoms of the common adverse effects seen with antimicrobial therapy.	1. The selection of an antimicrobial agent must be based on the sensitivity of the pathogen and the possible toxicity to the patient. If at all possible, infecting organisms should first be isolated and identified. In the inpatient setting, it is routine to obtain specimens of the infecting organisms from infected sites, then start therapy immediately with one or more antimicrobial agents that are most likely to stop the infection. The use of prophylactic antibiotics is recommended for patients at risk for the development of infective endocarditis prior to dental, gastric, and genitourinary surgery, and other invasive procedures.
3. Differentiate between gram-negative and gram-positive microorganisms, and anaerobic and aerobic properties of microorganisms.	2. Allergy: rash or skin reaction (e.g., hives with or without dyspnea, laryngeal edema, shock, stridor, and sternal retractions). Direct tissue damage: hepatotoxicity (liver damage) as noted by an elevation of AST, ALT, GGT, and alkaline phosphatase. Ototoxicity: dizziness, tinnitus, and progressive hearing loss. Nephrotoxicity [renal damage: as noted by an increase in serum creatinine, BUN, and by alterations in the urine (e.g., decrease in specific gravity, casts, or protein in the urine, and an excess of RBCs over 0–3)]. Secondary infection: stomatitis, glossitis, itching, vulvovaginitis, cold sores, or canker sores. See textbook, pp. 719-720, Blood Dyscrasias, and p. 719, Nausea, Vomiting, and Diarrhea.

4. Describe basic principles of patient care that can be implemented to enhance an individual's therapeutic response during an infection.

5. Review components of a baseline assessment to evaluate a patient's hydration status and assessments needed to detect renal or hepatic toxicity.

6. Identify significant data in a patient's history that could alert the medical team that the patient is more likely to experience an allergic reaction.

7. Describe the usual management of nausea, vomiting, and diarrhea when they occur in conjunction with antimicrobial therapy.

8. State the signs and symptoms of a secondary infection and actions that can be taken to minimize these effects.

9. Review techniques and procedures for parenteral administration and vaginal insertion of drugs.

10. Identify significant information relating to patient education when caring for a person receiving an antibiotic.

11. Cite the primary uses of aminoglycosides and the serious adverse effects that require close monitoring of the patient.

3. Classification of microorganisms as *gram-positive* or *gram-negative* refers to the type of staining properties of a bacterium. Cells with a cell wall retain stain and are referred to as *gram-positive* cells. Cells without a cell wall do not retain the gram stain, and are referred to as *gram-negative* cells. Broad-spectrum antibiotics are effective against many gram-positive and gram-negative organisms. Anaerobic bacteria grow in the absence of oxygen; aerobic bacteria require oxygen to reproduce.

4. Adequate rest, hydration, and nutrients. Teach personal hygiene measures (e.g., handwashing, proper techniques for changing dressings).

5. Hydration: skin turgor, intake and output, inspect mucous membranes for moisture or dryness, check firmness of eyeballs, check specific gravity of urine (see Table 42-1). Renal toxicity: decreasing urine output, increasing BUN and/or serum creatinine; check for presence of protein, blood, or casts in the urine. Hepatic toxicity: anorexia, nausea, vomiting, jaundice, hepatomegaly, splenomegaly, and abnormal (elevated) liver function tests (AST, ALT, LDH, GGT, alkaline phosphatase).

6. Before administering any antibiotic, check for any prior allergies to medications or foods or the presence of asthma. If the patient is allergic to anything, get details regarding the symptoms and previous treatment of the allergy.

7. Gather data relative to the patient's usual pattern of elimination (e.g., number of stools per day, consistency) and compare this information with the current data. Read individual drug monographs to identify antimicrobials that may cause diarrhea, nausea, or vomiting. Report these to the physician.

8. Be particularly alert for secondary infection in patients receiving broad-spectrum antibiotics and those patients who are immunosuppressed. Assess for white patches in the mouth, cold sores, canker sores, vaginal itching, diarrhea, and recurrent fever.

9. See Chapter 8, Percutaneous Administration; Chapter 10, Parenteral Administration: Safe Preparation of Parenteral Medications; Chapter 11, Parenteral Administration: Intradermal, Subcutaneous, and Intramuscular Routes; and Chapter 12, Parenteral Administration: Intravenous Route.

10. With the instructor's assistance, identify significant points relating to the prescribed drug therapy that should be taught to the patient for each class of antimicrobials ordered.

12. Identify precautions needed to prevent incompatibilities between aminoglycosides and other medications.

13. State the mechanism of action of aminoglycosides on the bacterial cell.

14. What premedication assessments should be made before aminoglycoside therapy?
15. What is the mechanism of action of carbapenems?

16. Prior to administration of a carbapenem, what premedication assessments should be performed?
17. Why is it essential to report the occurrence of severe diarrhea with antibiotic therapy?

18. Explain the admixture compatibility of carbapenems.
19. Cite the effectiveness of cephalosporins, according to generation, against gram-positive and gram-negative microorganisms.

11. Aminoglycosides are used to treat gram-negative bacteria causing meningitis, wound infections, chronic urinary tract infections, and life-threatening septicemia. Monitor the patient closely for ototoxicity and nephrotoxicity. If the patient has had anesthesia within 48–72 hours that included the administration of a skeletal muscle relaxant, withhold aminoglycoside and ask health care provider for further instructions.

12. Do not mix aminoglycosides in the same syringe or infuse these drugs simultaneously with other medications. Tag the chart of any patient going to surgery who is receiving an aminoglycoside. Respiratory depression may occur when these agents are combined with skeletal muscle relaxants.

13. Aminoglycosides inhibit protein synthesis of bacteria.

14. Baseline assessment of allergies, presenting symptoms, T, P, R, BP, and hydration status. Check for any hearing disorders or deficits or renal disease. If present, hold drug and notify physician. Check for patient having received any skeletal muscle relaxants within the past 72 hours. If taking aminoglycosides, check serum level. Check for laboratory results ordered by the health care provider (e.g., CBC with differential).

15. Carbapenems inhibit bacterial cell wall synthesis.

16. Check T, P, R, BP, and hydration status for preexisting gastric symptoms and any allergies (specifically to penicillin and cephalosporins), obtain laboratory studies, check for history of seizures and assess basic mental status and symptoms present.

17. Severe diarrhea with any antibiotic may indicate drug-induced pseudomembranous colitis.
18. See textbook, pp. 725-726.

20. What premedication assessments should be performed before therapy with cephalosporins?

21. State the mechanism of action of cephalosporins on the cell wall.

22. What types of infections can be treated effectively using cephalosporins?

23. What adverse effects from cephalosporins should be reported?

24. Why may hypoprothrombinemia occur with cephalosporin therapy?

25. What are the signs and symptoms of thrombophlebitis, which may occur with cephalosporin therapy?

26. What precautions should be instituted when cephalosporins are combined with probenecid or alcohol?

27. What is the difference between bacteriostatic and bactericidal?

28. What effect do cephalosporins have on oral contraceptives?

19. The first-generation cephalosporins have good activity against gram-positive bacteria and mild activity against gram-negative bacteria. The second-generation cephalosporins have somewhat increased activity against gram-negative bacteria but are much less active than the third-generation agents. The third-generation agents are less active than first-generation agents against gram-positive cocci. Some of the third-generation agents are also active against *Pseudomonas aeruginosa*, a very potent gram-negative microorganism. The third-generation cephalosporins have greater activity against gram-positive penicillinase-producing bacteria than first-generation cephalosporins. Fourth-generation cephalosporins are considered broad-spectrum, with both gram-negative and gram-positive coverage.

20. Baseline assessment of allergies, presenting symptoms, T, P, R, BP, and hydration status, symptoms of renal disease or bleeding disorder (hold drug and notify physician if present), and laboratory studies as ordered by physician (e.g., CBC with differential).

21. Interferes with synthesis of bacterial cell wall.

22. Respiratory, urinary, gastrointestinal, skin, and soft-tissue infections, septicemia, meningitis, osteomyelitis, and certain sexually transmitted diseases

23. Diarrhea, secondary infections, abnormal liver and renal function tests

24. Although rare, hypoprothrombinemia may develop in the older adult, debilitated, or otherwise compromised patient with borderline vitamin K deficiency. Treatment with broad-spectrum antibiotics eliminates enough gastrointestinal flora to cause a further reduction in vitamin K synthesis.

25. Report redness, warmth, tenderness to touch, or edema in the affected part. Homans' sign may be present in lower extremities.

26. Probenecid with cephalosporins may increase likelihood of toxicity. When combined with alcohol, cephalosporins may produce flushing, dyspnea, tachycardia, and hypotension. Do not ingest alcohol within 72 hours of taking cephalosporins.

27. Bactericidal agents kill the microorganism; bacteriostatic agents weaken the microorganism. Whether an agent is bacteriostatic or bactericidal depends on the organism and concentration of medication present.

29. What is the action of tigecycline (Tygacil)?

30. How is telithromycin (Ketek) used?

31. Identify the uses of macrolides.

32. What is the action of the oxazolidiones, linezolid (Zyvox)?

33. State the actions of penicillins on the bacterial cell.

34. Identify the clinical uses of penicillins.

35. For what types of adverse effects should a patient taking penicillin be monitored?

36. Cite questions that should be asked to screen a patient for a penicillin allergy before administration of the agent.

37. Identify precautions necessary to prevent an incompatibility between penicillin and other medications given intramuscularly or intravenously.

38. Briefly describe the mechanisms of action of the quinolones and fluoroquinolones.

28. Cephalosporins may interfere with the contraceptive activity of oral contraceptives. Oral contraceptives should not be discontinued, but counseling regarding use of additional methods of contraception should be planned.

29. Tigecycline is chemically related to the tetracyclines, but is not susceptible to the mechanisms that cause resistance to the tetracyclines. It acts by binding to the 30S ribosome, preventing protein synthesis. It is a bacteriostatic antibiotic effective against a broad spectrum of gram-positive, gram-negative, and anaerobic microorganisms. It is not effective against viruses.

30. Telithromycin is used to treat acute bacterial sinusitis, bronchitis, and pneumonia caused by susceptible strains of gram-positive bacteria. In an effort to slow the development of strains of bacteria resistant to telithromycin, it should be used only when the pathogen is resistant to other available antibiotics.

31. Macrolides are used for respiratory, gastrointestinal tract, skin and soft-tissue infections, and STDs, especially when penicillins, cephalosporins, and tetracyclines cannot be used.

32. Linezolid is the first of a new class of antimicrobial agents. It acts by inhibiting protein synthesis in bacterial cells. It is bactericidal in certain strains of bacteria and bacteriostatic in others.

33. Penicillins act by interfering with the synthesis of the bacterial cell wall. They are most effective against bacteria that are multiplying.

34. Treatment of middle ear infection, pneumonia, meningitis, urinary tract infections, syphilis, and gonorrhea; and as a prophylactic antibiotic before surgery or dental procedures for patients with a history of rheumatic fever.

35. Watch for diarrhea, abnormal liver and renal function tests, thrombophlebitis, and electrolyte imbalances from sodium or potassium types of penicillin. Older adult or debilitated patients with impaired renal function are more likely to develop adverse effects.

36. "Have you ever taken an antibiotic before?" "Do you have any known allergies to foods or medications?" If so, obtain further details, such as: "When you got sick while taking the medication, what symptoms did you have?" "What did the doctor tell you to do when this occurred?" "Do you have hay fever or asthma?"

37. Do not mix penicillin with other drugs in the same syringe or infuse together with other drugs.

39. Review the multiple uses of quinolones, and fluoroquinolones.

38. Quinolones act by interfering with replication of bacterial DNA. Quinolones are effective against gram-negative and gram-positive bacteria, including anaerobes. Fluoroquinolones act by inhibiting activity of DNA gyrase, an enzyme essential for the replication of bacterial DNA.

40. Why are the quinolones not used in children under the age of 12 years?

39. See textbook, pp. 735-736.

41. What premedication assessments should be made prior to beginning quinolone therapy?

40. Quinolones may cause permanent damage to cartilage in a pediatric patient.

42. Describe the effects of antacids, iron, and sucralfate on quinolones and the adaptations in scheduling required if both agents are prescribed concurrently.

41. Baseline assessment of allergies, presenting symptoms, T, P, R, BP, and hydration status, gastric symptoms present, baseline laboratory studies as ordered, check for pregnancy. Warn about possible photosensitivity with lomefloxacin.

43. Identify the drug interactions that may occur when quinolones are combined with concurrent use of NSAIDs.

42. Antacids, iron-containing products, and sucralfate may decrease the absorption of quinolones. The antibiotic should be scheduled 4 hours before or 4 hours after taking any of these medications.

44. What is the mechanism of action of the class of antibiotics known as *streptogramins*?

43. See textbook, p. 737.

45. What are the uses of streptogramins?

44. Streptogramins (quinupristin-dalfopristin) act by inhibiting protein synthesis in bacterial cell wall.

46. What precautions need to be used when reconstituting streptogramins or administering them IV?

45. These agents should be reserved for treatment of serious or life-threatening infections associated with vancomycin resistance.

47. Cite the mechanism of action of sulfonamides and the importance of monitoring following administration.

46. See textbook, p. 738.

48. State the effect of sulfonamides on people taking sulfonylurea oral hypoglycemic agents.

47. Sulfonamides inhibit bacterial biosynthesis of folic acid, leading to inadequate metabolism and cell death. People taking sulfonamides for 14 days or more need periodic monitoring of RBC and WBC (with differential) counts. All patients receiving sulfonamides need adequate hydration and should be encouraged to drink eight 12-oz glasses of water daily.

48. Sulfonamides may displace sulfonylurea oral hypoglycemic agents from their protein binding sites, potentially resulting in hypoglycemia. Have patients taking these two agents concurrently test their blood glucose 1/2 hour after meals and at bedtime to detect the development of a problem.

49. State the mechanism of action of tetracyclines.

49. Tetracyclines inhibit protein synthesis by bacterial cells.

50. List a minimum of two types of antibiotics that may cause photosensitivity.

50. Quinolones, tetracyclines, sulfonamides, and griseofulvin may cause photosensitivity. Patients taking these antibiotics should be cautioned to avoid exposure to sunlight and ultraviolet lights. Discourage the use of artificial tanning lights and instruct patients to wear clothing that provides adequate coverage of the body when in the sunlight.

51. Identify the effects of administering tetracyclines during pregnancy and at the age of tooth development.

52. Describe the dosage and administration considerations when tetracycline is prescribed.

53. Identify the causative organism and mode of transfer of tuberculosis.

54. Describe factors that need consideration to enhance a patient's response to antitubercular therapy.

55. Develop a teaching plan for patients receiving antitubercular agents.

56. Compare the mechanisms of action of ethambutol (Myambutol), isoniazid (INH), and rifampin (Rifadin).

57. Identify the effects of rifampin (Rifadin) on body secretions (e.g., urine, feces, saliva, and sputum).

58. What drug interaction does rifampin (Rifadin) have with oral contraceptives?

59. What is the mechanism of action of monobactams?

60. What is the mechanism of action of chloramphenicol?

61. State specific limitations for the use of chloramphenicol.

62. Identify specific nursing assessments needed to detect possible serious hematologic effects from chloramphenicol.

63. What is the mechanism of action of clindamycin (Cleocin)?

64. Describe effective treatment for severe diarrhea associated with clindamycin (Cleocin) therapy.

51. Do not administer tetracycline during the last half of pregnancy or to children through 8 years of age because it may cause enamel hypoplasia and permanent staining of the teeth. Do not administer to nursing mothers because it is secreted in breast milk.

52. Take medication 1 hour before or 2 hours after ingesting antacids; milk; dairy products; or products containing calcium, aluminum, magnesium (antacids), or iron (vitamins). Exception: doxycycline is not affected by food or milk.

53. *Mycobacterium tuberculosis* is spread by airborne droplets from the cough or sneeze of a person infected with the organism.

54. Personal hygiene, nutritional status, and stress reduction are factors that must be considered during the treatment of tuberculosis.

55. Review your teaching plan with the course instructor.

56. Ethambutol inhibits TB bacterial growth by altering cellular RNA synthesis and phosphate metabolism. The mechanism of action of isoniazid is unknown. It appears to disrupt the *M. tuberculosis* cell wall and inhibit replication. Rifampin acts against enzymes in the bacterial cell required to produce DNA.

57. Rifampin may tinge urine, feces, saliva, sweat, and tears a reddish-orange color.

58. Rifampin (Rifadin) interferes with the contraceptive activity of birth control pills. Alternate methods of birth control should be used during rifampin (Rifadin) therapy.

59. Monobactams are a new class of synthetic, bactericidal antibiotics that act by inhibiting cell wall synthesis.

60. Chloramphenicol acts by inhibiting bacterial protein synthesis.

61. Use only for serious infections; it is particularly effective in treating rickettsial infections, meningitis, and typhoid fever.

62. Check for sore throat, feelings of fatigue, elevated temperature, small petechial hemorrhages, and bruises of the skin. Report any of these symptoms immediately to the physician. Routine laboratory studies including RBC, WBC, and differential counts are scheduled for patients taking chloramphenicol 14 days or longer.

63. Clindamycin acts by inhibiting protein synthesis.

65. State the primary clinical uses for metronidazole (Flagyl).

66. What premedication assessments should be done whenever metronidazole (Flagyl) is to be administered?
67. What is the mechanism of action of spectinomycin (Trobicin)?
68. Identify the effectiveness of spectinomycin (Trobicin) against gonorrhea and syphilis.
69. Cite specific recommendations for intramuscular administration of spectinomycin (Trobicin).
70. Why should serology testing for syphilis be done prior to initiating therapy using spectinomycin (Trobicin)?
71. What is the primary therapeutic outcome expected from tinidazole (Tindamax) therapy?
72. What is the mechanism of action of vancomycin (Vancocin)?
73. Describe nursing assessments that may be used to detect ototoxicity.
74. Describe "red man syndrome" and identify the drug that is associated with its occurrence.

75. What type of dressings should be avoided with topical antifungal medications and what type of precautions should be taken to prevent accidental pregnancy when these drugs are administered intravaginally?
76. What is the mechanism of action of amphotericin B?

77. Cite the primary uses of amphotericin B.

78. Describe the adverse effect seen with intravenous administration of amphotericin B.
79. Identify the monitoring parameters used to detect nephrotoxicity.

64. The patient should report five or more stools per day to the health care provider. This may be an indication of drug-induced pseudomembranous colitis. Blood or mucus in the stool should also be reported to the health car provider. Warn the patient to not treat diarrhea themselves when taking this drug. The use of diphenoxylate, loperamide, or paregoric may prolong or worsen the condition.
65. Metronidazole is used to treat trichomoniasis, giardiasis, amebic dysentery, amebic liver abscess, and anaerobic bacterial infections.
66. See textbook, p. 747.

67. Spectinomycin acts by inhibiting protein synthesis.

68. Spectinomycin is used to treat gonorrhea in both males and females. It is not effective in treatment of syphilis.
69. Use a 20-gauge needle, and inject into upper outer quadrant of gluteal muscle. Causes pain at injection site.
70. This drug masks symptoms of syphilis.

71. Elimination of parasitic infection

72. Vancomycin (Vancocin) acts by preventing synthesis of bacterial cell walls.
73. Ototoxicity may initially manifest by dizziness, tinnitus, and progressive hearing loss. Assess the patient for difficulty in walking unaided and assess the level of hearing daily.
74. "Red man syndrome" or "redneck syndrome" is caused by rapid IV infusion of vancomycin; symptoms include sudden hypotension with or without maculopapular rash over face, neck, upper chest, and extremities.
75. Avoid occlusive dressings. Alternative forms of birth control should also be used when antifungal ointments are instilled intravaginally. Diaphragms and condoms may deteriorate with prolonged contact with petroleum-based ointment.
76. Amphotericin B disrupts the cell membrane of fungal cells resulting in loss of cellular content and death of the cell.
77. Amphotericin B is used primarily to treat systemic life-threatening fungal infections.
78. Patients receiving IV amphotericin B should be assessed for thrombophlebitis.

80. Cite specific dosage and administration characteristics associated with the use of amphotericin B.

81. Review procedures used to administer topical medications to the skin.

82. Describe the uses of fluconazole (Diflucan) and flucytosine (Ancobon).

83. Compare the premedication assessments needed for flucytosine (Ancobon), griseofulvin microsize (Grifulvin V), itraconazole (Sporanox), ketoconazole, and terbinafine (Lamisil).

84. What action prohibits the administration of itraconazole (Sporanox) to a patient with heart failure?

85. What are the therapeutic outcomes from administration of abacavir (Ziagen)?

86. Describe the mechanisms of action and uses of griseofulvin microsize (Grifulvin V).

87. State laboratory tests needed periodically to monitor renal, hepatic, and hematopoietic function when griseofulvin microsize (Grifulvin V) is administered.

88. State the mechanisms of action and types of fungal infections for which itraconazole (Sporanox), ketoconazole, and terbinafine (Lamasil) are used.

89. What are the therapeutic outcomes of abacavir (Ziagen), efavirenz (Sustiva), and lamivudine (Epivir)?

90. Identify the mechanism of action of acyclovir (Zovirax), didanosine (Videx), famciclovir (Famvir), and valacyclovir (Valtrex).

91. Cite the potential effects of acyclovir (Zovirax) on renal function.

---

79. Nephrotoxicity is indicated by increased excretion of uric acid, magnesium, oliguria, granular casts in urine, proteinuria, increased BUN, and serum creatinine. Report decrease in daily urine volume or changes in visual appearance of the urine.

80. See textbook, p. 753.

81. See Chapter 8, Percutaneous Administration.

82. Fluconazole is used for cryptococcal meningitis and oropharyngeal, esophageal, vulvovaginal, or systemic candidiasis. Flucytosine is effective against susceptible candidal septicemia, endocarditis, urinary tract infections, cryptococcal meningitis, and pulmonary infections.

83. See textbook, pp. 755-759.

84. Itraconazole (Sporanox) has the action of being a negative inotropic agent and may seriously aggravate a patient with heart failure.

85. Abacavir slows clinical progression of HIV-1 infection and reduces the frequency of opportunistic secondary infections.

86. Griseofulvin acts by stopping cell division and new cell growth and is used to treat ringworm of scalp, body, nails, and feet.

87. Hepatotoxicity (liver damage) is noted by an elevation in AST, ALT, GGT, and alkaline phosphatase. Nephrotoxicity (renal damage) is indicated by an increase in serum creatinine, BUN, and by alterations in the urine (e.g., decrease in specific gravity, casts or protein in the urine, and an excess of RBCs over 0–3). Hematologic: monitor for the development of sore throat, fever, purpura, jaundice, or excessive progressive weakness; check RBC, WBC, and differential counts.

88. Ketoconazole and itraconazole act by interfering with cell wall synthesis, causing leakage of cellular contents. Ketoconazole is used orally to treat candidiasis, chronic mucocutaneous candidiasis, oral thrush, coccidioidomycosis, histoplasmosis, chromomycosis, and paracoccidioidomycosis. Terbinafine is used to treat onychomycosis of the toenail or fingernail due to dermatophytes.

89. Abacavir, efavirenz, and lamivudine slow the progression of HIV-1 infection and reduce the frequency of opportunistic secondary infections.

90. These antiviral agents act by inhibiting the viral cell replication.

92. Identify the first antiviral agent that is effective against respiratory viruses.

93. What is the drug lamivudine (Epivir) used to treat?

94. What is oseltamivir (Tamiflu) used to treat?

95. Explain the administration of aerosol ribavirin powder using a small-particle aerosol generator (SPAG-2).

96. What is valacyclovir (Valtrex) used to treat?

97. What is the therapeutic outcome for zanamivir (Relenza)?

98. Cite the therapeutic outcomes of zidovudine (Retrovir).

99. Identify the hematologic tests that should be completed periodically during the use of zidovudine (Retrovir).

100. Describe the effect of zidovudine (Retrovir) transmission of HIV to others through sexual contact or blood contamination.

101. What is the mechanism of action of fosamprenavir (Lexiva)?

102. Review current Centers for Disease Control recommendations for handling body secretions and blood for all patients.

103. Which of the antiviral agents may reduce pulmonary function?

104. Study the antimicrobial tables throughout the chapter and identify common endings in the generic names of the antimicrobial agents.

91. Transient elevation of serum creatinine. Patients who are poorly hydrated, have low renal function, or who receive acyclovir by a bolus are susceptible to renal tubular damage.

92. Ribavirin (Virazole)

93. Lamivudine is combined with zidovudine in treating HIV-1 infection.

94. See textbook, p. 771.

95. See textbook, p. 773.

96. Acute herpes simplex virus (shingles)

97. Reduced symptomatology caused by influenza virus infection. It may also reduce the incidence of opportunistic secondary infections such as pneumonia.

98. Zidovudine slows the progression of HIV-1 infection and reduced the incidence of opportunistic secondary infections.

99. Monitor CBC with differential, platelets, hemoglobin, hematocrit, amylase, and liver function tests.

100. This drug does not reduce the risk of transmitting HIV to others through sexual contact or blood contamination.

101. Fosamprenavir is a prodrug of amprenavir. Amprenavir (APV) prevents maturation of viral particles by inhibiting HIV-1 protease. Immature viral particles are not infectious. Amprenavir is classified as a protease inhibitor.

102. Check with your instructor to obtain the latest recommendations or research the information on the CDC website.

103. Both ribavirin (Virazole) and zanamivir (Relenza) may affect pulmonary function.

104. See textbook Tables 46-1 through 46-9. Note: Because of the number of drugs included in these tables, ask the instructor to identify the more common drugs that will be encountered in the clinical site(s) where you are assigned.

Antimicrobial Agents

Learning Activities

FILL-IN-THE-BLANK

Finish each of the following statements using the correct term.

1. Antimicrobial agents that are derived from other living microorganisms are called _____.

2. Damage to the eighth cranial nerve, or _____, can occur from drug therapy, particularly from aminoglycosides.

3. Examples of antimicrobial agents that are potentially nephrotoxic include _____, _____, and _____.

4. When hypoprothrombinemia is present, the usual treatment is administration of vitamin _____.

5. Unless contraindicated by coexisting disease, patients taking antimicrobial agents should be encouraged to have an adequate fluid intake of _____ to _____ mL per 24 hours.

6. _____ were the first true antibiotics to be grown and used against pathogenic bacteria in human beings.

7. The _____ class of antibiotics should not be administered during the last half of pregnancy or while breastfeeding; do not administer to children until permanent teeth are in place (usually by age 8 years).

8. When antibiotics are described as "broad spectrum" in their clinical activity, it means that the antibiotic is generally effective against both _____ and _____ bacteria.

9. The _____ class is not considered a true antibiotic; its action is to inhibit biosynthesis of folic acid, which results in bacterial cell death.

10. The _____ class of antimicrobials is reserved for serious life-threatening infections that are vancomycin-resistant.

11. _____ is required for aerobic bacteria growth.

12. In general, a person who is allergic to sulfonamides should not take _____ oral hypoglycemic agents.

13. _____ agents kill bacterial pathogens.

14. Two major adverse effects associated with aminoglycoside antibiotics are _____ and _____.

MATCHING

Match the definition with the term that it best describes.

_____ 15. A microorganism that is able to grow and function without oxygen

_____ 16. Causing destruction or death of bacteria

_____ 17. A microorganism that lives and grows with oxygen present

_____ 18. Restrains or reduces the development or reproduction of bacteria

a. Bacteriostatic
b. Anaerobic
c. Bactericidal
d. Aerobic
e. Bacteremia

Match the definition with the term that it best describes.

_____ 19. Overgrowth of organisms resistant to current antibiotic therapy

_____ 20. Causes elevation in AST, ALT, LDH, and alkaline phosphatase

_____ 21. Causes increase in serum creatinine and BUN

_____ 22. Causes dizziness, tinnitus, and progressive hearing loss

a. Ototoxicity
b. Nephrotoxicity
c. Secondary infection
d. Pathogenic
e. Hepatotoxicity

Match the definition with the term that it best describes.

_____ 23. An inflammation of a vein

_____ 24. Reduction in formation and excretion of urine

_____ 25. Characterized by poor blood clotting

_____ 26. Increased albumin in urine

a. Thrombus
b. Phlebitis
c. Oliguria
d. Proteinuria
e. Hypoprothrombinemia

Match the generic drug name with its corresponding brand name. Each option will be used only once.

_____ 27. tolnaftate

_____ 28. ofloxacin

_____ 29. ampicillin

_____ 30. cefditoren

_____ 31. azithromycin

_____ 32. cephalexin

_____ 33. cefixime

_____ 34. cefaclor

_____ 35. ertapenem

_____ 36. neomycin

a. Zithromax
b. Invanz
c. Floxin
d. Suprax
e. Neo-Fradin
f. Tinactin
g. Spectracef
h. Keflex
i. Principen
j. Ceclor

TRUE OR FALSE

Write "T" for true and "F" for false for each statement. Correct all false statements.

_____ 37. The selection of the antimicrobial agent must be based on the sensitivity of the pathogen and the possible toxicity to the patient.

_____ 38. Antibiotics are usually given at even intervals over 24 hours to maintain cyclical blood levels of the medication.

_____ 39. Tetracyclines may be given with antacids, milk, and other dairy products or products containing calcium, magnesium, aluminum, magnesium, or iron.

_____ 40. Drugs such as sulfonamides require forcing fluids unless contraindicated by co-existing medical conditions.

_____ 41. Although serious reactions may occur with the first administration of a drug, repeated exposures to a previous sensitized substance can be fatal.

_____ 42. Patients with a sexually transmitted disease who are being treated with antimicrobial agents should be instructed to refrain from sexual intercourse during therapy.

_____ 43. Nursing mothers should remind their health care provider that they are breastfeeding so that antibiotics may be selected that will have no effect on the infant.

_____ 44. The sulfonamides are not true antibiotics because they are not synthesized by microorganisms.

_____ 45. Cephalosporins may be used as an alternative to penicillins for people allergic to penicillin.

_____ 46. Aminoglycosides cause hepatotoxicity.

_____ 47. Tetracyclines (except doxycycline) should not be taken concurrently with iron- or calcium-containing foods.

_____ 48. Patients receiving aminoglycosides should have a warning sign placed on the front of the chart before a procedure requiring a general anesthetic.

_____ 49. Diarrhea may be a symptom of secondary infection.

_____ 50. Chloramphenicol may cause fatal bone marrow depression.

_____ 51. Patient education for people taking antibiotics should stress taking all the prescribed medication.

_____ 52. Only drugs ending in "-mycin" are classified as macrolides.

_____ 53. Sulfonamides, when given to a patient taking sulfonylurea oral hypoglycemic agents, may cause hypoglycemia.

Antimicrobial Agents

Practice Questions for the NCLEX® Examination

_____ 1. Neomycin (Neo-Fradin) has been ordered for a patient who is scheduled for a colon resection. When the patient asks the nurse why an antibiotic is being administered before surgery, what is the nurse's reply?
1. "All patients requiring colon surgery are considered infectious."
2. "This drug will reduce the normal flora content of the intestine."
3. "You need this drug because you will develop an infection as soon as the surgeon opens the colon in the operating room."
4. "Any patient undergoing anesthesia must take neomycin."

_____ 2. When administering aminoglycosides to a patient, for what does the nurse assess? *(Select all that apply.)*
1. Anesthesia administration to the patient within the past 48–72 hours
2. Development of dizziness, tinnitus, and progressive hearing loss
3. Allergy to penicillin, because patients allergic to penicillin are allergic to aminoglycosides
4. History of renal disease
5. Hydration status

_____ 3. A patient taking an anticonvulsant for a seizure disorder has also been ordered a carbapenem antibiotic for an intra-abdominal infection. Which patient statement indicates that more teaching about this drug is necessary?
1. "If I should have blood and mucus in my stool, I should contact my health care provider."
2. "I should report any severe diarrhea to my health care provider and withhold the next dose of the antibiotic until I have approval to continue taking this drug."
3. "I should sit down if I feel dizzy until that feeling goes away."
4. "I should stop taking the anticonvulsant drug while taking my carbapenem antibiotic."

_____ 4. A patient has been ordered a cephalosporin for a respiratory tract infection. It is now 0900. The patient received the prescribed antacid at 0800. When is the earliest time the nurse will administer the cephalosporin?
1. 0900
2. 1000
3. 1100
4. 1200

_____ 5. Which statement does the nurse include when teaching a patient about macrolide therapy?
1. "If you use oral contraceptives, continue their use and ask your health care provider about additional methods of contraception."
2. "If you experience nausea when taking the drug, discontinue it immediately."
3. "If you experience diarrhea when taking this drug, take paregoric until it subsides."
4. "It is normal to have mucus in your stool when taking this drug."

_____ 6. Which statements about bacterial resistance to penicillin are true? _(Select all that apply.)_
1. Bacteria that become resistant to penicillin produce a protein called _penicil_ that affects the antibacterial activity of penicillins.
2. Penicillinase-resistant penicillins have been developed to maintain the antimicrobial activity of penicillin.
3. Many bacteria that are initially sensitive to penicillin develop a protective mechanism and become resistant to penicillin therapy.
4. The cause of resistance to penicillin is the bacteria's ability to secrete penicillinase which inactivates the penicillin antibiotics by splitting open the beta-lactam ring of the penicillin molecule.
5. There has been a dramatic decrease in the development of drug-resistant organisms.

_____ 7. Which drug class is preferred for treating patients exposed to anthrax?
1. Penicillin
2. Streptogramins
3. Quinolones
4. Tetracyclines

_____ 8. Which statements about tetracyclines are true? _(Select all that apply.)_
1. They are often used in patients allergic to penicillins.
2. They are particularly effective against acne.
3. Tetracyclines administered during the ages of tooth development may cause enamel hypoplasia and permanent yellow, gray, or brown staining of the teeth.
4. They do not enter the breast milk of lactating women, so nursing mothers on tetracycline therapy are encouraged to continue to breastfeed their infants.
5. They have no effect on the contraceptive activity of oral contraceptives.

_____ 9. Which medication is the drug of choice for tuberculosis prophylaxis?
1. Ethambutol (Myambutol)
2. Isoniazid (INH)
3. Rifampin (Rifadin)
4. Aztreonam (Azactam)

_____ 10. The nurse is teaching a patient about the use of isoniazid (INH) therapy for the treatment of active tuberculosis. Which statement made by the patient indicates that teaching has been effective?
1. "It is important that I take the pyridoxine pill with this drug."
2. "I will take this pill with food."
3. "If I develop tingling and numbness of my hands and feet, I will immediately discontinue treatment with this drug and discard any remaining pills I have, because this is a sign of an extreme allergic reaction."
4. "If I develop nausea and vomiting, I will immediately stop use of this drug."

_____ 11. When providing patient teaching to a 23-year-old woman who has been prescribed rifampin (Rifadin), which statements does the nurse include? *(Select all that apply.)*
   1. "You should use an alternative method of birth control if you are currently taking oral contraceptives."
   2. "If you wear soft contact lenses, they may become permanently discolored due to rifampin use."
   3. "You may expect your urine to turn green because of the adverse effects of rifampin."
   4. "You may experience nausea, vomiting, and anorexia when taking rifampin, but these symptoms will usually be mild and resolve with continued therapy."
   5. "If you experience abdominal cramps while taking this medication, immediately discontinue the drug."

_____ 12. Which statement about the administration of vancomycin (Vancocin) is true?
   1. Rapid IV administration may result in a severe hypertensive episode.
   2. Patients receiving IV vancomycin may develop red man syndrome.
   3. Patients receiving vancomycin must be placed on continuous electrocardiographic monitoring.
   4. Vancomycin may only be administered IV.

_____ 13. When teaching a patient about proper administration and use of a topical antifungal agent for treatment of a vaginal yeast infection, which statements does the nurse include? *(Select all that apply.)*
   1. "Wash the applicator after each use."
   2. "Use a pad to protect your clothing."
   3. "Discontinue use of the intravaginal antifungal if menstruation begins."
   4. "You should use contraception other than a diaphragm or condom while you are using the intravaginal antifungal."
   5. "Administer a saline douche every evening when taking this medication."

_____ 14. The nurse is teaching a patient about the use of oseltamivir (Tamiflu). Which statement made by the patient indicates teaching has been effective?
   1. "I can use this medication instead of the annual flu shot I usually get."
   2. "I must avoid use of any decongestants while taking this medication."
   3. "For this medication to be effective, it must be started within 2 days of any developed symptoms of the flu."
   4. "The main reason to take this medication is to prevent the spread of flu to other people."

15. A patient is ordered gentamicin 60 mg IV every 2 hours. The medication is available as 80 mg per 2 mL. How many mL of the medication does the nurse administer? _____ mL

16. A patient is ordered cephalexin (Keflex) 100 mg PO 4 times a day. The medication is available in suspension form, 250 mg per 5 mL. How many mL of the medication does the nurse administer? _____ mL

17. A patient is ordered azithromycin (Zithromax) 400 mg IV. The medication is available in a powdered vial, 500 mg. The directions on the side of the label state "constitute to 100 mg/mL with 4.8 mL of sterile water for injection." How many mL of the medication does the nurse administer? _____ mL

Nutrition

Review Sheet

The QUESTION column and the ANSWER column have been offset so that you can cover the answers while reading the questions, allowing you to assess your knowledge.

Question	Answer
1. What factors affect one's nutritional requirements?	
2. Summarize information related to nutrition on the My Pyramid guidelines.	1. See textbook, p. 781.
3. What do the Dietary Reference Intakes (DRIs) recommend concerning fat consumption? Describe the effects of consumption of various types of fats.	2. The pyramid recommends eating a variety of foods per day to receive the necessary nutrients while consuming an appropriate amount of calories to maintain health and weight. Daily servings of food groups are recommended along with reminders of the importance of physical activity. The new guidelines stress the importance of controlling weight.
4. What do the guidelines recommend for dairy product consumption?	3. The DRIs recommend obtaining 20% to 35% of the daily caloric intake from fats. Monosaturated fats decrease LDL and increase HDL and are considered to be cardioprotective. Polyunsaturated fats also lower LDL and raise HDL levels. Saturated fats raise both LDL and HDL and are thought to increase atherosclerotic plaque formation in the arteries. Only recently has it been recognized that trans fats may induce more heart disease than saturated fats because, in addition to raising LDL cholesterol, trans fats decrease HDL cholesterol and increase triglycerides as well as another undesirable blood fat, lipoprotein. Saturated fats and trans fats have no known beneficial nutritional effect and should be eliminated as much as possible from the diet.
5. What are the Dietary Reference Intakes (DRIs)?	4. The guidelines recommend drinking three glasses of low-fat milk or eating three servings of other dairy products per day to prevent osteoporosis. Calcium supplements have been shown to reduce the incidence of osteoporosis and do not add calories to the diet.
6. What are the Estimated Average Requirements (EARs) and Recommended Dietary Allowances (RDAs)?	5. The DRIs are a series of tables that provide quantitative estimates of nutrient intakes to be used in planning and assessing diets for healthy people.

7. What is the unit of measurement of energy requirements?

8. What are other names for simple carbohydrates?

9. What percent of calories of the total daily dietary intake of an adult is recommended to come from carbohydrates?

10. Carbohydrates supply _____ kilocalories of energy per gram, fats supply _____ kilocalories of energy per gram, and proteins supply _____ kilocalories of energy per gram.

11. What are the end products of protein metabolism?

12. How many water-soluble and fat-soluble vitamins are there to date?

13. Why are minerals essential to life?

14. Name three forms of malnutrition.

15. What laboratory studies can be used to assess lean body mass?

16. Differentiate between enteral and parenteral nutrition.

17. Explain components of a nutritional assessment.

18. What physical changes are related to a malnourished state?

19. What are the general routines used for checking tube placement and residuals of enteral feedings?

20. When is the use of enteral nutrition contraindicated?

21. What assessments should be performed prior to administering enteral nutrition?

22. Differentiate among bolus, intermittent, and continuous feedings.

23. How should prescribed medications be administered via a feeding tube?

24. List adverse effects of enteral feedings that should be reported to the health care provider.

25. What is the difference between peripheral parenteral nutrition solutions (PPN), and total parenteral nutrition (TPN) solutions?

6. The EAR is a nutrient intake value that is estimated to meet the requirements of half of the healthy individuals in a group. The most well-known component of the DRIs is the RDA.

7. Kilocalories (kcal)

8. Simple carbohydrates are known as *monosaccharides* and *disaccharides*.

9. 45% to 65%

10. Carbohydrates supply 4 kilocalories, fats supply 9 kilocalories, and proteins supply 4 kilocalories.

11. Nitrogenous products such as urea, uric acid, ammonia, carbon dioxide, and water.

12. Thirteen total vitamins; 9 water-soluble; 4 fat-soluble.

13. See textbook, p. 791.

14. Marasmus, kwashiorkor, and mixed kwashiorkor-marasmus.

15. Albumin, pre-albumin, retinol-binding protein, transferrin.

16. Enteral nutrition is administered orally; parenteral nutrition is given via venous access and implantable vascular access devices.

17. See textbook, p. 795.

18. Height, weight, muscle circumference, skin fold thickness, skin integrity, cardiovascular, respiratory, neurologic alteration, thyroid function, gastrointestinal symptoms.

19. See textbook, p. 796.

20. Enteral nutrition is contraindicated when the individual has intractable vomiting, a paralyzed ileum, or certain types of fistulas.

21. See textbook, p. 798.

22. See textbook, p. 799.

23. See textbook, p. 799.

24. Pulmonary complications (aspiration), diarrhea, constipation, nausea, vomiting, increased residual volume, rash, chills, fever, and respiratory difficulty.

26. List premedication assessments that should be performed before administering TPN or PPN.

27. List adverse effects of parenteral feedings that should be reported to the health care provider.

28. List key signs and symptoms of fat-soluble and water-soluble vitamin deficiencies.

25. PPN solutions consist of 2%–5% crystalline amino acid preparations and 5%–10% dextrose with electrolytes and vitamins. TPN consists of 15%–25% glucose, amino acids (3.5%–15%), fat emulsion (10%–20%), electrolytes, vitamins, and minerals. Due to high osmolality (see Chapter 12), TPN solutions must be administered through a central venous access line.

26. See textbook, p. 801.

27. Hypoglycemia, hyperglycemia, fluid imbalance, rash, chills, fever, respiratory difficulty, electrolyte imbalances, and hepatotoxicity.

28. See textbook, p. 802.

Nutrition

Learning Activities

FILL-IN-THE-BLANK

Finish each of the following statements using the correct term.

1. _____ are the only sugars capable of being used directly to produce energy for the body.

2. Complex carbohydrates such as starch, dextrin, and fiber are also known as _____.

3. _____ is a protein deficiency that develops when the patient receives adequate fats and carbohydrates in the diet, but little or no protein.

4. The equipment used to administer tube feedings are changed in accordance with the clinical facility's policy, which is usually every _____ hours.

5. Deficiencies of vitamin _____ are often associated with neurologic alterations.

6. Carbohydrates and proteins supply approximately _____ kilocalories of energy per gram.

7. Edema of the abdomen and subcutaneous tissue is a possible sign of _____ deficiency.

8. A _____ deficiency can increase the heart rate and heart size.

9. A pyridoxine deficiency can result in _____.

10. Vitamin _____ deficiency can result in anemia, depression, and delayed wound healing.

MATCHING

Match the generic drug name with its corresponding brand name. Each option will be used only once.

_____ 11. oral supplements

_____ 12. standard isotonic formulas

_____ 13. pediatric formulas

_____ 14. specialized formulas

a. Isocal
b. Boost
c. Glucerna
d. Similac

TRUE OR FALSE

Write "T" for true and "F" for false for each statement. Correct all false statements.

_____ 15. Fiber is recognized as a macronutrient, a separate factor necessary for complete nutrition and wellness.

_____ 16. Essential fatty acids (EFAs) are produced by the body.

_____ 17. Parenteral feedings are administered orally, either by drinking or instillation into the stomach by way of a feeding tube or feeding gastrostomy port.

_____ 18. Total parenteral nutrition (TPN) orders are formulated daily based on the patient's status, weight, and fluid and electrolyte balance.

_____ 19. Vitamins, whose name originally derived from the term "vital amines," are a specific set of chemical molecules that regulate human metabolism necessary to maintain health.

_____ 20. Patients receiving warfarin (Coumadin) should avoid herbal medicines that inhibit platelet aggregation.

Nutrition

Practice Questions for the NCLEX® Examination

_____ 1. What are advantages of enteral nutrition over parenteral nutrition? *(Select all that apply.)*
   1. Enteral nutrition provides gastrointestinal stimulation.
   2. Enteral nutrition has less chance of infection associated with its use.
   3. Enteral feedings are more expensive.
   4. Enteral nutrition is more physiologic.
   5. Enteral nutrition therapy does not require blood glucose assessment.

_____ 2. When administering drugs to a patient receiving an enteral feeding, what does the nurse do?
   1. Crushes enteric-coated tablets before administration via the feeding tube
   2. Crushes slow-release tablets before administration via the feeding tube
   3. Combines all drugs together and administers at the same time
   4. Administers the medicines on an empty stomach

_____ 3. The nurse teaches a patient to take calcium channel blockers with which liquids? *(Select all that apply.)*
   1. Milk
   2. Orange juice
   3. Grapefruit juice
   4. Carbonated soft drink
   5. Water

_____ 4. A patient is receiving total parenteral nutrition at a rate of 80 mL per hour. The TPN bag is due to be changed at 0900. The nurse enters the patient's room at 0845 and finds 300 mL of the TPN fluid remaining in the bag. What does the nurse do next?
   1. Continues the infusion of the current rate until it is complete
   2. Increases the rate of the TPN to 150 mL per hour to use up the remainder of fluid in the least amount of time
   3. Hangs an IV bag of normal saline if the next bag of TPN is not readily available
   4. Discards any TPN remaining in the current bag and hangs a new bag of TPN

_____ 5. A patient admitted with a diagnosis of malnutrition has been ordered total parenteral nutrition (TPN). In the initial stages of therapy, the nurse assesses for the development of which common adverse effect of TPN?
   1. Hyperglycemia
   2. Rash
   3. Diarrhea
   4. Abdominal cramping

_____ 6. When providing patient teaching about kwashiorkor, which statements does the nurse include? *(Select all that apply.)*
   1. "It occurs because of a fat deficiency in the diet."
   2. "Patients with this condition are often difficult to recognize because they appear to be well-nourished."
   3. "Patients with this condition receive adequate carbohydrates in the diet."
   4. "Patients with this condition receive adequate fat in the diet."
   5. "Patients are usually dehydrated when they have this condition."

_____ 7. Which routes can be used for administering enteral nutrition? *(Select all that apply.)*
   1. Central venous
   2. Nasogastric
   3. Intrathecal
   4. Nasojejunal
   5. Needle-catheter jejunostomy

_____ 8. A patient is ordered Ensure 1/4 strength 120 mL every 2 hours for 3 feedings. Ensure is available in 4- and 8-ounce cans. How many cans of Ensure are needed?
   1. One 4-ounce can
   2. One 8-ounce can
   3. One 4-ounce can AND one 8-ounce can
   4. Two 4-ounce AND two 8-ounce cans

9. A patient is ordered Boost 800 mL at 3/4 strength to infuse over 8 hours. Boost is available in 10 fluid ounce cans. How many mL of solvent does the nurse add? _____ mL

10. A patient is ordered 2/3 strength Ensure 6 fluid ounces over 3 hours. Ensure is available in 4 fluid ounce cans. How many ounces of water does the nurse add to the 4 fluid ounce can? _____ fl oz

Herbal and Dietary Supplement Therapy

Review Sheet

The QUESTION column and the ANSWER column have been offset so that you can cover the answers while reading the questions, allowing you to assess your knowledge.

Question	Answer
1. Define the key terms associated with this chapter.	
2. Describe the role of the Food and Drug Administration (FDA) in the regulation of herbal products.	1. See textbook, pp. 804 and 806.
3. What factors should be considered when recommending herbal products?	2. The FDA has no direct role in regulation of herbal products. The Dietary Supplement Health and Education Act (DSHEA) of 1994 governs the use of herbal medicines, vitamins, minerals, and amino acids. Under this Act, almost all herbal medicines, vitamins, minerals, amino acids, and other supplemental chemicals used for health were reclassified legally as dietary supplements, a food category. The labels and advertisements from the manufacturer must contain a statement that the product has not yet been evaluated by the FDA for treating, curing, or preventing any disease. The law does not prevent other people from making claims (founded or unfounded) about the therapeutic effects of supplement ingredients. The end result of the new law is that dietary supplements are not required to be safe and effective and unfounded claims of therapeutic benefit abound. There are now hundreds of herbal medicines and other dietary supplements being marketed in the United States as single- and multiple-ingredient products for an extremely wide variety of uses, all implying that they will improve one's health. The vast majority of the popular claims made for herbal medicines and dietary supplements are unproven. There are also no standardized manufacturing practices that control the manufacture of most of these products as there are with medicines approved by the FDA.
4. Prepare a list of herbal products listed in the chapter and insert the corresponding popular uses by lay people of these herbal products.	3. See Box 48-1, p. 805.

5. What questions as part of a medication history should elicit information regarding the use of herbal products and other alternative medicines?

4. *Herbal Product:*   *Use(s):*
   Aloe   See p. 806.
   Black cohosh   See p. 807.
   Chamomile   See pp. 807-808.
   Echinacea   See p. 808.
   Ephedra   See pp. 808-809.
   Feverfew   See p. 809.
   Garlic   See pp. 809-810.
   Ginger   See p. 810.
   Ginkgo   See pp. 810-811.
   Ginseng   See pp. 811-812.
   Goldenseal   See p. 812.
   Green tea   See pp. 812-813.
   Saw palmetto   See p. 813.
   St. John's wort   See pp. 813-814.
   Valerian   See p. 814.

   Other Dietary Supplements:
   Coenzyme Q_{10} See pp. 814-815.
   Creatine   See p. 815.
   Gamma-hydroxybutyrate
     (GHB)   See pp. 815-816.
   Lycopene   See p. 816.
   Melatonin   See pp. 816-817.
   Policosanol   See p. 817.
   Omega-3 fatty acids   See pp. 817-818.
   S-adenosylmethionine
     (SAM-e)   See pp. 818-819.

6. What potential drug interactions may occur with each herbal product listed?

7. What is the common use for aloe?

8. What is the most common drug interaction with aloe?

9. What is the common use for black cohosh?

10. When should black cohosh not be used?

11. What is the common use for chamomile?

12. What is echinacea commonly used for?

5. Consult with your instructor for assistance.

6. Review individual monographs throughout chapter.

7. Aloe has been used for arthritis, colitis, common cold, hemorrhoids, seizures, and glaucoma. Most recently, aloe gel has been marketed for topical use to treat pain, inflammation, and itching, and as a healing agent for sunburn, skin ulcers, psoriasis, and frostbite.

8. Patients who are diabetic should have their blood glucose monitored because there have been claims that when taken orally, aloe may have hypoglycemic effects.

9. Black cohosh is used to reduce symptoms of premenstrual syndrome (PMS), dysmenorrhea, and menopause.

10. Black cohosh should not be used in the first two trimesters of pregnancy because of its uterine relaxing effects.

11. Chamomile is used as a digestive agent for bloating, an antispasmodic and an anti-inflammatory in the gastrointestinal tract, an antispasmodic for menstrual cramps, an anti-inflammatory for skin irritation, and a mouthwash for minor mouth irritation or gum infections.

13. What is ephedra commonly used for?

14. When is the use of ephedra contraindicated?

15. What are the adverse effects of ephedra?

16. What is feverfew commonly used for?

17. What is garlic commonly used for?

18. What is ginger commonly used for?

19. What is ginkgo commonly used for?

20. What is ginseng commonly used for?

21. What is goldenseal commonly used for?

22. When should goldenseal not be taken?

23. What is green tea commonly used for?

12. Echinacea is a nonspecific immunostimulant that may prevent or treat viral respiratory tract infections such as the common cold or flu. It may be used to treat urinary tract infections and may be applied externally to difficult-to-heal superficial wounds.

13. Ephedra is used as a bronchodilator for asthma, a nasal decongestant, and a central nervous system (CNS) stimulant.

14. Ephedra is contraindicated in patients with heart conditions, hypertension, diabetes, and thyroid disease.

15. Ephedra elevates systolic and diastolic blood pressure and heart rate, causing palpitations. It also causes nervousness, headache, insomnia, and dizziness.

16. Feverfew is used to reduce the frequency and severity of migraine headaches. Its anti-inflammatory effects have also been used to treat rheumatoid arthritis.

17. The most frequent use of garlic supported by scientific literature is in reducing cholesterol and triglycerides. It has demonstrated antiplatelet activity similar to aspirin, and may also modestly lower blood pressure.

18. Ginger has been used for centuries to alleviate nausea and vomiting. It has also been found to be modestly effective in reducing inflammation associated with rheumatoid arthritis and muscle discomfort.

19. Ginkgo biloba extract is used primarily to increase cerebral blood flow, particularly in geriatric patients. Other uses include improved walking distance in patients with intermittent claudication, improvement in erectile dysfunction secondary to antidepressant therapy, improved peripheral blood flow in patients with diabetes mellitus, and improved hearing in patients with hearing impairment due to poor circulation to the ears.

20. Ginseng is not used as a cure for disease, but as an "adaptogen" in maintaining health.

21. Goldenseal is used topically as a tea for treatment of canker sores, sore mouth, and cracked and bleeding lips. It may help fight viral upper respiratory infections such as cold or flu. There is a common myth that goldenseal will mask assays for street drugs.

22. Goldenseal in high doses may have a uterine stimulant effect, so it should not be taken during pregnancy.

24. What is saw palmetto commonly used for?

25. What drug should not be used with saw palmetto?

26. What is St. John's wort commonly used for?
27. What are the adverse effects of St. John's wort?
28. What syndrome is use of St. John's wort associated with?
29. What is valerian commonly used for?
30. What is coenzyme Q_{10} commonly used for?

31. What is creatine commonly used for?

32. What is gamma-hydroxybutyrate (GHB) commonly used for?

33. What are the adverse effects of GHB?

34. What is lycopene commonly used for?

35. What is melatonin commonly used for?

23. Green tea is used to improve cognitive performance. It raises blood pressure, heart rate, and contractility, and acts as a diuretic. It has been shown to lower cholesterol, triglycerides, and low-density lipoprotein, and raise high-density lipoprotein. There is some evidence that green tea might reduce the risk of bladder, esophageal, and pancreatic cancer, and reduce or prevent the onset of parkinsonism. Green tea is also used to treat diarrhea.

24. Saw palmetto is used to treat the symptoms associated with benign prostatic hyperplasia (BPH), to reduce the risks associated with urinary retention, and to minimize the need for surgery associated with BPH.

25. Finasteride

26. St. John's wort is used to treat mild depression and to heal wounds.

27. St. John's wort may cause photosensitivity.

28. Serotonin syndrome
29. Valerian is used for restlessness and may promote sleep.
30. CoQ_{10} is primarily used as an adjunct therapy for chronic heart failure. It may also be used to treat other cardiovascular diseases, cancer, muscular dystrophy, periodontal disease, and AIDS.
31. Creatine supplementation is thought to enhance muscle performance for short periods of intense exercise. Patients with heart failure and muscular dystrophy might benefit from creatine supplementation.

32. In the late 1980s GHB was marketed and sold as a growth hormone stimulator. It was banned by the FDA in 1990 because of adverse reactions to the drug. Despite the FDA ban, GHB continues to be marketed as a dietary supplement. GHB is usually abused for its intoxicating, sedative, and euphoric properties, particularly at rave parties where it is used as a "date rape" drug. It is available as a prescription product for treating patients with narcolepsy.

33. The adverse effects of GHB are highly individualized; however, those that are potentially life-threatening include vomiting with aspiration to the lungs, respiratory depression, bradycardia, and hypotension.

34. There is some evidence to suggest that diets high in lycopene may reduce risk of prostate cancer. It has antioxidant properties that may lower LDL-cholesterol, thus protecting against heart attack and stroke. Lycopene may also protect against macular degeneration and cataracts.

36. What is policosanol commonly used for?

37. What are the omega-3 fatty acids primarily used for?

38. What is SAM-e commonly used for?

35. Melatonin is best known as a sleep aid and treatment for jet lag. It may also be helpful in patients withdrawing from benzodiazepine therapy.

36. Policosanol is used to treat dyslipidemia. It is also used as a platelet inhibitor for the treatment of intermittent claudication. Policosanol is also used to treat myocardial ischemia in patients with coronary artery disease.

37. Omega-3 fatty acids are primarily used for the prevention of myocardial infarction.

38. SAM-e is used for the treatment of depression, osteoarthritis, and fibromyalgia.

| Herbal and Dietary Supplement Therapy | chapter 48 |

Learning Activities

FILL-IN-THE-BLANK

Finish each of the following statements using the correct term.

1. _____ medicines are defined as natural substances derived from botanical or plant origin.

2. Concurrent consumption of large quantities of green tea with warfarin may _____ the anticoagulant effects of warfarin.

3. The most common use of ginger is to alleviate _____ and _____.

4. Most individuals using St. John's wort do so for its supposed ability to treat mild _____ and to heal _____.

5. There is some evidence to suggest that diets high in _____ may reduce the risk of prostate cancer.

MATCHING

Match each herb to the other name it is known by. Each option will be used only once.

_____ 6. valerian

_____ 7. St. John's wort

_____ 8. ginkgo

_____ 9. black cohosh

_____ 10. echinacea

_____ 11. aloe

_____ 12. goldenseal

a. squawroot
b. klamath weed
c. burn plant
d. maidenhair tree
e. amantilla
f. purple coneflower
g. yellow root

TRUE OR FALSE

Write "T" for true and "F" for false for each statement. Correct all false statements.

_____ 13. Under the Dietary Supplement Health and Education Act (DSHEA) of 1994, almost all herbal medicines, vitamins, minerals, amino acids, and other supplemental chemicals used for health were reclassified legally as dietary supplements, a food category.

_____ 14. Diet supplements should not be recommended for use by pregnant women, lactating mothers, infants, or young children without approval from the patient's primary care health provider.

_____ 15. Homeopathy employs the use of therapeutic doses of botanical drugs.

_____ 16. It is reported that SAM-e may reduce some of the adverse effects of levodopa used to treat parkinsonism, but it is also thought that SAM-e may reduce the beneficial effects of levodopa in the treatment of parkinsonism over time.

_____ 17. Ginseng has been shown to lower insulin levels in laboratory animals.

_____ 18. Chamomile has been shown to be an effective antidepressant.

_____ 19. Echinacea is a bacteriostatic and bactericidal agent.

_____ 20. There are essentially no drug interactions with ephedra.

_____ 21. Feverfew is used as an antiplatelet and antihypertensive agent.

_____ 22. Garlic affects platelet aggregation and therefore should be used with caution for patients taking antiplatelet medications.

_____ 23. Saw palmetto is used to treat symptoms of benign prostatic hyperplasia.

_____ 24. Ginseng may cause hyperglycemia.

_____ 25. Valerian is used as a sleep aid and as a mild tranquilizer.

Herbal and Dietary Supplement Therapy

Practice Questions for the NCLEX® Examination

_____ 1. A 62-year-old woman is on hormone replacement therapy to treat symptoms associated with menopause and to prevent osteoporosis. She also takes medication to control high blood pressure. She is interested in taking black cohosh and asks the nurse about it. What is the best response by the nurse?
  1. "Studies have found that black cohosh is an excellent herb for women to treat symptoms of menopause that are not controlled by hormone replacement therapy."
  2. "High blood pressure will be lowered with the use of black cohosh, so you won't need to take your high blood pressure pills any longer."
  3. "Black cohosh works by stimulating the body to produce its own natural testosterone."
  4. "Black cohosh may cause added antihypertensive effects when taken with medication to lower blood pressure. Consult your health care provider before adding black cohosh to your treatment regimen."

_____ 2. Which herb is most commonly used in the treatment of asthma?
  1. Ephedra
  2. Echinacea
  3. Chamomile
  4. Goldenseal

_____ 3. Which statements does the nurse include when teaching a patient about St. John's wort? _(Select all that apply.)_
  1. "The active ingredients of St. John's wort are unknown."
  2. "St. John's wort may cause photosensitivity, so individuals using it should avoid overexposure to the sun."
  3. "Patients who take other serotonin stimulants should not take St. John's wort without consulting their health care provider."
  4. "St. John's wort is a safe drug for anyone with depression."
  5. "There are no adverse effects associated with the use of St. John's wort."

_____ 4. Which conditions are possible indications for the use of S-adenosylmethinonine (SAM-e)? _(Select all that apply.)_
  1. Depression
  2. Osteoarthritis
  3. Diabetes mellitus
  4. Fibromyalgia
  5. Infection

_____ 5. Which herb is most commonly used for treating symptoms associated with benign prostatic hypertrophy?
  1. Valerian
  2. Feverfew
  3. Saw palmetto
  4. Ginseng

_____ 6. Which statements about herbal medicines and dietary supplements are correct? *(Select all that apply.)*
   1. Black cohosh is often taken in conjunction with antihypertensive medications.
   2. Patients taking platelet inhibitors should use garlic with caution.
   3. Ginseng has the potential to induce hyperglycemia.
   4. Patients taking melatonin should avoid alcohol.
   5. Goldenseal may turn urine a distinctive dark amber or brown color.

_____ 7. When a patient is taking aloe, it is most important for the nurse to assess the patient for the development of which condition?
   1. Infection
   2. Hypertension
   3. Hypokalemia
   4. Hypoglycemia

_____ 8. A patient with which condition is most likely to benefit from the administration of echinacea?
   1. Acquired immunodeficiency syndrome (AIDS)
   2. Multiple sclerosis
   3. Viral respiratory tract infection
   4. Systemic lupus erythematosus

Substance Abuse

Review Sheet

The QUESTION column and the ANSWER column have been offset so that you can cover the answers while reading the questions, allowing you to assess your knowledge.

Question	Answer
1. Define *substance-related disorders, substance abuse, impairment, dependence, addiction,* and *illicit substances.*	
2. Differentiate among the biologic model, psychological theories, and sociocultural factors that are associated with substance abuse.	1. See textbook, p. 821.

3. List sociologic signs of impairment associated with substance abuse.	2. Biologic model: caused by person's genetic profile.
	    Psychological theory: sees alcoholism as occurring in an individual who is fixated in the oral stage of development and is seeking oral gratification. This theory also recognizes a link to depression, anxiety, antisocial personality, and dependent personality.
	    Sociocultural: the individual is influenced by such things as attitudes, norms, values, nationality, religion, gender, family background, and social environment.

4. List four tests used to screen for alcohol and substance abuse.	3. Substance abuse first affects the family life, then social life, and finally results in physical and mental changes.
5. What is the prevalence of substance abuse by health care professionals?	4. See Table 49-2.
6. Cite legal considerations associated with substance abuse and dependence in health care providers.	5. See textbook, p. 827.
7. List three long-term goals of treatment of substance abuse as defined by the American Psychiatric Association.	6. See textbook, pp. 827-829; research laws governing nursing in the state where you are practicing.
8. Cite examples of organizations that promote the goals of abstinence from substance abuse.	7. Reduction or abstinence in use and effects of substances; reduction in frequency and severity of relapse; and improvement in psychologic and social functioning.
9. Compare the effects on the body of acute and chronic use of alcohol.	8. Alcoholics Anonymous (AA), Narcotics Anonymous (NA), and others.
10. Define *alcohol intoxication* and *alcohol withdrawal.*	9. See textbook, p. 830.

11. What drugs are used to treat alcohol withdrawal symptoms?
12. Describe components of an alcohol relapse prevention program.

13. Name three medications used to promote abstinence from alcohol use.
14. List commonly abused opiates.

15. List the signs and symptoms of opioid intoxication and opioid withdrawal.

16. What limitations does naltrexone (ReVia) have in the treatment of opioid addiction?
17. Name two forms of buprenorphine approved for opioid maintenance programs.
18. What effect does cocaine have on the CNS?

19. What is the difference between "freebase" and "crack" cocaine?

20. Describe the signs and symptoms of cocaine intoxication and withdrawal from cocaine.

21. List the nursing assessments that should be used when substance abuse is suspected or diagnosed.
22. What laboratory tests are routinely ordered for drug screening?
23. Study Table 49-1 to identify drugs, usage forms, possible adverse effects, signs of overdose, and long-term effects of drugs classified as stimulants, depressants, narcotics, cannabis, hallucinogens, and inhalants.

10. See textbook, pp. 830-831.

11. Benzodiazepines are used for detoxification. Long-acting chlordiazepoxide, diazepam, and clorazepate are the most commonly used protocol for alcohol withdrawal.
12. See textbook, p. 832.

13. Disulfiram (Antabuse), naltrexone (ReVia), and acamprosate (Campral).
14. Heroin, morphine, hydromorphone, codeine, oxycodone, and hydrocodone; opiate-like substances (e.g., meperidine, fentanyl, others).
15. See textbook, pp. 832-833.

16. Naltrexone does not block the desire to get "high;" it only blocks the "high" when an opioid is used.
17. Buprenorphine-only (Subutrex) and buprenorphine-naloxone (Suboxone).
18. Cocaine blocks the metabolism of catecholamines in the brain, bringing on a sudden CNS stimulation with euphoria or a "rush."
19. "Freebase" is cocaine hydrochloride mixed with ammonia and dissolved in ether. As ether evaporates, it forms a powder residue that can be smoked for its "high." "Crack" cocaine is cocaine hydrochloride mixed with baking soda that is heated to form "rocks" which are then smoked.
20. See textbook, p. 835.

21. See textbook, pp. 836-838.

22. See textbook, p. 838.

23. See Table 49-1.

Student Name _____

Substance Abuse

Learning Activities

FILL-IN-THE-BLANK

Finish each of the following statements using the correct term.

1. _____ _____ is defined as the periodic purposeful use of a substance that leads to clinically significant impairment.

2. If substance abuse behavior is not stopped, it leads to a more serious medical condition known as substance _____ or _____.

3. A(n) _____ substance is any chemical or mixture of chemicals that alters biologic function and is not required for the maintenance of health.

4. _____ is defined as the ingestion of ethanol to the point of clinically significant maladaptive behavioral or psychologic changes.

5. THC, hashish, and marijuana are classified as _____.

6. LSD and PCP are classified as _____.

7. Nicotine, caffeine, amphetamines, and cocaine are classified as _____.

8. Lack of coordination, sluggishness, slurred speech, and disorientation are possible adverse effects of the use of drugs classified as _____.

MATCHING

Match the common drug name with its corresponding medical name. Each option will be used only once.

_____ 9. sedatives

_____ 10. tranquilizers

_____ 11. opium

_____ 12. heroin

_____ 13. marijuana

a. Valium
b. tetrahydrocanabinol
c. paregoric
d. phenobarbital
e. diacetylmorphine

TRUE OR FALSE

Write "T" for true and "F" for false for each statement. Correct all false statements.

_____ 14. Even though substance abuse has been a condition of the human mind since prehistoric times, and very extensively studied, there is no one theory that accounts for why individuals abuse chemicals.

_____ 15. Substance abuse has been linked to several psychological traits, but there is no particular evidence that these traits cause the substance abuse.

_____ 16. The disease of substance impairment problems usually manifests first in social life then followed by family life.

_____ 17. There are twelve steps to the Alcoholics Anonymous program.

_____ 18. Withdrawal from opioids is uncomfortable but usually not life-threatening unless there are coexisting medical conditions.

Substance Abuse

Practice Questions for the NCLEX® Examination

_____ 1. Which signs/symptoms does the nurse expect to find upon assessment of a patient experiencing opioid withdrawal? *(Select all that apply.)*
   1. Pupillary constriction
   2. Rhinorrhea
   3. Increased blood pressure
   4. Diarrhea
   5. Anxiety

_____ 2. Patients being treated for recovery from opioid addiction would likely receive which drugs? *(Select all that apply.)*
   1. Meperidine (Demerol)
   2. Methadone
   3. Naltrexone (ReVia)
   4. Clonidine (Catapres)
   5. Buprenorphine (Subutex)

_____ 3. What is the first step to the Twelve Steps of Alcoholics Anonymous?
   1. "Make a list of all people harmed by use of alcohol."
   2. "Make a searching and fearless moral inventory of yourself."
   3. "Become entirely ready to have God remove all defects of your character."
   4. "Admit that you are powerless over alcohol and that your life has become unmanageable."

_____ 4. When working with a patient who is withdrawing from long-term use of amphetamines, the nurse expects the patient to exhibit which signs/symptoms? *(Select all that apply.)*
   1. Severe depression
   2. Fatigue
   3. Loss of memory
   4. Inability to manipulate information
   5. Insomnia

_____ 5. When providing teaching about the effects of substance use and abuse with pregnancy, which statements does the nurse include? *(Select all that apply.)*
   1. "Using alcohol and drugs while pregnant has a strong likelihood of harming the baby after birth."
   2. "Infants of drug addicts must be monitored closely for symptoms of withdrawal after delivery."
   3. "Using alcohol and drugs during pregnancy has a high likelihood of causing the need for induction of pregnancy due to the fetus being post-term."
   4. "Alcohol and drug use during pregnancy has been associated with potentially fatal bleeding disorders."
   5. "Babies of mothers who used alcohol during pregnancy have a higher incidence of behavioral problems later in life."

6. A patient is ordered naltrexone hydrochloride (ReVia) 50 mg/day PO. The medication is available in 50-mg tablets. The patient received a 90-day supply of the medication. On day 38 of treatment, how many tablets of the prescription should remain? _____ tablets

7. An order reads methadone hydrochloride (Methadone) 15 mg IM every day. The medication is available as 10 mg/mL. How many mL of the medication does the nurse administer? _____ mL

8. A patient is ordered disulfiram (Antabuse) 125 mg/day PO. The medication is available as 250 mg/tablet. How many tablets does the patient receive in a 7-day period? _____ tablets

Miscellaneous Agents

Review Sheet

The QUESTION column and the ANSWER column have been offset so that you can cover the answers while reading the questions, allowing you to assess your knowledge.

Question	Answer
1. What is the therapeutic outcome of the use of acamprosate (Campral)?	
2. What are the serious adverse effects with the use of acamprosate (Campral)?	1. The primary therapeutic outcome expected from acamprosate is improved adherence with an alcohol treatment program by abstinence from alcohol.
3. What is the action and primary use of allopurinol (Zyloprim)?	2. Monitor alcohol-dependent patients, including those patients being treated with acamprosate for the development of symptoms of negative thoughts, feelings, behaviors, depression, or suicidal thinking. Alert families and caregivers of patients being treated with acamprosate of the need to monitor for the emergent nature of these symptoms and to report such symptoms to the patient's health care provider.
4. What are common adverse effects of allopurinol (Zyloprim) therapy?	3. Allopurinol blocks the terminal steps in uric acid formation by inhibiting the enzyme xanthine oxidase. This agent can be used to treat primary gout or gout secondary to antineoplastic therapy.
5. What is the primary therapeutic outcome of colchicine therapy?	4. Patients should be told that the frequency of gout attacks may increase for the first few months of therapy. The patient should continue therapy without changing the dosage during the attacks. Nausea, vomiting, diarrhea, dizziness, and headache are usually mild and tend to resolve with continued therapy.
6. In which patient groups should colchicine be used with extreme caution?	5. Elimination of joint pain secondary to acute gout attack.
7. Via which routes should colchicine *not* be administered?	6. Older adults or debilitated patients, and patients with impaired renal, cardiac, or gastrointestinal function should be extremely cautious with colchicine.
8. What is disulfiram (Antabuse) used for?	7. Subcutaneously or intramuscularly
9. How is a disulfiram (Antabuse) reaction manifested?	8. Disulfiram is used in alcohol rehabilitation programs for chronic alcohol patients who want to maintain sobriety.

Copyright © 2010, 2007, 2004, 2001, 1997 by Mosby, Inc., an affiliate of Elsevier Inc. All rights reserved.

10. What is the therapeutic outcome of donepezil (Aricept)?

11. What are the serious adverse effects for patients taking donepezil (Aricept) therapy?

12. What is the action of lactulose (Cephulac)?

13. What are the therapeutic outcomes of lactulose (Cephulac) therapy?

14. What is the primary therapeutic outcome of memantine (Namenda)?

15. What are the drugs that interact with memantine (Namenda)?

16. What is the primary therapeutic outcome of probenecid?

17. Who should not receive probenecid therapy?

18. What is the action of tacrine (Cognex)?

19. What are the common adverse effects of tacrine (Cognex) therapy?

9. Disulfiram reaction is manifested by nausea, severe vomiting, sweating, throbbing headache, dizziness, blurred vision, and confusion.

10. Improved cognitive skills

11. The health care provider should be notified if the patient's heart rate is fewer than 60 beats per minute.

12. Lactulose is a sugar that acidifies the colon, thus preventing the absorption of ammonia.

13. Improved orientation to surroundings and a gentle laxative effect with formed stool.

14. Improved cognitive skills

15. Acetazolamide and sodium bicarbonate

16. The primary therapeutic outcome of probenecid is prevention of acute attacks of gouty arthritis.

17. Patients with histories of blood dyscrasias or uric acid kidney stones should not receive probenecid.

18. Tacrine is an acetylcholinesterase inhibitor that allows acetylcholine to accumulate at cholinergic synapses causing a prolonged and exaggerated cholinergic effect.

19. Nausea, vomiting, dyspepsia, and diarrhea